# FUNDAMENTALS OF EPIDEMIOLOGY

## LAUREN CHRISTIANSEN-LINDQUIST, PhD, MPH

Dr. Christiansen-Lindquist is an Assistant Professor and Director of Graduate Studies for MPH and MSPH programs in the Department of Epidemiology at Emory University's Rollins School of Public Health. She teaches epidemiologic methods at the introductory, intermediate, advanced, and doctoral levels, and was selected as the 2023 recipient of the Society for Epidemiologic Research's Noel Weiss & Tom Koepsell Excellence in Education Award. She is well known for her unique pedagogical techniques that make complicated concepts more accessible. Her research focuses on stillbirth in the United States, with particular interests in surveillance, data quality, prevention, and improving the care families receive after a loss.


## KRISTIN M. WALL, PhD, MS

Dr. Wall is an Associate Professor in the Department of Epidemiology at Emory University's Rollins School of Public Health. She teaches epidemiologic methods to undergraduate and graduate students, junior faculty, and clinicians. Dr. Wall also mentors masters and doctoral students along with junior epidemiologists and public health clinicians in several countries on research and analysis methods, scholarship, and dissemination and implementation of results. Her research focuses on evidence-based decision-making to improve sexual and reproductive health by exploring effective and cost-effective interventions and programs both in the United States and in limited-resource settings.

# FUNDAMENTALS OF EPIDEMIOLOGY

LAUREN CHRISTIANSEN-LINDQUIST, PhD, MPH

KRISTIN M. WALL, PhD, MS

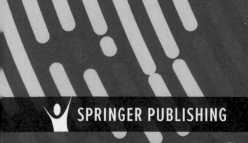

Springer Publishing Company, LLC
902 Carnegie Center, Suite 140, Princeton, NJ 08540
www.springerpub.com
connect.springerpub.com

*Acquisitions Editor*: David D'Addona
*Senior Content Development Editor*: Lucia Gunzel
*Production Editor*: Dennis Troutman
*Compositor*: Amnet

*ISBN*: 978-0-8261-6693-7
*ebook ISBN*: 978-0-8261-6694-4
*DOI*: 10.1891/9780826166944

SUPPLEMENTS:

A robust set of instructor resources designed to supplement this text is located at http://connect.springerpub.com/content/book/978-0-8261-6694-4. Qualifying instructors may request access by emailing textbook@springerpub.com.

INSTRUCTOR MATERIALS:
LMS Common Cartridge Instructions
LMS Common Cartridge With All Instructor Resources
Instructor Manual: 978-0-8261-6699-9
Instructor Test Bank: 978-0-8261-6695-1
Instructor PowerPoints: 978-0-8261-6696-8
Instructor Image Bank: 978-0-8261-6697-5
Sample Syllabus: 978-0-8261-6692-0

STUDENT MATERIALS:
Answers to Chapter Exercises and Practice Problems: 978-0-8261-6698-2

24 25 26 27 / 5 4 3 2 1

Library of Congress Cataloging-in-Publication Data

Names: Christiansen-Lindquist, Lauren, author. | Wall, Kristin M., author.
Title: Fundamentals of epidemiology / Lauren Christiansen-Lindquist, Kristin M. Wall.
Description: New York, NY : Springer Publishing Company, LLC, [2024] |
   Includes bibliographical references and index.
Identifiers: LCCN 2023027843 (print) | LCCN 2023027844 (ebook) |
   ISBN 9780826166937 (paperback) | ISBN 9780826166944 (ebook) |
   ISBN 9780826166999 (instructor's manual) | ISBN 9780826166951 (instructor's test bank) |
   ISBN 9780826166968 (instructor's PowerPoints) | ISBN 9780826166975 (instructor's image bank) |
   ISBN 9780826166982 (student materials)
Subjects: MESH: Epidemiologic Methods | Epidemiology
Classification: LCC RA651 (print) | LCC RA651 (ebook) | NLM WA 950 | DDC
   614.4—dc23/eng/20230727
LC record available at https://lccn.loc.gov/2023027843
LC ebook record available at https://lccn.loc.gov/2023027844

Contact sales@springerpub.com to receive discount rates on bulk purchases.

*Publisher's Note:* New and used products purchased from third-party sellers are not guaranteed for quality, authenticity, or access to any included digital components.

Printed in the United States of America by Gasch Printing.

*To Ethan, Reid, Collin, and Matt.*
–LCL

*To Leona, Onva, Brazos, and Annita.*
–KMW

# CONTENTS

List of Reviewers     ix

Foreword *Timothy L. Lash, DSc, MPH*     xi

Preface     xiii

How to Use This Book     xv

Acknowledgments     xvii

Springer Publishing Resources     xix

**CHAPTER 1**    Introduction to Public Health and the Fundamentals of Epidemiology    1

**CHAPTER 2**    Descriptive Epidemiology, Surveillance, and Measures of Frequency    23

**CHAPTER 3**    Introduction to Analytic Epidemiologic Study Designs and Measures of Association    55

**CHAPTER 4**    Randomized Controlled Trial Designs    89

**CHAPTER 5**    Cohort Designs    117

**CHAPTER 6**    Case-Control Designs    139

**CHAPTER 7**    Cross-Sectional Designs    171

**CHAPTER 8**    Effect Measure Modification and Statistical Interaction    191

**MIDDLE MATTER**    215

**CHAPTER 9**    Error in Epidemiologic Research and Fundamentals of Confounding    221

**CHAPTER 10**    Selection Bias    265

**CHAPTER 11**    Information Bias and Screening and Diagnostic Tests    293

**CHAPTER 12**    Random Error in Epidemiologic Research    327

**CHAPTER 13**    Introduction to Epidemiologic Data Analysis    361

Glossary     397

Index     405

# LIST OF REVIEWERS

The following instructors reviewed early drafts of the chapters and provided valuable feedback:

**Raed Ba Helah, MD, PhD, MPM, and TM**
Assistant Professor of Public Health, Baldwin Wallace University, Berea, Ohio

**Sandie Ha, PhD, MPH**
Assistant Professor, Public Health, Chair, Public Health Undergraduate Education, University of California-Merced, Merced, California

**Ernesto Moralez, PhD, MPH, CHES**
Assistant Professor of Public Health, Co-Coordinator of the Public Health Minor, St. Lawrence University, Canton, New York

**Megan Quinn, DrPH, MSc**
Associate Professor, Department of Biostatistics and Epidemiology, East Tennessee State University College of Public Health, Johnson City, Tennessee

# FOREWORD

Historically, the science of epidemiology has most often been taught in graduate courses offered by schools and programs of public health. The curricula were built on knowledge and skills gained in undergraduate education, including mathematics and the scientific method. Early epidemiology textbooks were often brief, at least in relation to the length of a typical chemistry, biology, physics, or calculus text. The first edition of *Modern Epidemiology*, often viewed as one of the first intermediate textbooks about the science of epidemiology, was only approximately 350 pages long, whereas my undergraduate calculus text clocked in at nearly 1,000 pages. Epidemiology has caught up; the fourth edition of *Modern Epidemiology* includes nearly 1,200 pages and there are now comprehensive textbooks on the specialized methods of epidemiology applied to social determinants of health, genetic epidemiology, and many topics in between.

This expansion, however, has largely focused on more complex writing about more complex methods geared toward graduate students or practicing epidemiologists. There are many introductory textbooks, mostly used for a first course in graduate curricula and often divorced from the biostatistics curriculum that many students learn in tandem. There has been little reach by textbook authors toward undergraduate education in epidemiology, despite the recent emergence of many undergraduate programs in public health.

It is these gaps in the available textbooks that have been expertly filled by the present text. The text presents a logical flow of epidemiologic concepts and methods. Each chapter builds on what came before, as key concepts are reinforced, then used to expand into new ideas, which are in turn reinforced by active exercises. This paradigm maps to modern education theory and will allow students to readily learn topics many find challenging. More importantly, Drs. Wall and Christiansen-Lindquist are ideally suited as authors of a text with this approach to teaching. They have each taught undergraduate, introductory graduate, and advanced graduate courses in epidemiologic and biostatistical methods. Their experiences in successfully conveying this content show through in the writing and in the approach. Color coding of key concepts within tables and figures so readers can easily keep track of how variables are used in an analysis, and the use of a primary example carried through each chapter, are just two examples of their attention to detail and their empathy for the learner. Call-out sections summarize key concepts, opportunities to practice reinforce learning through active engagement, and segments that dig deeper explain the nuances of some topics so that students can avoid unlearning of overly simplified concepts often taught at an introductory level.

*Fundamentals of Epidemiology* is a valuable new introductory text, ideally suited to undergraduate and graduate instruction in epidemiology, and optimized for modern teaching approaches that engage students with active learning and that seek to convey complex epidemiologic and biostatistical concepts clearly and without simplifications that will later need to be unlearned. The field has needed such a text for as long as I can remember; it is exciting to finally see just such a text become available.

*Timothy L. Lash, DSc, MPH*
*O. Wayne Rollins Distinguished Professor of Epidemiology*
*Chair, Department of Epidemiology*
*Rollins School of Public Health*
*Emory University*
*Atlanta, Georgia*

# PREFACE

We believe now more than ever that the fundamentals of epidemiology provide an essential critical thinking framework to help navigate the constant flow of health (mis)information. While we would be thrilled if all our readers joined the epidemiologic workforce, we have written this text with the goal of being accessible to future epidemiologists as well as those who will pursue careers in anything from the arts to zoology.

We have strived to produce a resource that has a wealth of examples that reflect the diversity of the field and the populations that we serve. To the best of our knowledge, the language that we have used in this book is what is currently considered the most accurate and inclusive; however, we are keenly aware that our understanding and language are constantly evolving. The language used in this book looks very different from earlier texts in epidemiology, and we anticipate that future texts will differ from this one as well. We are committed to the life-long process of learning how to improve ourselves and the work that we do.

Some of the examples we will discuss in this text, from cancer to depression to the health effects of racism, may be sensitive topics for many readers. We selected our examples to reflect key public health issues of today as well as topics of interest to our students. While many reasons for poor human health can be difficult to discuss, we believe that only by increasing awareness and conversation about these topics can they begin to be addressed.

Finally, as you embark on a journey to learn about the fundamentals of epidemiology, we remind readers to keep the big picture in view. As reflected in the cover art of this text, every data point reflects a real person with a real story; we must never lose the people, or the challenges and health disparities they may face, in the numbers.

*Lauren Christiansen-Lindquist*
*Kristin M. Wall*

# HOW TO USE THIS BOOK

Over a combined 20 years of experience teaching epidemiology, we have had a front row seat to the discoveries and questions of thousands of students exploring this incredible field. As epidemiologists, we couldn't help but notice patterns in the questions asked and mistakes made by learners of epidemiology at both introductory and more advanced levels. We saw writing this text as an opportunity to share our approach to teaching epidemiologic methods while also addressing common questions and misconceptions head-on. We have used a scaffolding approach where each chapter builds upon the one that came before, and connections are frequently made within and between chapters. We have incorporated **Pause to Practice** segments throughout each chapter, which afford readers the opportunity to practice as they move along. Given the way that the concepts build upon one another, this practice-as-you-go approach allows learners to build a solid foundation. Throughout the book you will see call-out boxes that highlight common errors new learners of epidemiology make, and the reasons why these mistakes miss the mark. We have also included summary tables in the middle of the book (**Middle Matter**) as a resource to help readers remember the key features discussed throughout this text. Finally, to help synthesize what has been covered, each chapter also includes **Highlights**, which are periodic summaries of the main concepts.

Another unique feature of this text is the consistent color coding used in the tables and figures. Working through epidemiologic problem sets can sometimes feel like an exercise in reading comprehension rather than an application of the epidemiologic concepts of interest. We have employed a color-coding strategy to assist readers in distinguishing between key variables and populations of interest, a technique we have found to be very effective in the classroom. Examples of how the color coding is used in the tables, figures, and boxes are shown in **Figure M.1**, located in the **Middle Matter** section of this book.

One of the challenges of writing this book is that epidemiologic concepts are often described using the metaphor of an onion: as we peel back the layers, it becomes evident that these topics are much more complicated than they appear on the surface. There is a delicate balance between presenting introductory material in a way that is both accurate and accessible versus teaching things so simplistically that they must be "unlearned" in future courses as the material becomes more complex. We have done our best to preview where learners can expect to find more nuanced details in future courses using **Digging Deeper** segments. The chapters have been written so that those using this text at the most introductory level can skip over these sections without losing the thread of the chapter. We have also been intentional about the order in which the topics are presented so that commonly confused concepts are less likely to be conflated and to emphasize the prioritization of certain topics.

# ACKNOWLEDGMENTS

This book would not be possible without the enthusiasm and dedication of our epidemiology students and teaching assistants over the years. They have helped us grow as instructors through their insightful questions in pursuit of addressing major public health problems around the world.

We are grateful to Rebecca Nash, Chrystelle Kiang, and Meredith Dixon for preparing the accompanying PowerPoints, test bank questions, and for their careful review of the chapters.

Thanks to Meghna Ray for her helpful review of the text from the perspective of a student not pursuing a degree in epidemiology.

We give special thanks to Tim Lash for the profound influence that he has had on our understanding and teaching of epidemiologic methods, and his thoughtful review of Chapter 12: Random Error in Epidemiologic Research.

Notably, we would not be the instructors we are today without Mike Goodman, David Kleinbaum, Mitch Klein, and Cecile Janssens, all of whom share our passion for teaching.

LCL would like to thank Carol Hogue and SD for their mentorship and guidance.

KMW is grateful for the invaluable mentorship of Surangani Dharmawardhane, Susan Allen, and Patrick Sullivan.

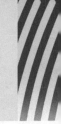

# SPRINGER PUBLISHING RESOURCES

 A robust set of instructor resources designed to supplement this text is located at **http://connect.springerpub.com/content/book/978-0-8261-6694-4.** Qualifying instructors may request access by emailing **textbook@springerpub.com.**

## INSTRUCTOR RESOURCES

- LMS Common Cartridge (With All Instructor Resources and Instructions)
- Instructor Manual and Sample Syllabi
- Test Bank
- PowerPoint Slides
- Instructor Image Bank

## STUDENT RESOURCES

- Answers to "Pause to Practice" Exercises
- Solutions to End of Chapter Problem Sets

# CHAPTER 1

# INTRODUCTION TO PUBLIC HEALTH AND THE FUNDAMENTALS OF EPIDEMIOLOGY

## KEY TERMS

| | | |
|---|---|---|
| determinants | ethics | levels of prevention |
| endemic | exposure | pandemic |
| epidemic | health-related outcome | public health |
| epidemiologic transition | human subjects | social determinants of health |

## LEARNING OBJECTIVES

1.1  Define epidemiology.

1.2  Define and distinguish between the terms endemic, epidemic, pandemic, and syndemic.

1.3  Define the three levels of prevention in public health.

1.4  Describe how changes in the leading causes of mortality are related to the epidemiologic transition.

1.5  Describe some of the major achievements in public health, and describe how they are relevant to health today.

1.6  Describe the ethical foundations of human subjects research and how they have evolved.

1.7  Describe how social determinants of health are related to epidemiology.

## EPI ... DEMI ... WHAT?!

Epidemiology was launched into the global spotlight after SARS-CoV-2, the novel coronavirus that causes COVID-19, was first reported in Hubei Province, China, in 2019. The onset of the pandemic launched epidemiology into the common lexicon, making it a topic of discussion on the news and at dinner tables—but this was not always the case. Prior to the COVID-19 pandemic, epidemiologists were often confused with dermatologists, under the assumption that the "epi" in "epidemiology" stood for "epidermis." If epidemiologists don't study skin, what do we do?

Epidemiology is one of the core disciplines of **public health**, which is an art and science broadly dedicated to promoting and protecting the health of human populations. While health practitioners, such as physicians and nurses, attend to the health of *individuals*, public health practitioners focus on the patterns of health and disease in *populations* with the goal of applying the lessons learned to improve population health.

Other core disciplines of public health include health policy and management; social, behavioral, and health education sciences; environmental health sciences; and biostatistics. These interrelated disciplines are broadly defined in **Figure 1.1**. Throughout this textbook, you will read examples that touch on each of these disciplines and will have an opportunity to think about how they relate to epidemiology. For reasons you will soon discover, epidemiology is often viewed as the foundational science of public health.

Broadly, epidemiologists apply scientific and quantitative methods to understand the distribution and causes of health and disease in human populations. Whether you realize it or not, you are consuming information rooted in epidemiology all the time. And it can be confusing—do the potential risks of drinking coffee outweigh the possible benefits? How should the latest data about the impact of climate change on human health be interpreted? Are societies prepared for the next global pandemic? Given the immense accessibility of health-related information and the increasing threat of health misinformation, it is more important than ever to critically evaluate such questions. Epidemiology provides an invaluable framework for critical thinking that is applicable to everyone, regardless of your aspirations to become an epidemiologist yourself. As you read this book, we encourage you to keep in mind that we are building a toolkit of skills that will make you better poised to evaluate health-related data both in the scientific literature and in the popular media.

In this chapter, we will provide a broad overview of epidemiology and discuss how it relates to the other public health disciplines. We will also explore a brief history of epidemiologic and public health advances and ethical principles—after all, we can't know where we're going if we don't know where we've been.

## FIGURE 1.1 CORE DISCIPLINES OF PUBLIC HEALTH

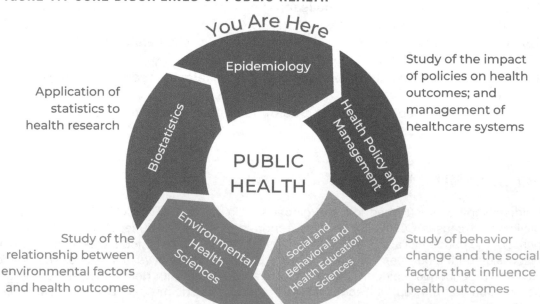

## WHAT IS EPIDEMIOLOGY? (LEARNING OBJECTIVE 1.1)

Epidemiology is the study of the **distribution** and **determinants** of **health-related states or events** in **specified populations** and the **application** of study findings to improve public health.

The key components of this definition, bolded in this definition and summarized in **Figure 1.2**, are discussed in the text that follows.

**Health-related states or events.** It is helpful to begin parsing out the definition of epidemiology by thinking about the health-related states or events (often called **health-related outcomes**) that might be of interest. These outcomes are broadly defined as any event that impacts population well-being. In epidemiology, the health-related outcomes of interest are often **diseases**, or conditions that impair normal functioning that typically manifest with distinct signs and symptoms.[1] In epidemiology, the manifestation of disease can be classified into one of two categories: morbidity and mortality. Diseases may result in illness in a population, which is referred to as **morbidity**. Diseases may also result in death in a population, which is referred to as **mortality**. Researchers are also often interested in health-related outcomes that are *not* diseases, such as the use of health services or survival.

Regardless of whether you are studying a disease or some other outcome that is related to health, it is critical to establish a rigorous **case definition** that details the criteria needed to determine whether someone has your outcome of interest. For example, the case definition for gonorrhea used in the United States and defined by the U.S. Centers for Disease Control and Prevention includes detailed information about the identification of the bacteria using different types of laboratory tests.[2] Case definitions are described further in **Chapter 2, "Descriptive Epidemiology, Surveillance, and Measures of Frequency."**

**Distribution.** Calculating the distribution, or **frequency**, of health-related outcomes involves not just *counting* the number of instances of the outcome, but also putting their occurrence into context. If we describe the frequency of health-related outcomes relative to the size of a population, we can make appropriate comparisons across populations. For example, suppose

## FIGURE 1.2 BREAKING DOWN THE DEFINITION OF EPIDEMIOLOGY

# ep·i·de·mi·ol·o·gy

The study of the **distribution** and **determinants** of **health-related states or events** in **specified populations** and the **application** of study findings to improve public health.

| | | |
|---|---|---|
| **distribution** | How **common** is the health outcome? **Who** is affected? **Where** and **when** are the health outcomes occurring? | Identify the **frequency** of the health outcome - not just *how many* cases, but also the size of the population (**Chapter 2**). Often consider person, place, and time characteristics. |
| **determinants** | **Why** is the health outcome occurring? | Identify the **causes** of the health outcomes - these causes are often referred to as **exposures** (**Chapter 3**). |
| **health–related states or events** | **What** is the health outcome of interest? | Establish a **case definition** (**Chapter 2**) for the health outcomes impacting population well-being. |
| **specified populations** | **Who** is affected? | Identify the populations of interest (**Chapters 1, 4-7, & 10**). |
| **application** | What next? | Take action to **improve public health** (**Chapters 2, 3, 4-8**). |

researchers observe 100 cases of a rare cancer in two different populations. Without knowing the size of each of these populations, public health officials do not have enough information to evaluate the scope of the problem across these two groups. One-hundred cases of this rare cancer in China (population ~1.4 billion as of 2023) would be interpreted very differently from 100 cases of the same rare cancer in Vatican City (population ~800 as of 2023). This example emphasizes the importance of **denominators** when interpreting the frequency of health outcomes and for making comparisons across populations. We need to know how many cases of an outcome have occurred as well as the size of the population that those cases came from.

Epidemiologists use **descriptive epidemiology** (the focus of **Chapter 2, "Descriptive Epidemiology, Surveillance, and Measures of Frequency"**) to calculate the distribution of health-related outcomes in populations. Often, researchers will observe how health outcomes are distributed according to demographic, geographic, or temporal factors, referred to in epidemiology as **person**, **place**, and **time** characteristics. For example, researchers may be interested in evaluating the frequency of an outcome among certain age groups (a person characteristic), in certain countries (a place characteristic), or across several decades (a time characteristic). Examples of common person, place, and time characteristics are shown in **Figure 1.3**.

**FIGURE 1.3 EXAMPLES OF PERSON, PLACE, AND TIME CHARACTERISTICS THAT MAY BE USED TO DESCRIBE THE DISTRIBUTION OF HEALTH OUTCOMES**

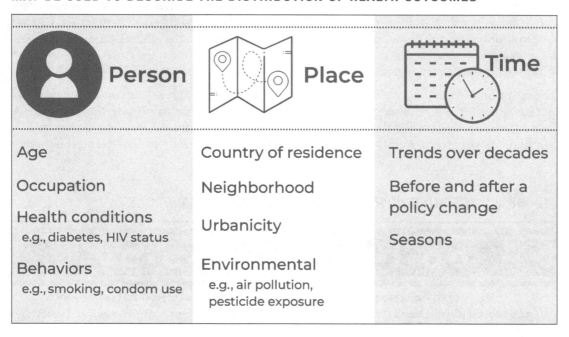

| Person | Place | Time |
|---|---|---|
| Age | Country of residence | Trends over decades |
| Occupation | Neighborhood | Before and after a policy change |
| Health conditions e.g., diabetes, HIV status | Urbanicity | Seasons |
| Behaviors e.g., smoking, condom use | Environmental e.g., air pollution, pesticide exposure | |

## Endemic, Epidemic, Pandemic, and Syndemic Diseases (LEARNING OBJECTIVE 1.2)

Diseases can be described as endemic, epidemic, pandemic, or syndemic. Diseases that are **endemic** to a certain population are regularly occurring with some endemic, or expected, frequency. For example, malaria is currently endemic to Uganda, with 219 cases occurring per 1,000 individuals in 2018, which is roughly the expected frequency of cases in Uganda.[3]

An **epidemic** occurs when the frequency of a disease *exceeds* the expected level in a population. For example, if Uganda were to experience a surge in malaria cases, say 500 cases per 1,000 individuals, this would be considered a malaria epidemic.

It is important to note that whether a disease is classified as endemic or epidemic depends on the location and time period being considered—a disease that is endemic in one population may be considered an epidemic in another. For example, if 219 cases of malaria per 1,000 individuals (roughly the current endemic level in Uganda) occurred in the United States in 2023, this would be considered an epidemic in the United States because this frequency is much higher than expected (locally transmitted malaria cases are currently very rare in the United States).[4] Similarly, a disease that is considered endemic in a particular location at one point in time could later be classified as an epidemic and vice versa.

A **pandemic** is defined as an epidemic that occurs across various geographically distant populations, for example, across international borders. COVID-19 is a recent example of a pandemic disease that has affected the entire globe.

A **syndemic** describes the occurrence of two simultaneous epidemics which work together to exacerbate health outcomes. For example, some researchers have hypothesized that there is a syndemic of COVID-19 and malaria.[5,6]

**Determinants.** Health-related outcomes rarely occur randomly, meaning by chance alone. Instead, they typically occur because of **determinants**, also called **exposures**, which are factors that cause an outcome to occur. Broadly speaking, **analytic epidemiology** (described in **Chapter 3, "Introduction to Analytic Epidemiologic Study Designs and Measures of Association"**) is used to estimate associations between exposures and outcomes and to quantify their strength.

Some well-studied exposure-outcome associations are shown in **Table 1.1**. As shown in this table, the association between an exposure and a health outcome can be described as either **positive** or **negative**. Positive associations, such as the relationship between smoking and lung cancer, are associations where increases in exposure frequency lead to *increases* in outcome frequency. On the other hand, negative associations, such as the relationship between handwashing and respiratory disease infection, are associations where increases in exposure frequency lead to *decreases* in outcome frequency.

**Specified populations.** While health practitioners, such as physicians and nurses, attend to the health of individuals, public health researchers focus on the patterns of health and disease in specified populations to improve health on a larger scale. The particular population will depend on the research question of interest. For example, returning to some of the examples shown in **Table 1.1**, findings from a study on smoking prevention measures would ideally be applicable to a population of smokers. However, findings from studies of more ubiquitous exposures like water sanitation and air pollution would ideally be applicable to everyone who lives in a particular area.

**Application.** Epidemiologic data should be disseminated to improve the health of the specified population. Often this takes the form of informing public health prevention, treatment, control programs, and public health policy. It is not enough to conduct epidemiologic studies

**TABLE 1.1 EXAMPLES OF EXPOSURE AND OUTCOME ASSOCIATIONS**

| Determinants (Exposures) | Health-Related States or Events (Outcomes) |
|---|---|
| **Positive Associations**—Increases in the exposure lead to increases in the outcome. | |
| Unprotected sex | HPV infection |
| Air pollution | Infertility |
| Smoking | Lung cancer |
| **Negative Associations**—Increases in the exposure lead to decreases in the outcome. | |
| Handwashing | Respiratory disease infection |
| Water sanitation | Cholera infection |
| Smallpox vaccination campaign | Smallpox infection |
| U.S. Supplemental Nutrition Assistance Program (SNAP) | Childhood malnutrition |
| Birth control access | Abortion |

to increase knowledge among academics. Findings from epidemiologic studies should be shared with the appropriate public health practitioners, agencies, and the general public. Without dissemination of study findings, there can be no action to ultimately improve public health. Importantly, public health is a science that sometimes cannot wait for perfect evidence to take action. Rather, we must make recommendations based on the best available evidence and public health need. These recommendations are then updated over time if new evidence comes to light. For example, once COVID-19 vaccines were approved for nonpregnant adults in 2020, many institutions, including the U.S. CDC, recommended that pregnant persons receive the vaccine despite limited data at the time in that group given the higher morbidities associated with COVID-19 among pregnant versus nonpregnant persons (subsequent data have found no adverse events associated with COVID-19 vaccination during pregnancy, with benefits outweighing any potential risks).[7]

## PREVENTION IN PUBLIC HEALTH (LEARNING OBJECTIVE 1.3)

Epidemiologists often focus on improving public health through prevention or treatment of outcomes that have a negative impact on health. **Prevention** not only keeps negative outcomes from occurring, but it also avoids the physical, emotional, and financial costs of illnesses. An emphasis on preventing negative health outcomes has been strongly emphasized by public health practitioners, including former U.S. Surgeon General Dr. Regina Benjamin, who wrote in 2011: "Prevention is the foundation of public health.… If we want to truly reform health care in this country, we need to prevent people from getting sick in the first place and stop disease before it starts."[8] Public health prevention is often categorized into three levels: primary prevention, secondary prevention, and tertiary prevention (**Figure 1.4**).

### FIGURE 1.4 LEVELS OF PREVENTION IN PUBLIC HEALTH

The goal of each level of prevention is to keep individuals from moving to the next stage in this continuum

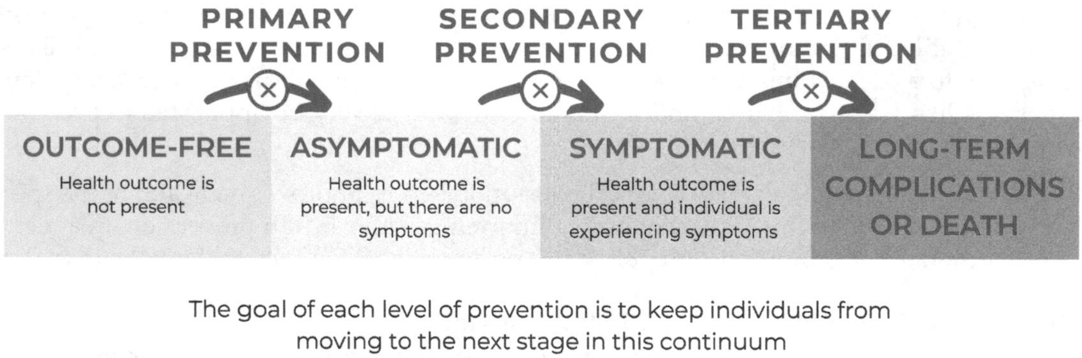

## Primary Prevention

When you think about disease prevention, **primary prevention** is likely what comes to mind. This level of prevention is aimed at keeping negative health outcomes from occurring at all. Primary prevention can occur either passively or actively. **Passive prevention** strategies, which are often driven by policy decisions, require little or no participation on the part of the population of interest. For example, two large-scale passive primary prevention strategies are fluoridation of water to reduce cavities and folic acid fortification of foods to reduce neural tube defects. In many countries, widespread consumption of tap water and fortified foods like bread and cereal means that individuals do not have to change their behavior to reap the benefits of these prevention measures. In contrast, **active prevention** requires participation from the population of interest. Returning to prevention of cavities and neural tube defects, active prevention strategies may require individuals to brush their teeth with fluoridated toothpaste and regularly take folic acid supplements, respectively.

## Secondary Prevention

The next line of defense is **secondary prevention**, which addresses the health of those who are already affected by a negative health outcome but are not experiencing symptoms (also called **asymptomatic**). The goal of secondary prevention is to decrease morbidity or mortality using interventions such as screening and early detection. Mammography-based breast cancer screening programs are a great example of secondary prevention; they can be used to detect cases of breast cancer early, often prior to the onset of symptoms, to reduce cancer morbidity and mortality.

## Tertiary Prevention

Finally, **tertiary prevention** seeks to reduce long-term complications and death from health-related outcomes in those with established disease. Interventions that focus on treatment, management of comorbidities and complications, rehabilitation, and palliative care are all considered tertiary prevention strategies.

Now that you have been introduced to the **levels of prevention**, it is worth considering that when most people think about "prevention," they typically only have primary prevention in mind. In the earlier quote, Dr. Benjamin is really only referring to primary prevention by stating that "we need to prevent people from getting sick in the first place." It is well worth noting that when public health, particularly primary prevention activities, are working well, the populations served may not realize that epidemiologists and other public health professionals are there at work! As a result, it can sometimes be difficult to demonstrate the value of the time and money spent on prevention efforts to the public and policy makers because we cannot observe what *didn't* happen.

## LEADING CAUSES OF MORTALITY AND THE EPIDEMIOLOGIC TRANSITION (LEARNING OBJECTIVE 1.4)

The leading causes of death today are quite different from what they were centuries, or even decades, ago. Most countries are experiencing or have experienced an **epidemiologic transition,** which is characterized by a shift from relatively high mortality among infants and children (largely attributable to **communicable diseases**, also known as **infectious diseases**—diseases that can be transmitted from one individual to another) to higher morbidity and mortality among older adults (largely attributable to **noncommunicable diseases**—diseases that *cannot* be transmitted from one individual to another). In fact, by 2030, noncommunicable health conditions are projected to account for three-fourths of global deaths.[9]

Global deaths among children aged 0 to 4 years have declined considerably, with children accounting for 40% of deaths in 1955,[9] 25% in 1990, to under 10% in 2017.[10] At the same time, many populations have experienced a shift toward older average populations with increased life expectancies.[11] It is remarkable that the average global human life expectancy increased *22 years* between 1955 and 2020, from 50 to 72 years of age.[12] Much of the increase in life expectancy can be attributed to advances in both public health and medicine; many of the key successes in these domains are described in the text that follows. Unfortunately, COVID-19 triggered dramatic changes to mortality trends, and caused a decline in life expectancy in many countries around the globe.[13]

**TABLE 1.2 10 LEADING CAUSES OF DEATH GLOBALLY, 2000 AND 2019**

| Rank | 2000 (Number of Cases in Millions) | 2019 (Number of Cases in Millions) |
|------|------------------------------------|-------------------------------------|
| 1 | Ischemic heart disease (6.8) | Ischemic heart disease (8.9) |
| 2 | Stroke (5.5) | Stroke (6.2) |
| 3 | Neonatal conditions* (3.2) | Chronic obstructive pulmonary disease (3.2) |
| 4 | Lower respiratory infections* (3.1) | Lower respiratory infections* (2.6) |
| 5 | Chronic obstructive pulmonary disease (3.0) | Neonatal conditions* (2.0) |
| 6 | Diarrheal diseases* (2.6) | Trachea, bronchus, lung cancers (1.8) |
| 7 | Tuberculosis* (1.7) | Alzheimer disease and other dementias (1.6) |
| 8 | HIV/AIDS* (1.4) | Diarrheal diseases* (1.5) |
| 9 | Trachea, bronchus, lung cancers (1.2) | Diabetes mellitus (1.5) |
| 10 | Road injury (1.2) | Kidney disease (1.2) |

*Communicable diseases
*Source*: World Health Organization. Leading causes of death and disability: a visual summary of global and regional trends. n.d. https://www.who.int/data/stories/leading-causes-of-death-and-disability-2000-2019-a-visual-summary

To get an idea of how the leading causes of death have shifted over recent decades, the leading global causes of death in 2000 and 2019 are shown in **Table 1.2**. As more countries experience the epidemiologic transition, deaths from noncommunicable diseases rise. In 2019, three non-communicable conditions (Alzheimer disease and other dementias, diabetes, and kidney disease) newly reached the top 10 causes of death worldwide. Although ischemic heart disease and stroke, also noncommunicable diseases, topped the lists in both 2000 and 2019, they are responsible for a larger number of deaths in 2019. In contrast, communicable diseases are on the decline: by 2019, the ranking of deaths due to neonatal disorders and diarrheal diseases fell, and tuberculosis and HIV/AIDS dropped out of the top 10 causes of mortality altogether. Lower respiratory infections and neonatal conditions were the leading causes of death from communicable diseases in both years, though the absolute number of deaths from both causes decreased by 2019. After the onset of the COVID-19 pandemic, COVID-19 ranked the third leading cause of death in the U.S. (after heart disease and cancer) in 2020 and 2021, and dropped to the fourth leading cause of death (behind unintentional injury) in 2022.[14-16]

**TABLE 1.3 10 LEADING CAUSES OF DEATH IN LOW- AND HIGH-INCOME COUNTRIES, 2019**

| Rank | Low-Income Countries | High-Income Countries |
|------|----------------------|------------------------|
| 1 | Neonatal conditions* | Ischemic heart disease |
| 2 | Lower respiratory infections* | Alzheimer disease and other dementias |
| 3 | Ischemic heart disease | Stroke |
| 4 | Stroke | Trachea, bronchus, lung cancers |
| 5 | Diarrheal diseases* | Chronic obstructive pulmonary disease (COPD) |
| 6 | Malaria* | Lower respiratory infections* |
| 7 | Road injury | Colon and rectum cancers |
| 8 | Tuberculosis* | Kidney disease |
| 9 | HIV/AIDS* | Hypertensive heart disease |
| 10 | Cirrhosis of the liver | Diabetes |

*Communicable diseases
The World Bank uses the following four income categories based on gross national income to categorize countries: low, lower-middle, upper-middle, and high income.
Not showing results from lower-middle or upper-middle income countries
*Source*: World Health Organization. The top 10 causes of death. December 9, 2020. https://www.who.int/news-room/fact-sheets/detail/the-top-10-causes-of-death

While the data in **Table 1.2** provide important insight into the distribution of the leading causes of death worldwide, they conceal many important differences, including those for low-versus high-income countries. As shown in **Table 1.3**, leading causes of death in low-income countries in 2019 included communicable diseases like neonatal conditions, malaria, tuberculosis, HIV/AIDS, and diarrheal diseases.[17] In contrast, nine of the top 10 leading causes of death in high-income countries were due to noncommunicable diseases.

In the section that follows, we will provide an overview of several major public health achievements that have contributed to the epidemiologic transition. These examples will also highlight some reasons why differences remain between low- and high-income countries.

## MAJOR ACHIEVEMENTS IN EPIDEMIOLOGY AND PUBLIC HEALTH
### (LEARNING OBJECTIVE 1.5)

To better understand why there has been a shift in the distribution of the leading causes of death, we will turn our attention to some key milestones in epidemiology and public health which have improved human health and increased life expectancy.

**Water, sanitation, and hygiene.** John Snow, a British physician, is often credited as one of the founders of epidemiology due to his investigation of the 1840s and 1850s cholera epidemics, during which tens of thousands of people in England died.[18] Snow noted that cholera patients' initial symptoms were digestive and thus hypothesized that the disease was waterborne and related to sanitation and hygiene. Prior to his landmark study in London, in which he mapped cases of cholera per household along with where each household received its water, it was thought that cholera was transmitted via the air or "atmospheric miasma." Though many doctors and scientists were resistant to Snow's hypothesis, the data he collected provided strong support that cholera is indeed a waterborne disease.

Some of the principles that Snow used (such as hypothesis generation based on previous observations, contact tracing, and mapping of exposures and outcomes) are still used today in epidemiology to identify the distribution and determinants of many health outcomes. Modern water treatment services (an example of primary passive prevention) have practically eliminated cholera in many countries. Broadly, over the last 200 years, our understanding of the relationships between water, sanitation, hygiene, and poor health outcomes has improved, and advancements in access to clean water and education about sanitation and hygiene have drastically reduced deaths due to communicable diseases (though disparities remain, especially in low- and middle-income countries). This has led to a substantial reduction in child mortality and contributed to the epidemiologic transition.

**Vaccination**. Vaccines, an example of primary active prevention, save millions of lives globally each year. The impact of vaccines on childhood morbidity and mortality has been especially immense, also contributing to the epidemiologic transition.

The story of smallpox eradication provides an excellent example of the immense impact vaccines can have on public health. Some reports indicate that inoculation for smallpox, a viral infectious disease that is primarily airborne or transmitted via fomites, was practiced in China and India thousands of years ago, possibly by putting fluid from smallpox pustules into cuts made in healthy people's skin.[19] In the 1790s, British doctor Edward Jenner documented that English milkmaids (who had frequent contact with cows that had cowpox) believed that infection with cowpox provided them with protection from smallpox. Jenner decided to test this hypothesis by inoculating milkmaids, who had previously been infected with cowpox, with smallpox. He found they had no subsequent symptoms of smallpox. Jenner then went on to inoculate more people with material from a cowpox pustule—these individuals were later exposed to smallpox and did not become ill. Some ridiculed Jenner for his methods (many of which are unethical by today's standards), and he was unable to publish his findings at the Royal Society because his peers felt more proof was needed. Despite these setbacks, Jenner ultimately self-published a report of smallpox resistance among 25 individuals with a history of cowpox.[20] These early advancements in our understanding of smallpox immunity and vaccination helped set the stage for the long road to smallpox eradication. In 1959, the World Health Organization implemented a vaccination strategy to eradicate smallpox globally, which was achieved in 1977.[21]

Today, vaccines for communicable diseases such as polio, measles, mumps, rubella, hepatitis, influenza, tetanus, diphtheria, human papillomavirus (HPV), pneumococcal disease, meningococcal disease, and pertussis are recommended in the United States along with many other countries to prevent cases of disease and future epidemics. The pace of vaccine development has increased dramatically over the years, exemplified by the unprecedented speed with which COVID-19 vaccines were able to move into human trials in 2020 without sacrificing methodologic rigor.[22]

## Pause to Practice 1.1

### Linking Epidemiology to Social and Behavioral Sciences

Social and behavioral scientists seek to understand why humans behave as they do, devoting their studies to various models and methodologies to understand decision-making about health. Epidemiologists often work with behavioral scientists to understand determinants of health outcomes which are related to human behavior. Behavioral scientists are experts in **qualitative research** which involves the collection and analysis of non-numeric data such as a narrative of individuals' health experiences. Epidemiologic studies, which make use of quantitative data are often informed by information generated by qualitative research.

For example, vaccine hesitancy is often an important determinant of vaccine-preventable disease frequency in populations. People who have concerns about vaccination are often less likely to get vaccinated and, thus, are more likely to acquire diseases that vaccines are designed to prevent. Behaviors related to vaccine uptake may also be influenced by the media, demonstrated by an (ultimately retracted) study by Andrew Wakefield and colleagues which suggested a link between measles, mumps, and rubella (MMR) vaccination and autism.[23] Though this link was refuted by several large studies, and the ethics of retracted study called into question, much damage had already been done in terms of public perception of the safety of the MMR vaccine,[24] and this continues to influence behaviors related to vaccine uptake more generally.

1. What other examples can you think of that link behavioral sciences and epidemiology? Think about how specific behavioral determinants (exposures) may be associated with certain health outcomes.

**Malaria prevention and control.** Malaria, a parasite transmitted by mosquitos, is a serious disease that leads to substantial morbidity and mortality (**Table 1.3**), particularly in warm, tropical locales. Thanks to a coordinated global response that included both financial and political support, malaria cases have decreased significantly over time. This response included broad implementation of both preventive and therapeutic measures, including distribution of insecticide-treated bed nets, removal of standing water and mosquito breeding sites, drainage improvements, spraying, rapid diagnosis, treatment, and prophylaxis (i.e., drugs taken for the purposes of primary disease prevention). Although malaria is not currently endemic in the United States, it was endemic at one time and affected both Presidents Washington and Lincoln.[25] In fact, the United States "Communicable Disease Center," now known as the U.S. CDC, was established in Atlanta, Georgia, in 1946 to combat malaria during World War II. At that time, most malaria transmission occurred in the Southeastern United States, which includes the state of Georgia. Malaria was endemic in the United States until it was considered eliminated there in 1951.[26]

**HIV prevention and control.** HIV, a viral infectious disease that is primarily bloodborne, remains a major global health threat and is the ninth leading cause of death in low-income countries where endemic levels remain high (**Table 1.3**). As with malaria, the number of new HIV cases globally is decreasing due to a coordinated global response, including increased access to condoms, HIV testing, counseling and education, sterile injection equipment, antiretroviral therapy, and enhanced blood supply safety procedures. Early in the HIV epidemic, people living with HIV did not live very long after diagnosis. Fortunately, treatments have extended the life expectancy of people living with HIV to be almost equivalent to that of persons not living with HIV.

**Cancer prevention and control.** While some cancers are still a leading cause of mortality worldwide (**Table 1.2**), several public health interventions have led to decreased numbers of new cancer cases as well as a reduction in cancer-related morbidity and mortality. These include primary prevention measures such as HPV vaccination for cervical cancer prevention; secondary prevention measures such as access to early screening for colorectal, breast, and cervical cancers; and tertiary prevention measures such as curative or palliative cancer treatments.

## Pause to Practice 1.2

### Linking Epidemiology to Health Policy and Management

Epidemiologists recognize that the distribution and determinants of diseases and other health outcomes are often closely tied to health policy. Health policy and management experts study the management of healthcare delivery, quality, and costs, as well as policies and regulations affecting entire public health systems. For example, reductions in lung cancer rates can be attributed to a wide range of tobacco control policies over the last several decades, including raising taxes and/or prices on tobacco, smoke-free laws in public places, restrictions on tobacco advertising, educational campaigns, age restrictions for purchasing tobacco, and graphic warning labels.

As a more recent example, beginning in 2019, the U.S. CDC began investigating an epidemic of lung injuries associated with vaping or e-cigarette use. Cases of e-cigarette-associated lung injuries peaked in September 2019 and have since continued to decrease.[27] An important policy response to this epidemic was a 2020 United States Food and Drug Administration (FDA) policy which banned unauthorized flavored e-cigarettes that appeal to children, such as mint and fruit flavors.[28]

1. What other examples can you think of that link health policy and epidemiology? Think about how specific health-policy determinants (exposures) may be associated with certain health outcomes.

**Public health preparedness.** Our ability to successfully address future public health emergencies is dependent upon having the infrastructure and resources to plan and respond in a timely manner. Public health preparedness is critical to combat new pandemics and natural disasters. In partial response to bioterrorism threats, the early 2000s saw large improvements in public health preparedness to implement coordinated public health responses. This included increased laboratory, epidemiology, and surveillance response capabilities. The importance of public health preparedness has been evident during the COVID-19 pandemic: countries without robust public health preparedness systems and those lacking strong, coordinated responses fared much worse than those with greater preparedness and a more coordinated response. Just as it can be challenging to demonstrate the value of prevention activities when you cannot observe what *didn't* happen, it can also be challenging to gain the political and social backing that is required to prepare for a range of public health emergencies that *might* occur. For this reason, much work remains to ensure that we are ready to respond to whatever the next crisis might be. Additional information on this important topic is available elsewhere.[29]

## Pause to Practice 1.3

### Public Health Preparedness

A U.S. CDC report[30] describes the importance of public health preparedness during the H1N1 flu pandemic:

> As a result of [public health preparedness and response] efforts, the global response to the 2009 influenza A (H1N1) pandemic, which affected more than 214 countries and territories, was the most rapid and effective response to an influenza pandemic in history. The pandemic virus was rapidly identified and characterized. Epidemiologic investigations were conducted to characterize the severity and risk groups, and surveillance data were used to estimate the burden of disease and guide the response in real time. Within weeks of detecting the pandemic virus, diagnostic reagents were provided to laboratories in 146 countries, and laboratory and clinical training were provided, in collaboration with partners, to more than 6,100 health professionals in 34 countries. A vaccine was developed within 20 weeks of virus detection, and through an international donation program, made available to 86 countries. The lessons and experiences of the 2009 H1N1 response continue to inform preparedness efforts for future influenza pandemics as well as future public health emergencies.

Public health preparedness systems are only as strong as the political will and funding for these systems. For example, prior to and during the COVID-19 pandemic, many scientists were concerned about the impact that funding cuts for public health and preparedness in the United States would have on the trajectory of the pandemic.[31]

1. What other examples can you think of that link public health preparedness and epidemiology?

The previously noted key advances in public health were selected because they have significantly impacted mortality and/or the epidemiologic transition; however, this list is certainly not exhaustive. There have been many other major accomplishments attributable to improvements in public health, including advancements in occupational safety (e.g., workers' safety laws), neglected tropical disease control and prevention (including Guinea worm disease, onchocerciasis, and lymphatic filariasis, all of which have been targeted for elimination), road safety (e.g., seatbelts, vehicle and road design, safety laws, and public transport, and targeting alcohol impaired driving), tuberculous (TB) prevention and control (e.g., directly observed therapy initiatives), and ischemic heart disease prevention and control (e.g., reductions in hypertension, cholesterol, and smoking, and improved treatments). The achievements discussed in this chapter have helped shape the course of public health and highlight the interplay between epidemiology and other core public health disciplines.

## ETHICAL FOUNDATIONS OF HUMAN SUBJECTS RESEARCH
### (LEARNING OBJECTIVE 1.6)

Throughout this text, you will learn about the scientific methods that are foundational to the study of epidemiology. As important as these methods are, they must be accompanied by an understanding of and commitment to the conduct of ethical research in **human subjects**. Many textbooks confine the discussion of ethics to the discussion of clinical trials (described in **Chapter 4, "Randomized Controlled Trial Designs"**). Although there are ethical considerations pertinent to clinical trials, it is imperative that ethics and the history of medical research be kept at the forefront of *all* epidemiologic research with human subjects.

One of the oldest foundational ideals in human subjects research ethics is found within the Hippocratic Oath[32]—an oath taken by physicians—to "first, do no harm." This statement encapsulates the concept of **nonmaleficence**. Unfortunately, there have been, and continue to be, instances where both medical practices and research have failed to live up to this ideal.

Figure 1.5 illustrates a timeline beginning in the 1900s of major, though not exhaustive, examples of ethical violations of human subjects research according to today's standards, along with guidelines and regulations designed to improve the protection of human subjects. Some of the public health ethics violations are discussed in the text that follows in relation to the ethical guidelines which they spurred; however, we encourage readers to seek out additional resources to learn about each event indicated in Figure 1.5.

**The Nuremberg Code.**[33] The Nuremberg Code was developed after the 1946–1947 Nuremberg trials of Nazi doctors for committing atrocious medical experiments on Jewish people and others during World War II. A description of key principles from the Nuremberg Code is provided in **Table 1.4**. After you review these principles, consider how relatively recently they were established. For example, there were no requirements for voluntary consent of human subjects prior to 1946. The Nuremberg Code has been foundational in shaping current public health ethics.

**U.S. Kafauver–Harris Amendments.** Thalidomide, a drug with sedative effects, was prescribed in some countries in the 1950s to help with pregnancy-related nausea. Due to a lack of safety data, Dr. Frances Oldham Kelsey, a medical officer at the U.S. FDA, refused to approve the drug for use in the United States.[34] However, in places where thalidomide was introduced, it was found that the drug caused severe, and often fatal, birth defects in affected fetuses.[35]

In response to this tragedy, which ultimately affected tens of thousands of children worldwide, the United States passed the Kafauver–Harris Amendments, which are still used today by the FDA. These amendments require pharmaceutical companies to provide scientific evidence of drug safety *prior* to receiving FDA approval; disclose accurate information about side effects to users during marketing; and market generic drugs as existing, rather than new, medications. This amendment was a landmark achievement in protecting consumers and providing accurate information to allow the public to make informed decisions about their healthcare. Importantly, dietary supplements, such as multivitamins and probiotics, are regulated as foods, not drugs, and do not require FDA approval.[36] This means that dietary supplements have considerably less oversight in terms of establishing their safety and effectiveness before they are marketed compared to prescription or over-the-counter medications.

**Declaration of Helsinki.**[37] This declaration, first adopted in 1964, expanded on the Nuremberg Code with the goal of providing guidelines for human subjects research. The key principles from the Declaration of Helsinki are outlined in **Table 1.5**.[38]

The Declaration of Helsinki continues to shape ethics in many countries, and at the time of this writing it has been amended eight times to reflect advancements in our understanding of public health ethics (key amendments are also indicated in **Table 1.5**). This highlights that public health ethics are evolving and, in some cases, still debated. An important recent debate considers the ethics related to using placebo controls in clinical trials and ensuring all participants can access any treatments found to be effective once the trial ends—we will discuss this in **Chapter 4, "Randomized Controlled Trial Designs."**

As technologies evolve, so must research ethics: The 2000 Helsinki amendment included information about the need for informed consent from donors of biospecimens that could be linked to identifiable personal information. Consider the famous case of Henrietta Lacks, a Black woman with cervical cancer who died in 1951 at the age of 31. When seeking care,

# FIGURE 1.5 A TIMELINE OF SELECTED STUDIES VIOLATING TODAY'S PUBLIC HEALTH ETHICAL STANDARDS AND ETHICAL GUIDELINES AND REGULATIONS, 1932 TO 2010

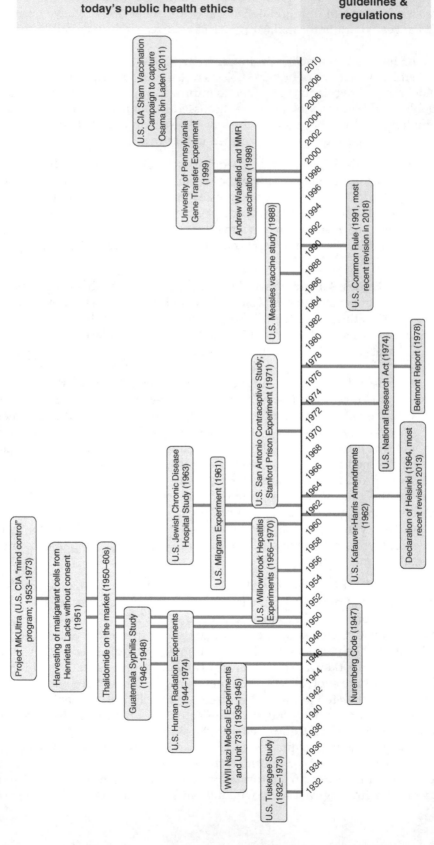

CIA, Central Intelligence Agency; MMR, measles, mumps, and rubella.

**TABLE 1.4 THE NUREMBERG CODE: SUMMARY OF KEY PUBLIC HEALTH ETHICAL PRINCIPLES**

| Voluntary Consent | • Potential study participants must have the legal capacity and knowledge of the study elements to decide whether to be involved in a study without coercion. |
|---|---|
| Benefit to Society | • Research using human subjects should not be conducted simply for the sake of acquiring new knowledge; rather, the study should be used to produce findings that benefit society. |
| Preliminary Data | • The study should be based on preliminary data (i.e., there should be some existing evidence base that supports the proposed study). |
| Risk Minimization | • The study should be designed to limit physical and mental suffering of the participants. |
| No Anticipated Death or Disability | • Researchers should not anticipate disability or death of the participants as a result of the study. |
| Benefits Outweigh Risks | • The expected benefits of the study to improve human health should outweigh any anticipated risks for the study participants. |
| Protection From Risks | • Systems must be in place to protect participants from any possible harm that could occur during the study. |
| Qualified Researchers | • The researchers must be scientifically qualified to conduct the study. |
| Participant Discontinuation | • Participants can leave the study at any point if they so choose. |
| Early Termination | • Researchers must be prepared to stop the study at any point if there is reason to believe that study participants may experience harm. |

**TABLE 1.5 THE DECLARATION OF HELSINKI: SUMMARY OF KEY PUBLIC HEALTH ETHICAL PRINCIPLES AND AMENDMENTS**

| General Principles<br>*2000 Amendment* | • The health of patients must be prioritized above research knowledge to be gained and protected.<br>• Respect for all human subjects must be ensured. |
|---|---|
| Benefits Outweigh Risks | • The expected benefits of the study to improve human health should outweigh any anticipated risks for the study participants. |
| Risk Minimization<br>*1975 Amendment* | • The study should be designed to assess, manage, and minimize risks to participants.<br>• Participants who are harmed should be compensated and/or treated. |
| Vulnerable Groups and Individuals<br>*2004 Amendment* | • Special protections should be provided for vulnerable groups who are at an increased risk of harm during the study.<br>• Research among vulnerable populations is only justifiable if the research is responsive to the health needs of this group *and* if the research cannot be carried out in nonvulnerable populations. |
| Scientific Requirements and Research Protocols<br>*1975 Amendment* | • The study must be conducted by qualified researchers.<br>• Study design and conduct must be justified and described in a research protocol which adheres to Declaration of Helsinki principles, as well as other generally accepted scientific principles. |
| Research Ethics Committees<br>*1975, 1989, & 2000 Amendments* | • The study protocol must be approved in advance by a transparent, independent, research ethics committee that is knowledgeable of the Declaration of Helsinki's guidance along with relevant international and local laws and regulations.<br>• This committee must also have the right to monitor the study and protocol amendments while it is ongoing. |
| Privacy and Confidentiality<br>*1975 Amendment* | • Efforts must be taken to maintain participant privacy and confidentiality of their personal information. |
| Informed Consent | • For individuals *capable* of giving informed consent, participants must be informed of the study elements, made aware that they can refuse to participate or withdraw consent at any time without penalty, and voluntarily provide (preferably written) informed consent to participate.<br>• For individuals *incapable* of giving informed consent, informed consent can be obtained from a legally authorized representative under certain circumstances. Such study participants may additionally be able to provide *assent* to certain aspects of the study.<br>• *2000 amendment*—For research using identifiable human material or data, researchers should seek to obtain, if possible, informed consent for its collection, storage, and use. |

*(continued)*

**TABLE 1.5 THE DECLARATION OF HELSINKI: SUMMARY OF KEY PUBLIC HEALTH ETHICAL PRINCIPLES AND AMENDMENTS** (*continued*)

| | |
|---|---|
| **Use of Placebo Groups**<br>*1996, 2000, & 2004 Amendments* | • When evaluating a new health intervention, the intervention should generally be compared to the best evidence-based intervention, if one exists.<br>• If no such intervention exists, researchers may use placebo controls (more on this in Chapter 5, "Cohort Designs") |
| **Post-trial Provision of Care**<br>*2000 & 2013 Amendments* | • In clinical trials, protocols must specify how all participants can access interventions found to be beneficial upon study completion. |
| **Research Registration, Publication, and Dissemination of Results**<br>*1975, 2000, 2008, & 2013 Amendments* | • Studies involving human subjects must be registered in a publicly available database prior to recruitment.<br>• Researchers have ethical obligations regarding the publication and dissemination of all findings to the public. |

her malignant cervical cancer cells were harvested and, due to their ability to survive and reproduce, were used for research without her consent. These became the first human cells successfully cloned for mass production, leading to millions of metric tons of cells. These cells have been used in thousands of studies including by Jonas Salk during the development of a polio vaccine, and more recently in research for COVID-19 vaccines. The use of HeLa (named for **H**enrietta **La**cks) cells has also sparked debate about confronting past healthcare injustices experienced disproportionately by people of color and evolving privacy issues—for example, the Lacks family contested the unauthorized publication of the HeLa cell.[39] The question of whether researchers should be allowed to use biospecimens without consent, even if that specimen is *not* identifiable with personal information (though it could be identifiable via genetic testing), is still being debated in the United States. In August 2023, the Lacks family reached a confidential settlement with Thermo Fisher Scientific, the biotech company that profitted extensively from the unauthorized use of Henrietta Lacks' cells.[39]

**The U.S. National Research Act and the Belmont Report.** In 1932, the U.S. Public Health Service and the Tuskegee Institute undertook a study in which researchers enrolled 399 Black men with syphilis—a serious bacterial infection that is typically sexually transmitted—and 201 Black men without syphilis.[40] These men did not provide informed consent, were not informed of the real purpose of the study, and did not receive treatment for their syphilis when penicillin became available in 1947. The atrocious Tuskegee syphilis experiments were conducted over 40 years—39.5 years longer than planned—and were finally exposed and halted in 1972.

Several hearings on unethical human subjects research, including the Tuskegee study, led the United States Congress to pass the 1974 **National Research Act**, which authorized federal agencies to develop human research regulations and ethical guidelines. The regulations required that institutions form **Institutional Review Boards (IRBs)**, which are boards of expert, independent reviewers, to review human subjects research studies to protect the welfare of study participants. The **U.S. Belmont Report**, also developed in response to the Tuskegee syphilis study, was written in 1978 by a commission established by the National Research Act. The Belmont Report established basic ethical principles in human subjects research. The key principles of the Belmont Report are:

- **Respect for persons:** Individuals should be treated autonomously and those with limited autonomous should be protected.

- **Beneficence:** A favorable risk–benefit ratio in which benefits are maximized and harms are minimized.

- **Justice:** Selection of subjects such that the burdens and benefits of research are equitably distributed.

**U.S. Common Rule.** The Common Rule is a federal policy for the protection of human subjects codified for use across U.S. federal institutions in 1991.[41] The main components include requirements for informed consent, IRBs, compliance across research institutions, and treatment of **vulnerable populations**. Key 2018 revisions to the Common Rule include:

- **Informed consent:** Informed consent forms must begin with a synthesis of all key information about the study for ease of understanding by study participants and must also specify if/when findings will be shared with study participants.

- **IRB monitoring for studies of minimal risk:** Studies that pose minimal risk to participants may be able to undergo less frequent IRB review.

- **Single IRBs:** Studies conducted at multiple research sites must have a single primary IRB that oversees the study to promote consistent compliance with ethical standards.

### Populations Requiring Additional Protections in Human Subjects Research

Some populations are at higher risk of harm when participating in a research study and thus require additional protection. These populations include fetuses, children, pregnant persons, those who are incarcerated, and those with impaired decision-making capacity. Depending on the particular study, other groups of individuals might be considered vulnerable, such as non-English speakers in a U.S.-based study, minoritized populations, or undocumented immigrants. It is important that these groups are protected during the study and that they are not coerced into participating. Both the Declaration of Helsinki and the Common Rule make specifications regarding the inclusion of these populations, sometimes called vulnerable populations, in human subjects research.

The ethical fundamentals described in this textbook are based on the current best practices in public health and medicine. It is critical to understand that public health ethics have evolved in leaps over time, often in response to atrocities committed through research, and recognize that these practices will continue to evolve. Researchers in public health and medicine must acknowledge these previous wrongdoings and work to *earn* (and, in many cases, *repair*) the trust of the communities we serve, many of whom have been historically mistreated and marginalized.

## EPIDEMIOLOGY AND SOCIAL DETERMINANTS OF HEALTH
### (LEARNING OBJECTIVE 1.7)

As demonstrated by the previous examples, epidemiology is not conducted in a vacuum—we must be mindful of the historical, ethical, and political contexts in which health-related outcomes occur. **Social determinants of health** are defined by the U.S. CDC as "conditions in the places where people live, learn, work, and play that affect a wide range of health risks and outcomes."[42] These determinants include access to quality healthcare and education, social and community context, and socioeconomic status. These determinants are often intertwined—as an example, poverty impacts access to good nutrition, safe living conditions, and education, all of which influence many different health outcomes.

Often, social determinants of health lead to **health inequities**, which occur when health outcomes are more frequent in some groups than in others. Findings from epidemiologic studies can be used to identify these inequities and inform the equitable allocation of resources to improve the health of those with the greatest need. Indeed, it is the ethical responsibility of public health researchers to study and address these inequalities.

Though researchers may be well-intentioned, they must be mindful that their experiences may differ from those of the communities that they aim to serve. For this reason, it is imperative that researchers acknowledge that they do not have all the answers and work closely with relevant communities and stakeholders to establish their trust and understand their unique strengths and struggles. By seeking to understand social determinants of health and applying what we learn, researchers can improve population health and promote **health equity**, which occurs when all people can achieve their health potential regardless of their social circumstances.

## ROADMAP FOR WHERE WE WILL GO FROM HERE

You now know what epidemiology is. You realize that we aren't dermatologists—but that we study the distribution and determinants of health-related outcomes such as diseases in order to improve human health. This text will provide you with a toolkit containing the foundational knowledge that is required to study any health outcome from asthma to Zika virus infection. We will also attempt to highlight throughout this text the importance of keeping the people and stories behind the numbers at the forefront.

Up next, we will differentiate between descriptive (**Chapter 2, "Descriptive Epidemiology, Surveillance, and Measures of Frequency"**) and analytic (**Chapter 3, "Introduction to Analytic Epidemiologic Study Designs and Measures of Association"**) epidemiologic study designs. We will then provide detailed information about the most common analytical epidemiologic study designs (**Chapter 4, "Randomized Controlled Trial Designs"; Chapter 5, "Cohort Designs"; Chapter 6, "Case-Control Designs"; and Chapter 7, "Cross-Sectional Designs"**). It turns out that an exposure might have a different effect on a health outcome for different groups of people—we'll explore this phenomenon, in **Chapter 8, "Effect Measure Modification and Statistical Interaction."** As you can guess, there are a lot of ways that errors can influence an epidemiologic study—we'll be sure to point these out and describe how to avoid common pitfalls (**Chapter 9, "Error in Epidemiologic Research and Fundamentals of Confounding"; Chapter 10, "Selection Bias"; and Chapter 11, "Information Bias and Screening and Diagnostic Tests"**). Next, we will discuss the role that random error plays in epidemiologic studies (**Chapter 12, "Random Error in Epidemiologic Research"**). Finally, this text will conclude with an introduction to more advanced epidemiologic analyses with an emphasis on how to interpret results from the published literature (**Chapter 13, "Introduction to Epidemiologic Data Analysis"**). As you read this text, you will see how epidemiology provides a framework for critical thinking that is needed not just for public health professionals but for everyone to be a responsible consumer of health-related information.

## END OF CHAPTER PROBLEM SET

1. What is the definition of epidemiology?

2. Are the following examples of endemic, epidemic, or pandemic diseases?
   a. In 2009, H1N1 influenza ("swine flu") unexpectedly affected millions of people around the globe.
   b. In the past several years, an average of 10 bubonic plague cases have been reported in the United States each year.
   c. A cook spread typhoid to over 100 New Yorkers in the early 1900s.

3. For each prevention activity noted in the following list, indicate whether it is an example of passive primary prevention, active primary prevention, secondary prevention, or tertiary prevention.
   a. Chemotherapy for cancer patients
   b. Improvement of air quality through required vehicle emissions testing
   c. Implementation of regular colonoscopy screening programs
   d. Enactment of seatbelt laws

4. How do the leading causes of mortality relate to the epidemiologic transition?

5. What are the key principles of the Belmont Report?

6. Provide at least three examples that link specific environmental exposures to their related health outcome(s).

7. Recall that social determinants of health are defined by the U.S. CDC as "conditions in the places where people live, learn, work, and play that affect a wide range of health risks and outcomes." Provide at least three examples of social determinants of health and their related health outcome(s).

8. In late summer of 2021, breakthrough cases of COVID-19 among fully vaccinated individuals started raising concern for some about the effectiveness of the vaccines. While no COVID-19 vaccine is 100% effective at preventing infection, those licensed in the United States have strong demonstrated benefits.
   Importantly, the vaccines licensed in the United States as of mid-2021 have also been shown to be effective at preventing hospitalizations and death after COVID-19 infection. According to the CDC, as of September 13, 2021, a total of 12,750 fully vaccinated individuals were hospitalized with a COVID-19 infection, and 3,040 fully vaccinated individuals had died from a COVID-19 infection. What additional data are needed to help support the underlined statement?

9. Revisit **Table 1.2,** which illustrates the 10 leading causes of death globally in the years 2000 and 2019. These data provide important insights into changes in the leading causes of mortality over *time,* but there may be some *person* and *place* characteristics that would also be useful to explore. What person and place characteristics might you be interested in to better understand patterns in causes of death?

10. Revisit **Table 1.3,** which compares the 10 leading causes of mortality in low- and high-income countries from 2019. What is your best guess (i.e., hypothesis) to explain the difference between the ranking of each of the following causes of death for low- and high-income countries:
    a. Diarrheal diseases
    b. Alzheimer disease and other dementias
    c. Road injury

# REFERENCES

1. Merriam-Webster. Disease. Updated May 22, 2023. https://www.merriam-webster.com/dictionary/disease?utm_campaign=sd&utm_medium=serp&utm_source=jsonld

2. Centers for Disease Control and Prevention. Gonorrhea (*Neisseria gonorrhoeae infection*) 2023 case definition. 2023. https://ndc.services.cdc.gov/case-definitions/gonorrhea-neisseria-gonorrhoeae

3. World Health Organization, Global Health Observatory Data Repository, and World Health Statistics. Incidence of malaria (per 1,000 population at risk)—Sub-Saharan Africa, Uganda. 2018. https://data.worldbank.org/indicator/SH.MLR.INCD.P3?locations=ZG-UG

4. Centers for Disease Control and Prevention. Malaria transmission in the United States. 2018. https://www.cdc.gov/malaria/about/us_transmission.html

5. Shi B, Zheng J, Xia S, et al. Accessing the syndemic of COVID-19 and malaria intervention in Africa. *Infect Dis Poverty.* 2021;10(1):Article 5. https://doi.org/10.1186/s40249-020-00788-y

6. Gutman JR, Lucchi NW, Cantey PT, et al. Malaria and parasitic neglected tropical diseases: potential syndemics with COVID-19? *Am J Trop Med Hyg.* 2020;103(2):572–577.

7. Centers for Disease Control and Prevention. COVID-19 vaccines while pregnant or breastfeeding. October 20, 2022. https://www.cdc.gov/coronavirus/2019-ncov/vaccines/recommendations/pregnancy.html#anchor_1628692520287

8. Benjamin R. Dr. Regina Benjamin's story: promoting health and wellness for all Americans. February 23, 2011. https://obamawhitehouse.archives.gov/blog/2011/02/23/dr-regina-benjamins-story-promoting-health-and-wellness-all-americans

9. World Health Organization. *World Health Statistics 2008.* Author; 2008. https://www.who.int/docs/default-source/gho-documents/world-health-statistic-reports/en-whs08-full.pdf

10. Ritchie H, Spooner F, Roser M. *Causes of death.* Our World in Data. Updated December 2019. https://ourworldindata.org/causes-of-death

11. McKeown RE. The epidemiologic transition: changing patterns of mortality and population dynamics. *Am J Lifestyle Med.* 2009;3(1 suppl):19S–26S. https://doi.org/10.1177/1559827609335350

12. United Nations. *World Population Prospects 2022.* 2022. https://population.un.org/wpp/Download/Standard/Mortality/

13. Schöley J., Aburto JM, Kashnitsky I. et al. Life expectancy changes since COVID-19. *Nat Hum Behav.* 2022;6:1649–1659. https://doi.org/10.1038/s41562-022-01450-3

14. Murphy, SL, Kochanek, KD, Xu, J, Arias, E. Mortality in the United States, 2020. NCHS Data Brief No. 427, December 2021. U.S. Department of Health and Human Services. https://www.cdc.gov/nchs/data/databriefs/db427.pdf

15. Xu, J, Murphy, SL, Kochanek, KD, Arias, E. Mortality in the United States, 2021. NCHS Data Brief No. 427, December 2022. U.S. Department of Health and Human Services. https://www.cdc.gov/nchs/data/databriefs/db456.pdf

16. Ahmad, FB, Cisewski, JA, Xu, J, Anderson, RN. Provisional Mortality Data - United States, 2022. U.S. Department of Health and Human Services, May 2023. https://www.cdc.gov/mmwr/volumes/72/wr/pdfs/mm7218a3-H.pdf

17. World Health Organization. The top 10 causes of death. December 9, 2020. https://www.who.int/news-room/fact-sheets/detail/the-top-10-causes-of-death

18. Ramsay MAE. John Snow, MD: anaesthetist to the Queen of England and pioneer epidemiologist. *Proceedings.* 2006;19(1):24–28. https://doi.org/10.1080/08998280.2006.11928120

19. Boylston A. The origins of inoculation. *J R Soc Med.* 2012;105(7):309–313. https://doi.org/10.1258/jrsm.2012.12k044

20. Smith KA. Edward Jenner and the small pox vaccine. *Front Immunol.* 2011;2:21. https://doi.org/10.3389/fimmu.2011.00021

21. Centers for Disease Control and Prevention. History of smallpox. 2016. https://www.cdc.gov/smallpox/history/history.html

22. Kim YC, Dema B, Reyes-Sandoval A. COVID-19 vaccines: breaking record times to first-in-human trials. *npj Vaccines.* 2020;5(1):34. https://doi.org/10.1038/s41541-020-0188-3

23. Wakefield AJ, Murch SH, Anthony A, et al. Ileal-lymphoid-nodular hyperplasia, non-specific colitis, and pervasive developmental disorder in children. *Lancet.* 1998;351(9103):637–641. https://doi.org/10.1016/s0140-6736(97)11096-0

24. Dobson R. Media misled the public over the MMR vaccine, study says. *BMJ.* 2003;326(7399):1107. https://doi.org/10.1136/bmj.326.7399.1107-a

25. Institute of Medicine Committee on the Economics of Antimalarial Drugs. A brief history of malaria. In: Arrow KJ, Panosian C, Gelband H, eds. *Saving Lives, Buying Time: Economics of Malaria Drugs in an Age of Resistance.* National Academies Press; 2004:125–135. https://doi.org/10.17226/11017

26. Centers for Disease Control and Prevention. *CDC's origins and malaria.* 2018. https://www.cdc.gov/malaria/about/history/history_cdc.html

27. Editorial. The EVALI outbreak and vaping in the COVID-19 era. *Lancet Respir Med.* 2020;8(9):831. https://www.ncbi.nlm.nih.gov/pmc/articles/PMC7428296/. https://doi.org/10.1016/S2213-2600(20)30360-X.

28. U.S. Food and Drug Administration. FDA finalizes enforcement policy on unauthorized flavored cartridge-based e-cigarettes that appeal to children, including fruit and mint. January 2, 2020. https://www.fda.gov/news-events/press-announcements/fda-finalizes-enforcement-policy-unauthorized-flavored-cartridge-based-e-cigarettes-appeal-children

29. Centers for Disease Control and Prevention. Office of Readiness and Response: what we do. 2021. https://www.cdc.gov/cpr/whatwedo/index.htm

30. Centers for Disease Control and Prevention. Ten great public health achievements—worldwide, 2001–2010. *MMWR Morb Mortal Wkly Rep.* 2011;60(24):814–818. https://www.cdc.gov/mmwr/preview/mmwrhtml/mm6024a4.htm

31. Devi S. US public health budget cuts in the face of COVID-19. *Lancet Infect Dis.* 2020;20(4):415. https://doi.org/10.1016/S1473-3099(20)30182-1

32. Jones WHS. The Hippocratic oath—Ludwig Edelstein: the Hippocratic oath. Text, translation, and interpretation. *Classical Rev.* 1945;59(1):14–15. https://philpapers.org/rec/JONTHO-3

33. *The Nuremberg Code (1947). BMJ.* 1996;313(7070):1448. https://media.tghn.org/medialibrary/2011/04/BMJ_No_7070_Volume_313_The_Nuremberg_Code.pdf

34. U.S. Food and Drug Administration. Frances Oldham Kelsey: medical reviewer famous for averting a public health tragedy. 2018. https://www.fda.gov/about-fda/virtual-fda-history/frances-oldham-kelsey-medical-reviewer-famous-averting-public-health-tragedy

35. Franks ME, Macpherson GR, Figg WD. Thalidomide. *Lancet.* 2004;363(9423):1802–1811. https://doi.org/10.1016/S0140-6736(04)16308-3

36. U.S. Food and Drug Administration. Dietary supplements. 2020. https://www.fda.gov/consumers/consumer-updates/dietary-supplements

37. World Medical Association. *Declaration of Helsinki.* 2021. https://www.wma.net/what-we-do/medical-ethics/declaration-of-helsinki

38. World Medical Association. World Medical Association Declaration of Helsinki. Ethical principles for medical research involving human subjects. *Bulletin of the World Health Organization.* 2001;79(4), 373–374. World Health Organization. https://apps.who.int/iris/handle/10665/268312

39. Nuwer, R. Scientists published Henrietta Lacks' genome without the consent of her family. *Smithsonian,* March 26, 2013. https://www.smithsonianmag.com/smart-news/scientists-published-henrietta-lacks-genome-without-the-consent-of-her-family-9022347/

40. Centers for Disease Control and Prevention. The Untreated Syphilis Study at Tuskegee. The Tuskegee Timeline. 2020. https://www.cdc.gov/tuskegee/timeline.htm

41. U.S. Department of Health and Human Services Office for Human Research Protections. Federal Policy for the Protection of Human Subjects ('Common Rule'). 2016. https://www.hhs.gov/ohrp/regulations-and-policy/regulations/common-rule/index.html

42. Centers for Disease Control and Prevention. Social determinants of health at CDC. 2020. https://www.cdc.gov/socialdeterminants/about.html

# CHAPTER 2

# DESCRIPTIVE EPIDEMIOLOGY, SURVEILLANCE, AND MEASURES OF FREQUENCY

## KEY TERMS

case definition

case report

case series

descriptive epidemiology

measures of frequency

prevalence

rate

risk

surveillance

## LEARNING OBJECTIVES

2.1 Define descriptive epidemiology.

2.2 Differentiate between well-defined and poorly defined case definitions of health outcomes.

2.3 Define descriptive epidemiologic designs: case reports and case series.

2.4 Define surveillance programs.

2.5 Define and calculate epidemiologic measures of frequency: risk, rate, and prevalence.

2.6 Describe health outcomes by person, place, and time characteristics and explain how this information can be used to generate hypotheses.

## SANDY FORD: A HERALD OF THE AIDS EPIDEMIC

In 1981, Sandra (Sandy) Ford, a U.S. Centers for Disease Control and Prevention (CDC) drug technician, played a major role in heralding the beginning of the HIV/AIDS epidemic. She noticed an increase in requests for pentamidine isethionate—a drug that was available in the United States only through the CDC for treatment of Pneumocystis pneumonia (PCP). Sandy kept meticulous records of the drugs she dispensed and knew that those typically diagnosed with and treated for PCP were immunocompromised and/or immuno-suppressed. After further communication with the treating physicians, she learned that all of these patients were otherwise healthy men who had sex with men. She knew that PCP cases in this population were highly unusual and reported her concerns. This set off an investigation into what would become the HIV/AIDS epidemic. Although Sandy had no formal epidemiologic training, she thought like an epidemiologist. She noticed an increase in drug requests to treat PCP in a population that did not usually experience this disease.[1] As stated in the book *And the Band Played On* by Randy Shilts, "That was how the thorough GS-7 drug technician in Room 161 of the Centers for Disease Control's Building 6 alerted the federal government to the new epidemic."(p. 66)

## WHAT IS DESCRIPTIVE EPIDEMIOLOGY? (LEARNING OBJECTIVE 2.1)

Recall that epidemiology is defined as the study of both the *distribution* and the *determinants* of health-related states and events, and the application of study findings to improve public health. Captured within this definition are two broad categories of epidemiology: descriptive epidemiology and analytic epidemiology (**Figure 2.1**).

In **descriptive epidemiology**, the focus of this chapter, investigators measure the *distribution* of health-related states or events (often called "health-related outcomes," or simply "outcomes"). These outcomes represent the *what* in epidemiologic studies. Descriptive epidemiology is used to identify the *frequency* of these outcomes and to help us understand *who* is affected, along with *where* and *when* the outcome is occurring. This is in contrast to analytic epidemiology, the focus of **Chapter 3, "Introduction to Analytic Epidemiologic Study Designs and Measures of Association,"** which seeks to explain *why* health-related outcomes occur (**Figure 2.1**).

### FIGURE 2.1 DESCRIPTIVE AND ANALYTIC EPIDEMIOLOGY: THE WHO, WHAT, WHERE, WHEN, AND WHY

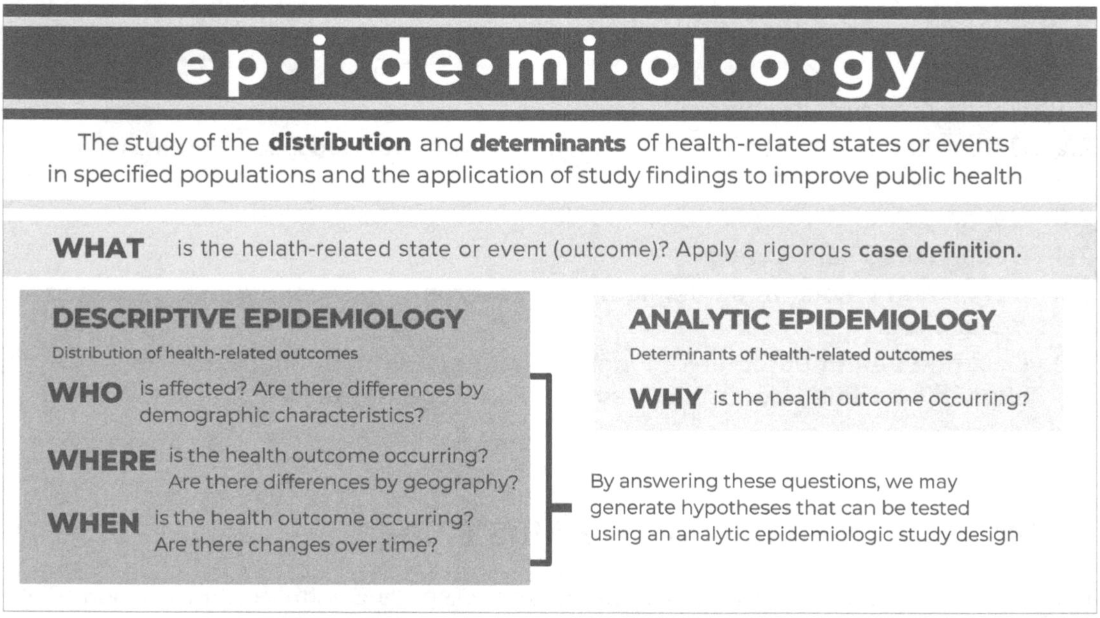

**ep·i·de·mi·ol·o·gy**

The study of the **distribution** and **determinants** of health-related states or events in specified populations and the application of study findings to improve public health

**WHAT** is the helath-related state or event (outcome)? Apply a rigorous **case definition**.

**DESCRIPTIVE EPIDEMIOLOGY**
Distribution of health-related outcomes

**WHO** is affected? Are there differences by demographic characteristics?

**WHERE** is the health outcome occurring? Are there differences by geography?

**WHEN** is the health outcome occurring? Are there changes over time?

**ANALYTIC EPIDEMIOLOGY**
Determinants of health-related outcomes

**WHY** is the health outcome occurring?

By answering these questions, we may generate hypotheses that can be tested using an analytic epidemiologic study design

Descriptive epidemiology is the backbone of epidemiologic research—to understand why patterns of health and disease are occurring, we must first understand which populations are affected as well as whether there are any important patterns of health-related outcomes over time and by geography. Epidemiologists use one or more **measures of frequency** (risk, rate, and prevalence, defined later in this chapter) to quantify the occurrence of health-related outcomes in populations that are often defined by person, place, or time characteristics. For example, if our outcomes of interest are cervical human papillomavirus (HPV) infection and cervical dysplasia (precancerous cells on the cervix), descriptive epidemiologic data can be used to illustrate how the proportion of people affected by these outcomes has decreased in the United States over the past several years. Mapping this to our considerations of person, place, and time characteristics, **Figure 2.2** illustrates the frequency of cervical HPV infection and cervical dysplasia among young women (person) in the United States (place) between 2003 and 2014 (time).

Although descriptive epidemiology does not evaluate *why* health outcomes occur, it can be used to generate hypotheses about the potential determinants, or causes, of outcomes. For example, the data in **Figure 2.2** may lead researchers to hypothesize that the decreasing frequency of HPV infection and cervical dysplasia over time is, in part, due to the increasing availability and uptake of the HPV vaccine, which was approved in the United States for females in 2006 and for males in 2011.

In contrast, analytic epidemiology (described in **Chapter 3, "Introduction to Analytic Epidemiologic Study Designs and Measures of Association"**) focuses on answering *why* health outcomes occur by quantifying the effect of determinants (often called "exposures") on health outcomes. Determinants can be any number of factors that are possibly associated with an outcome. For example, previous research has shown that determinants of cervical dysplasia may include younger age at first sexual intercourse, smoking, and not receiving the HPV vaccine.[2] As you will learn in **Chapter 3, "Introduction to Analytic Epidemiologic Study Designs and Measures of Association,"** to study the association between an exposure and a health outcome, we first develop testable hypotheses regarding the association between the two. Data from descriptive studies may help us generate hypotheses to be tested in an analytic study. For example, an analytic epidemiologic study may ask the question, "Is HPV vaccination uptake associated with decreasing rates of cervical dysplasia among women in the United States?" Data from descriptive studies may help us generate hypotheses to be tested in an analytic study.

## FIGURE 2.2 PROPORTION OF YOUNG WOMEN IN THE UNITED STATES WITH (A) CERVICAL HUMAN PAPILLOMAVIRUS INFECTION AND (B) CERVICAL DYSPLASIA

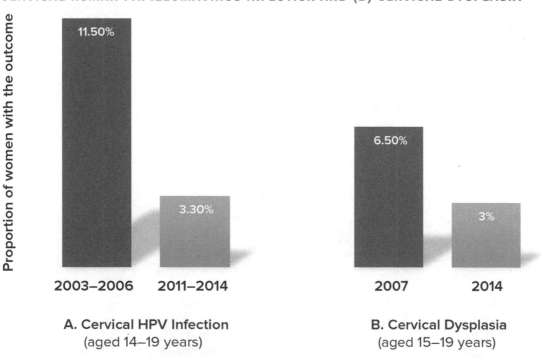

A. Cervical HPV Infection
(aged 14–19 years)

B. Cervical Dysplasia
(aged 15–19 years)

*Source:* https://prescancerpanel.cancer.gov/report/hpvupdate/HPVCancers.html

## DEFINING HEALTH OUTCOMES: CASE DEFINITIONS (LEARNING OBJECTIVE 2.2)

As mentioned in **Chapter 1, "Introduction to Public Health and the Fundamentals of Epidemiology,"** health-related outcomes are often, but not always diseases. Regardless of whether your outcome is a disease or some other health-related event, it is critical to establish a rigorous definition of the outcome, called a **case definition**. The case definition includes criteria that must be met for an individual to be classified as having the outcome of interest. This definition should be consistently applied within your study and, ideally, is one that has been consistently applied across prior studies.

### Fundamentals of Case Definitions

Depending on the outcome of interest, case definitions may contain a combination of clinical (e.g., blood pressure) and laboratory (e.g., total cholesterol) criteria and may be further categorized as suspect, probable, or confirmed. These classifications reflect different degrees of certainty in the classification of a health outcome—with the most certainty given to cases classified as "confirmed." The current U.S. CDC case definition for gonorrhea is shown in the text that follows as an example.

### U.S. Centers for Disease Control and Prevention 2023 Case Definition for Gonorrhea

#### Clinical Description

Gonorrhea is a sexually transmitted infection caused by the bacterium Neisseria gonorrhoeae. Gonococcal infection can result in urethritis, epididymitis, cervicitis, acute salpingitis, proctitis, pharyngitis, or other syndromes when sexually transmitted; however, infections at the endocervix, pharynx, and rectum are often asymptomatic.

#### Laboratory Criteria

Confirmatory laboratory evidence:
Isolation of Neisseria gonorrhoeae by culture of a clinical specimen, minimally with isolation of typical gram-negative, oxidase-positive diplococci,

OR

Detection of Neisseria gonorrhoeae by nucleic acid amplification (e.g., Polymerase Chain Reaction [PCR]) or hybridization with a nucleic acid probe in a clinical specimen.
Presumptive laboratory evidence:
Observation of gram-negative intracellular diplococci in a urethral or an endocervical smear.

#### Case Classification

Probable
Meets presumptive laboratory evidence in the absence of confirmatory laboratory evidence.
Confirmed
Meets confirmatory laboratory evidence.

*Source:* Adapted from the CDC website, accessed August 2023. Centers for Disease Control and Prevention. https://ndc.services.cdc.gov/case-definitions/gonorrhea-neisseria-gonorrhoeae[3]

The International Classification of Diseases (ICD) is a commonly used system to classify and report many diseases and other health outcomes in a standardized way. The first edition of the ICD was published in 1893 and focused on causes of death. ICD case definitions are now much broader and enable standardized reporting of many health-related outcomes across countries over time.

When a health-related outcome does not have a national or international standard case definition, it can be helpful to review the published literature to see how other researchers have defined the outcome. It may also be helpful to consult relevant experts in the field to develop a rigorous case definition.

## What Happens When a Case Definition Is Too Narrow?

Challenges can arise when case definitions are **insensitive**, meaning that they may not identify those who actually have a health outcome of interest. For example, if a case definition for a health outcome requires that an individual have a symptom that is seen in only 10% of those who truly have that health outcome, it is likely that individuals will be classified as *not* having the outcome when they actually *do* (these instances are called "false negatives").

## What Happens When a Case Definition Is Too Broad?

Challenges can also arise when case definitions are not **specific**, meaning that they may classify individuals as *having* a health outcome when they actually *do not*. For example, a case definition that only includes having fever and cough, very common symptoms associated with many diseases, would be unspecific. Using this case definition, it is likely that many people would be classified as having a given outcome when they actually do not (these instances are called "false positives").

We will discuss the use of case definitions with varying levels of sensitivity and specificity when we discuss screening and diagnostic programs in **Chapter 11, "Information Bias and Screening and Diagnostic Tests."** Once an appropriate case definition has been identified, it must then be consistently applied to identify individuals with that particular health outcome. We strive to capture everyone who meets these criteria and not accidentally classify someone as having the outcome when they do not.

### Pause to Practice 2.1

#### Real-World Challenges When Applying Case Definitions

Case definitions for some outcomes may be most rigorously defined using a combination of behavioral, clinical, and laboratory criteria. However, some gold standard (i.e., the best available) laboratory diagnostics may not be available in certain settings due to limited resources or logistical constraints. For example, in much of sub-Saharan Africa, molecular testing (a highly sensitive and specific method) for diagnosis of sexually transmitted infections (STIs) is not currently available in most government-run health facilities. For this reason, STI cases are commonly defined syndromically (i.e., only using clinical signs and symptoms, without laboratory criteria), which is not as accurate as molecular testing.

1. If the syndromic case definition for the STI gonorrhea in men was highly *sensitive*, what impact would this have on the accuracy of case identification?

2. If the syndromic case definition for the STI gonorrhea in men was not very *specific*, what impact would this have on the accuracy of case identification?

## What Happens When a Case Definition Changes Over Time?

It is important to note that case definitions may change over time, often due to improved understanding of the etiology of health-related outcomes or advancements in diagnostic testing. The ICD is currently in its 11th edition, which was released by the World Health Organization (WHO) in 2018 and included many substantive changes to some case definitions (https://icd.who.int/en). An historic update in this revision was the reclassification of gender incongruence from being classified as a mental health condition to classification as a condition related to sexual health.[4] Many experts and advocates had challenged the classification of gender in-congruence as a mental health disorder for many years, noting that the etiology is not, in fact, related to mental health conditions, and that incorrectly classifying it as such was stigmatizing and affected access to care. Such changes to case definitions over time also affect measures of outcome frequency; if researchers were conducting a study to measure *all* mental health dis-orders in a population, their case definition would have changed in 2018. The key takeaway is that, when looking at health outcome data collected over time, it is important to know whether there have been substantive changes in accepted case definitions in order to correctly interpret trends in the data. If a substantial change has been made to a case definition, direct compari-sons of the frequency of the health outcome before and after the change may be flawed.

The key considerations for case definitions are summarized in **Figure 2.3**.

## FIGURE 2.3 KEY CONSIDERATIONS FOR CASE DEFINITIONS

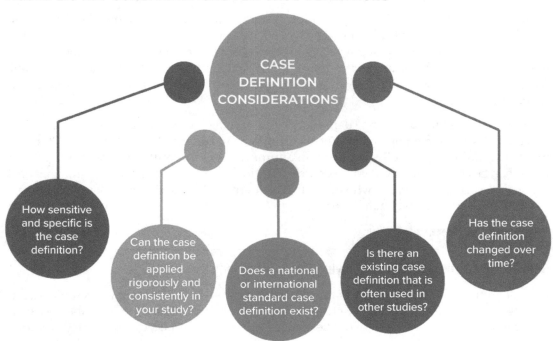

## DESCRIPTIVE EPIDEMIOLOGIC STUDY DESIGNS

We now know that descriptive epidemiology helps us understand how to define health out-comes (the *what*) along with the landscape to help address the questions of *who* is affected and *when* and *where* the outcome is occurring. Next, we will turn our attention to the different types of descriptive epidemiologic study designs, which include **case reports** and **case series**. Surveillance programs, though not a descriptive design per se, are also used to generate de-scriptive data and will be discussed later in this chapter.

### Case Reports and Case Series (LEARNING OBJECTIVE 2.3)

A **case report** is a detailed description of a single person with a particular health-related outcome of interest. Case reports are typically conducted when a new health-related outcome arises or a known outcome presents in an unexpected way. Case reports are prepared as a detailed story of the case and describe the main diagnosis, signs and symptoms, therapeutic interventions, clini-cal and laboratory diagnostic findings, follow-up assessments, and future health outcomes (e.g., prognosis). The **E**nhancing the **QUA**lity and **T**ransparency **O**f health **R**esearch (EQUATOR)

Network (www.equator-network.org), an international initiative that publishes guidelines for reporting different types of epidemiologic studies, created the CARE guidelines for reporting case reports. These guidelines help ensure that case reports are presented in a standardized way for consistency and comparability across reports. A collection of case reports for multiple individuals with the same unexpected health-related outcome is called a **case series**.

While case reports and case series can be helpful in describing a new health outcome or surprising signs and symptoms, they cannot be used to understand the outcome's frequency since we don't know the size of the population that these cases came from. Recall the importance of denominators for interpreting the frequency of health outcomes and making comparisons across different populations discussed in **Chapter 1, "Introduction to Public Health and the Fundamentals of Epidemiology."**

## Pause to Practice 2.2

### Case Series and the Identification of HIV/AIDS

Arguably one of the most famous case series was published in the *Morbidity and Mortality Weekly Report (MMWR)*, a publication from the U.S. CDC. On June 5, 1981, clinicians in Los Angeles, California, reported five cases of *Pneumocystis* pneumonia, a rare form of pneumonia, in formerly healthy young adult men who had had sex with men.[5] These cases occurred between October 1980 and May 1981. This clustering of cases, diagnosed in three Los Angeles hospitals, was unexpected; until that time, *Pneumocystis* pneumonia was almost exclusively diagnosed in older and immunosuppressed patients. This case series was fundamental in leading to the hypothesis that these patients were suffering from an unknown, underlying immunodeficiency that was later determined to be caused by the virus now known as human immunodeficiency virus (HIV).

Use the information from this case series description to answer the following descriptive epidemiologic questions.

1.  *What* is the health outcome of interest?
2.  *Who* is affected?
3.  *When* are the health outcomes occurring?
4.  *Where* is the health outcome occurring?

## PUBLIC HEALTH SURVEILLANCE (LEARNING OBJECTIVE 2.4)

**Public health surveillance,** a foundation of public health practice, is the systematic, ongoing collection of health-related data in a specified population that is disseminated in a timely manner to improve the health of populations (**Figure 2.4**).[6] Surveillance systems, though not epidemiologic study designs per se, are programs that generate descriptive epidemiologic data. Surveillance systems should be designed to meet well-defined objectives and are often used to:

*   Estimate the *frequency* of health-related outcomes in a population.
*   Identify *subgroups* with elevated frequency of health-related outcomes.
*   Identify *trends* such as new or worsening public health problems, epidemics, and changes in health-related behavior.
*   Support *contact tracing* programs for infectious diseases.
*   Facilitate public health *program planning.*
*   Evaluate the *effectiveness* of public health programs.
*   Generate research *hypotheses.*

**FIGURE 2.4 KEY CHARACTERISTICS OF A PUBLIC HEALTH SURVEILLANCE SYSTEM**

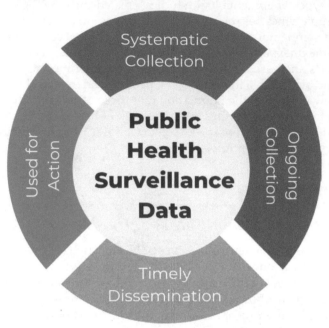

### Contact Tracing

Contact tracing is an important component of public health surveillance for some infectious diseases and is much like detective work. Once an individual has been identified as having a health outcome, public health officials provide them with information about how they can protect themselves and those around them while also asking about any individuals with whom they have been in contact. The definition of a contact depends on the disease. For example, for COVID-19, a close contact has been defined as anyone who was within 6 feet (2 meters) of an infected person for 15 minutes or more over a given 24-hour period.[7] Public health officials may then reach out to individuals who have been identified as close contacts and explain what precautions they should take to keep themselves and those around them safe. This process should maintain the confidentiality of all parties and should happen quickly to prevent further spread of the disease.

There are two main types of public health **surveillance**: passive and active. In **passive surveillance**, health-related outcomes are reported by hospitals, laboratories, physicians, or other relevant groups (called "reporting sites") to health agencies. Passive surveillance is relatively simple, inexpensive, and useful for routine, long-term surveillance activities. However, it relies on reporting by people and institutions, which can reduce data completeness and quality. As a result, passive surveillance systems often underreport the number of cases of a given health outcome.

In contrast, **active surveillance** requires proactive and regular contact by health agencies to obtain information about certain health outcomes that typically pose a high risk to public health. Active surveillance systems generally have better data completeness and quality than passive systems but are more expensive and resource intensive. Due to their higher cost, active surveillance systems are often shorter-term; for example, they are utilized during outbreaks or to monitor seasonal diseases such as influenza.

**Sentinel surveillance** is a type of active surveillance in which a limited number of reporting sites are selected for reporting. These sites typically have a high frequency of the health outcome of interest, robust staffing, and requisite laboratory facilities. Sentinel surveillance is useful when high-quality data are needed, and/or detailed case investigations are warranted.

## Notifiable Conditions

Some health outcomes are required to be reported to relevant health agencies. These are called *notifiable conditions*. The United States uses the CDC's National Notifiable Diseases Surveillance System (NNDSS; www.cdc.gov/nndss/index.html) to collect data on roughly 120 diseases. Some of the current nationally notifiable diseases in the United States include anthrax, botulism, cancer, measles, plague, and now COVID-19. Internationally notifiable diseases are reportable in compliance with the WHO's regulations. Lists of notifiable conditions are typically updated as new conditions emerge and their distributions change.

Public health surveillance data should be disseminated to, or shared with, relevant audiences including healthcare providers, public health personnel, policy makers, government officials, community-based organizations, and the public. This should happen in a timely manner to allow for public health action, including informing treatment and control programs as well as shaping policy. Public health surveillance programs are a vast topic in epidemiology, and indeed, entire textbooks and resources are dedicated to this subject.[8,9] We encourage readers who are interested in additional details about public health surveillance to explore these references.

## Pause to Practice 2.3

### SARS-CoV-2 Surveillance and Public Health Impact

Severe acute respiratory syndrome coronavirus-2 (SARS-CoV-2) is the virus responsible for the coronavirus disease (COVID-19) pandemic. In the United States, COVID-19 cases are reportable to the CDC, and standardized COVID-19 surveillance data come from multiple sources, including ILINet, which actively conducts surveillance for influenza-like illness. Surveillance data on U.S. COVID-19 cases, along with basic patient characteristics, are publicly available.[7]

1. What public health actions could COVID-19 surveillance data be used for?

## Highlights

### Descriptive Epidemiologic Study Designs and Surveillance

- **Case reports** and **case series** are two main descriptive epidemiologic study designs:
  - Case series are a collection of case reports on the same health outcome.
  - They are useful to learn about new health outcomes or health outcomes that are appearing in a new way.
  - They cannot be used to estimate outcome frequency since they lack information about the population from which the cases came.
- **Surveillance** is used to assess the health status of a population through standardized and routine data collection to ultimately improve the health of populations.
  - Surveillance systems generate data that are used for descriptive analyses.
  - Surveillance systems are used to estimate the frequency of health outcomes when the size of the population from which the cases came is known.

# EPIDEMIOLOGIC MEASURES OF FREQUENCY (LEARNING OBJECTIVE 2.5)

Once a case definition has been established and is applied in a research study, medical practice, or surveillance system, researchers can begin tabulating the number of health outcomes in a population. These **counts** provide one important piece of information used to describe the frequency of health outcomes in a population. Although it can be useful to know how many health outcomes have occurred, a count alone is often insufficient to appropriately describe the burden of a health outcome in a given population. Counts lack important contextualizing information regarding the size of the population in which these health outcomes occurred. Suppose that we only knew that 990 cases of a health outcome had occurred. The magnitude of this problem would be very different if these cases arose in a population of 1,000 versus a population of 100,000,000.

In epidemiology, the measures that quantify the occurrence of a health outcome, while also providing important context regarding the population, are called **measures of frequency**. Broadly speaking, measures of frequency are calculated by dividing the count of a given health outcome by a relevant denominator. The key measures of frequency are **risk**, **rate**, and **prevalence**. Risk and rate are used to describe the occurrence of *new*, or **incident**, health outcomes, whereas prevalence is used to describe the occurrence of *existing*, or **prevalent**, health outcomes. Measures of incidence and prevalence are discussed in further detail in the text that follows.

## Measures of Incidence

### RISK (CUMULATIVE INCIDENCE)

The **risk** (also called **cumulative incidence**) of a health-related outcome is defined as the proportion of at-risk individuals who develop a newly occurring outcome during a specified time-period.

$$\text{Risk} = \frac{\text{Number of newly occurring outcomes during a follow-up period}}{\text{Number of at-risk people observed during a follow-up period}} \tag{2.1}$$

Let's examine the key components of this definition.

**Proportion.** A proportion is a ratio that relates a part (the numerator) to a whole (the denominator). Proportions (and therefore risks) can be expressed as either a decimal or percentage and thus can range from 0 to 1 or 0% to 100%. A risk of 0 (or 0%) means that no one developed the outcome during the follow-up period. Whereas a risk of 1 (or 100%) means that everyone developed the outcome during the follow-up period.

**Newly occurring.** First, it is important to note that risk describes the frequency of newly occurring or *incident* outcomes (this is in contrast to existing, or prevalent, cases of an outcome, which we explore in detail later). For this reason, the numerator contains the number of *new* cases of a health outcome that developed during a specified period of time.

**At-risk.** To estimate the proportion of people who *develop* a newly occurring outcome during a specified time period, we should include only those who are at-risk of developing the health outcome in the denominator. Another way to think about this is that anyone included in the denominator must be at-risk of being (or eligible to be) counted in the numerator. For example, a newly occurring case of multiple sclerosis (MS; a disease of the central nervous system that is currently incurable) cannot occur in someone who already has MS. Since someone with MS is no longer at-risk for developing a new case of MS, they should not be included in the denominator of a risk calculation. As another example, individuals without prostates are not at-risk of developing prostate cancer, and thus they should not be included in the denominator of a calculation aimed to identify the risk of prostate cancer.

**Follow-up period.** To observe newly occurring cases of an outcome, and thus obtain a measure of the outcome's incidence, at-risk individuals must be followed (or observed) for some specified period of time. The period during which at-risk individuals are followed is called follow-up time, the follow-up period, or the risk period. This period must be specified when interpreting a measure of risk.

Let's work through an example of calculating and interpreting risk. Assume a group of 2,000 individuals who did not have MS were enrolled in a study and each person was followed for up to 20 years. Assume that none of the 2,000 individuals were **lost to follow-up**, meaning that they were all followed until either 1) they developed MS or 2) the study ended after 20 years. If during the 20 years of follow-up, seven new cases of MS developed in this population, what is the 20-year risk of MS?

$$\text{Risk} = \frac{7}{2,000} = 0.0035 = 0.35\%$$

This risk can be interpreted in words as: *The 20-year risk of MS in this population is 0.0035, or 0.35%.* Said differently, 0.35% of this population developed MS during the 20-year follow-up period.

## How Many Decimal Places to Report?

We advise against reporting quantitative results with too many significant digits when you report your findings. Different fields and journals recommend reporting different numbers of significant digits; in general, we recommend rounding your findings to between one and three significant digits. Reporting extraneous significant digits can overstate how confident we are in our estimates and also becomes difficult to read.

Some examples of reporting too many decimal places are shown below:

✗ Risk = 0.012345
✗ Risk = 1.2345%

Some examples of how to report an appropriate number of decimal places are shown below:

✓ Risk = 0.012
✓ Risk = 1.23%
✓ Risk = 1.2%

Note that the risk gives no indication of *when* the outcomes occurred during the follow-up period. Individuals may have developed MS early in the 20-year follow-up period, or they may have developed it closer to the 20-year mark. It is possible that those who experience new outcomes *earlier* in the follow-up period may be different in important ways from those who experience new outcomes *later* in the follow-up period. One way to determine whether there are patterns over time would be to split the follow-up time into smaller intervals and calculate the risk within each of the intervals (e.g., what is the risk of MS during the first 10 years of follow-up? What is the risk of MS during the second 10 years of follow-up?).

It is critical to specify the length of the follow-up period when interpreting a risk. The importance of including the follow-up period in the interpretation is underscored when estimating the risk of death—an outcome that is inevitable over a long enough follow-up period. Let's consider the risk of death for a healthy 25-year-old. Their risk of death during the next 5 minutes is likely to be very small (e.g., 0.00005% risk of death during the next 5 minutes). However, as the length of follow-up time increases, that same person's risk of death will increase (e.g., 5% risk of death during the next 10 years; 20% risk of death during the next 25 years). Barring major medical breakthroughs, this person's risk of death during the next 200 years will be 100%. Thus, we would never interpret the risk of death without indicating the period of time to which we are referring. For example, we would say that the *25-year* risk of death for a healthy 25-year-old is 20%.

## Reoccurring Outcomes

If the outcome of interest can reoccur (for example, treatable STIs, some cancers, and many other outcomes that may resolve but reoccur at a later point in time), investigators must decide how to handle recurrent outcomes. Sometimes, either for the sake of simplicity or because a second occurrence of an outcome is not different in important ways from the first, researchers will define their outcome as the first event to occur during the study period. If there is an interest in studying repeated occurrences of an outcome, there are advanced analytic techniques beyond the scope of this text that allow for these considerations.[10]

## Challenges in Calculating Risk

To accurately calculate risk, we must know the outcome status for everyone in the population by the end of the follow-up period. Unfortunately, this doesn't always happen, for two possible reasons:

- **Loss to follow-up:** Loss to follow-up can occur because an individual has changed their contact information or no longer wants to participate in the study. Researchers don't know whether an individual got the outcome of interest because they were not able to re-contact the participant.

- **Competing risks:** Study participants experienced an event, like death, during follow-up that prevented the outcome of interest from occurring. Thus, we do not know if the outcome *would have* occurred had the competing event *not happened*.

Loss to follow-up or competing risks is more likely to occur when the follow-up period is very long, when the study population is highly mobile, or when the study population experiences high rates of morbidity or mortality.

Let's examine the impact that loss to follow-up could have on our risk calculation in the MS study. Suppose that during the 20 years of follow-up, four individuals who developed MS moved to a new address and could not be contacted before their MS diagnosis occurred. The 20-year risk would then be incorrectly calculated as:

$$\text{Risk} = \frac{(7-4)}{2,000} = \frac{3}{2,000} = 0.0015 = 0.15\%$$

In this example, we would underestimate the true risk of MS in the population. In short, if a study is impacted by loss to follow-up or competing risks, it can be difficult, if not impossible, to accurately calculate risk without advanced statistical techniques that are beyond the scope of this text.[11] Another alternative is to use a different measure of incidence that accounts for loss to follow-up and varying amounts of follow-up time: the incidence rate.

### RATE (INCIDENCE DENSITY)

The **rate** (also called **incidence rate** or **incidence density**) is a measure of how *quickly* new health-related outcomes occur in an at-risk population during a follow-up period.

$$\text{Rate} = \frac{\text{Number of outcomes newly occurring during a follow-up period}}{\text{Total \textbf{person-time} among at-risk individuals}} \qquad (2.2)$$

Like the risk, the rate is a measure of the *incidence* of health outcomes; thus, the numerator of a rate also includes the number of new cases of a health outcome that occurred in the study population during the follow-up period. Where the rate differs from the risk is in the construction of the denominator. Rather than summing the number of at-risk *individuals* followed in your study, the rate's denominator sums the total amount of *time* that the at-risk individuals contributed during your study. This summation of time is called **person-time** and it allows researchers to more accurately incorporate information from everyone enrolled in the study, regardless of how long they were followed.

It is often the case that participants will enter and leave studies at different time points. To conceptualize person-time, consider **Figure 2.5**, which illustrates how different participants might contribute different amounts of time during a study. This figure depicts five participants from a study population in which subjects could have been followed for up to 5 years (from January 1, 2020, to January 1, 2025).

**FIGURE 2.5 A SNAPSHOT OF AN EPIDEMIOLOGIC STUDY WITH VARYING AMOUNTS OF PERSON TIME**

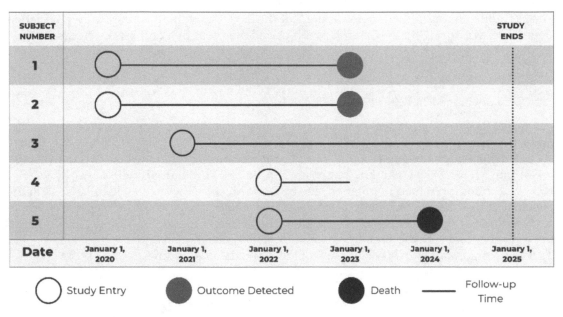

In this example, subjects #1 and #2 entered the study in 2020, while subject #3 entered in 2021, and subjects #4 and #5 didn't enter until 2022. Two subjects experienced the outcome of interest (subjects #1 and #2), one subject made it to the end of the study period without experiencing the outcome (subject #3), one subject was lost to follow-up (subject #4), and one subject died (subject #5). We can find the total person-time for these study participants by summing the number of years that each person contributed to the study:

$$\text{Person-years} = 3 \text{ years}_{(\#1)} + 3 \text{ years}_{(\#2)} + 4 \text{ years}_{(\#3)} + 1 \text{ year}_{(\#4)} + 2 \text{ years}_{(\#5)}$$
$$= 13 \text{ person-years}$$

Notice that a participant stops accumulating person-time as soon as they complete the study, are lost to follow-up, experience a competing risk, or experience the outcome of interest. There may be times when researchers continue to track person-time for someone after they have experienced the outcome—for example, when researchers are interested in studying outcome recurrence, or when they are also following participants for some other outcome (e.g., death). However, for the purposes of this textbook, we will only consider the person-time that someone contributes before they have their first occurrence of the outcome.

We can use this information to calculate the rate of the outcome in this study:

$$\text{Rate} = \frac{2 \text{ cases}}{13 \text{ person-years}} = 0.154 \text{ cases per person-year}$$

$$= \frac{2 \text{ cases}}{13 \text{ person-years}} \times \frac{100}{100} = 15.4 \text{ cases per 100 person-years}$$

Equivalent ways to interpret this rate include:

- An average of 0.15 cases of this health outcome occurred per person per year.
- An average of 15 cases of this health outcome occurred per 100 people per year.
- In every 100 people, an average of 15 cases of the health outcome occurred each year.

Presenting the rate as 0.15 cases per person-year is mathematically correct but isn't very easy to interpret. Instead, the convention is to scale the rates by multiplying both the numerator and denominator by a factor of 10 (e.g., 10, 100, 1,000, 10,000, 100,000, or even 1,000,000) to yield a value that reflects at least one whole case of the outcome.

Let's return to our MS example, where 7 of the 2,000 individuals in the study population developed MS during the 20-year follow-up period. Suppose that of these seven cases:

- Two developed MS after 4 years.
- Three developed MS after 9 years.
- Two developed MS after 12 years.

Further, assume that all 1,993 individuals who did not develop MS were followed for the entire 20-year study period.

To calculate a rate, we must only consider the person-time that participants contributed when they were *at-risk* for an MS diagnosis. For the 1,993 individuals who never developed MS, we can multiply their population size by 20 years since they were all still at-risk at the conclusion of the follow-up period. However, we cannot assign 20 years of person-time to each of those who *did* develop MS, since they are no longer at-risk for MS once it has developed. Instead, we sum the amount of person-time they accumulated prior to developing MS. The total person-time for this example would be calculated as follows:

$$\text{Person-years} = (1{,}993 \text{ people} \times 20 \text{ years}) + (4 \text{ years}) + (4 \text{ years}) + (9 \text{ years})$$

$$+ (9 \text{ years}) + (9 \text{ years}) + (12 \text{ years}) + (12 \text{ years})$$

$$= 39{,}919 \text{ person-years}$$

We can then use this information to calculate the rate of MS in this population:

$$\text{Rate of MS} = \frac{7 \text{ cases}}{39{,}919 \text{ person-years (PY)}}$$

$$= 0.000175 \text{ cases per person-year}$$

We could report the **rate of multiple sclerosis per 10,000 person-years** as follows:

$$\text{Rate of MS per 10,000 person-years} = \frac{7 \text{ cases}}{39{,}919 \text{ PY}} \times \frac{10{,}000}{10{,}000}$$

$$= 1.75 \text{ cases per } \mathbf{10{,}000} \text{ person-years}$$

We could equivalently report the **rate of multiple sclerosis per 100,000 person-years** as:

$$\text{Rate of MS per 100,000 person-years} = \frac{7 \text{ cases}}{39{,}919 \text{ PY}} \times \frac{100{,}000}{100{,}000}$$

$$= 17.5 \text{ cases per } \mathbf{100{,}000} \text{ person-years}$$

Rates do not always have to be reported using person-years. We can consider other units of time, like months or days. To report the rate of MS in our population using person-months, we would calculate our person-time as follows:

$$\text{Person-months} = \frac{12 \text{ months}}{1 \text{ year}} \times \left( \left[ 2 \text{ people} \times 4 \text{ years} \right] + \left[ 3 \text{ people} \times 9 \text{ years} \right] \right.$$

$$\left. + \left[ 2 \text{ people} \times 12 \text{ years} \right] + \left[ 1,993 \text{ people} \times 20 \text{ years} \right] \right)$$

$$= 479,028 \text{ person-months}$$

If we were to use this denominator in our calculation, we would report the rate of MS per 100,000 person-months (PM) as:

$$\text{Rate of MS per 100,000 person-months} = \frac{7 \text{ cases}}{479,028 \text{ Person-Months}} \times \frac{100,000}{100,000}$$

$$= 1.46 \text{ cases per } \mathbf{100,000 \text{ person - months}}$$

Although these rate calculations appear different, it is important to note that they are all equivalent. There is no "right" or "wrong" selection for the units of the person-time denominator. What is important is to be consistent in your selection in order to compare rates across groups, as discussed in **Chapter 3, "Introduction to Analytic Epidemiologic Study Designs and Measures of Association."**

## Incidence: Risk, Rate, and What to Watch Out For

Risk and rate are both measures of *incidence*, meaning that they are used to describe the frequency of *new* cases of a health outcome. To calculate measures of incidence, participants must have been observed during some follow-up period, and all individuals must have been *at-risk* of the outcome at the start of that period.

The numerator for measures of risk and rate are the same. Where these measures of incidence differ is in the construction of their denominator:

• Risk denominator: Total number of at-risk individuals

• Rate denominator: Total person-time contributed by all at-risk individuals

This distinction is important because there are times when it is not appropriate to calculate a risk, such as when there is substantial loss to follow-up or competing risks. Imagine the following scenario:

• A study population of 3,000 people was followed for up to 5 years.

• A total of 1,000 participants were lost to follow-up after 2 years.

• There were 1,700 participants who did not develop the outcome and were followed for all 5 years.

• There were 300 participants who developed the outcome of interest:

  – One hundred developed the outcome after 2 years.

  – Two hundred developed the outcome after 4 years.

The risk of the outcome in this situation would be calculated as:

$$\text{Risk} = \frac{300 \text{ cases}}{3,000 \text{ at-risk individuals}} = 0.1 = 10\%$$

The 5-year risk of 10% is likely an underestimate of the true risk in the study population since it assumes that all 1,000 people who were lost to follow-up did *not* develop the outcome of interest (i.e., all 1,000 people who were lost to follow-up appear in the denominator; however, they cannot appear in the numerator even if they develop the outcome after the second year because they have been lost to follow-up). The result is that our numerator, and thus the risk, are likely smaller than they should be.

The rate provides a more accurate alternative, which is calculated as follows:

$$\text{Rate} = \frac{300 \text{ cases}}{(1,000 \text{ people} \times 2 \text{ years}) + (1,700 \text{ people} \times 5 \text{ years}) + (100 \text{ people} \times 2 \text{ years}) + (200 \text{ people} \times 4 \text{ years})}$$

$$= \frac{300}{11,500 \text{ PY}} \times \frac{1,000}{1,000}$$

$$= 26 \text{ cases per } 1,000 \text{ person-years}$$

### Caution With Vocabulary

The terms *risk* and *rate* each have their own unique meaning in epidemiology, yet they are often used incorrectly. These terms are sometimes used interchangeably, which is both incorrect and confusing. Additionally, some authors may just refer to the "incidence" of an outcome, without specifying whether they are referring to a risk (cumulative incidence) or a rate (incidence rate). As you come across descriptions of measures of outcome frequency in epidemiologic studies, we encourage you to pay attention to the context that is provided to understand whether the authors included at-risk *people* in the denominator to calculate a risk, or included at-risk *person-time* in the denominator to calculate a rate.

## Measures of Prevalence

The **prevalence** (sometimes called **point prevalence**) of a health outcome is the proportion of individuals in a specified population who have an existing outcome at a particular point in time.

$$\text{Prevalence} = \frac{\text{Number of existing outcomes observed at a point in time}}{\text{Total population size at a point in time}} \tag{2.3}$$

Unlike the risk and rate, prevalence does not require a follow-up period; rather, prevalence provides a "snapshot" of the burden of disease at a *particular moment in time*. Importantly, the population included in the denominator should only be those who could plausibly have the outcome of interest.

Let's take a look back at the example shown in **Figure 2.5**. We can use these data to calculate prevalence by considering a single date. For example, what is the prevalence of the outcome on January 1, 2023?

$$\text{Prevalence} = \frac{2}{5} = 0.4 = 40\%$$

The interpretation for this measure is that 40% of the study population has the health outcome of interest on January 1, 2023.

What is the prevalence of the health outcome on January 1, 2020?

$$\text{Prevalence} = \frac{0}{2} = 0.0 = 0\%$$

Notice that the denominators for these measures of prevalence differ from one another. The denominator should only include individuals who were included in the assessment of the outcome *at the time* that the measure was taken. There were only two people who had available data on January 1, 2020; in contrast, there were five people who had available data on January 1, 2023.

The prevalence of a health outcome can be influenced by several factors. The schematic in **Figure 2.6** illustrates some of these factors, where the individuals in the classroom represent those with the health outcome (i.e., prevalent cases, or those who make up the numerator of the prevalence calculation) in some population of fixed size (i.e., we are assuming that the prevalence denominator remains the same). The number of individuals in the classroom, and thus the prevalence, will *increase* as people enter the room through the blue door on the left. The number of people in the room may increase because the incidence of the outcome is increasing in the population you are studying, the duration of the health outcome is increasing, or more people with the health outcome are moving into the population (i.e., immigration of those with the outcome). Similarly, the number of individuals in the classroom will *decrease* as people exit the room through the red door on the right. People may exit because mortality among those with the outcome is increasing, more people with the outcome are recovering, or more people with the outcome are leaving the population (i.e., emigration). If there are more people entering the classroom than exiting, the prevalence of the outcome will increase. On the other hand, if there are more people exiting the classroom than entering, the prevalence of the outcome will decrease.

**FIGURE 2.6 FACTORS THAT INFLUENCE THE NUMBER OF PREVALENT CASES OF A HEALTH OUTCOME IN A POPULATION**

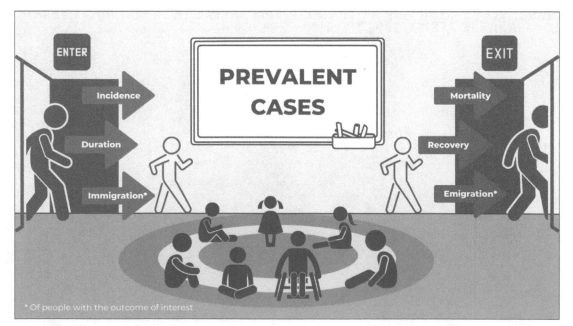

TABLE 2.1 **FACTORS THAT INFLUENCE PREVALENCE**

| | | Impact on Numerator | Impact on Denominator |
|---|---|---|---|
| If all else is equal, what causes prevalence in the population you are studying to *increase*? | | | |
| Incidence | More people are acquiring the outcome. | ↑ | None |
| Duration | The duration of the health outcome increases. | ↑ | None |
| Immigration | More people with the health outcome move into the population you are studying. | ↑ | Likely minimal increase |
| If all else is equal, what causes prevalence in the population you are studying to *decrease*? | | | |
| Mortality | Life-expectancy among those with the health outcome decreases. | ↓ | Likely minimal decrease |
| Recovery | The duration of the health outcome decreases. | ↓ | None |
| Emigration | More people with the health outcome leave the population you are studying. | ↓ | Likely minimal decrease |

Additional information about the factors that influence prevalence are detailed in **Table 2.1**. This table also provides information about how these factors can influence the size of the numerator and denominator of the prevalence calculation. There are some instances where the expected change to the denominator is likely to be minimal. These are instances where we have movement in the numerator that will also affect the denominator. For example, when more people with the health outcome immigrate into a population, it leads to an increase in both the numerator and the denominator. However, proportionally, the change to the denominator will have less impact on the prevalence because we typically study large populations, and the addition of a few people will have a relatively small influence on the size of the denominator.

An important illustration of the relationship between incidence and prevalence comes from the trajectory of the HIV/AIDS epidemic in sub-Saharan Africa, which is illustrated in **Figure 2.7**. At the beginning of the epidemic, the incidence of HIV/AIDS increased but began to drop around 1998. The decreased incidence of HIV was driven by evidence-based interventions such as condom use programs (implemented in the late 1990s) and large scale antiretroviral treatment programs (ART, a treatment that increases life expectancy among those living with HIV and also reduces infectiousness, was implemented around 2003).[12] Although fewer

**FIGURE 2.7 RELATIONSHIP BETWEEN HIV/AIDS PREVALENCE AND INCIDENCE IN SUB-SAHARAN AFRICA, 1990 TO 2017**

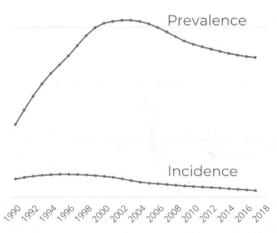

*Source:* Global Burden of Disease Collaborative Network. *Global Burden of Disease Study 2017 (GBD 2017) Results.* Seattle, United States: Institute for Health Metrics and Evaluation (IHME), 2018; https://data.worldbank.org/indicator/SP.POP.TOTL?end=2019&locations =ZG&start=1960&view=chart

individuals were becoming infected, the *prevalence* of HIV *increased* as life expectancy among those living with HIV/AIDS increased. With even greater reductions in the incidence of new HIV cases, the prevalence of HIV began to decline just prior to 2005.

Since prevalence is affected by many factors, it is not always useful for identifying the determinants, or causes, of health outcomes. Despite this limitation, prevalence is a useful measure of frequency for measuring the current burden of disease in a population which can, for example, inform how to best distribute limited public health resources.

## Digging Deeper

## Period Prevalence

A slightly different measure of prevalence, called period prevalence, can also be used to describe the frequency of a health outcome, though it is much less commonly used than (point) prevalence. *Period prevalence* is a measure that incorporates both prevalent (existing) and incident (new) cases occurring during a follow-up period and is calculated as:

$$\text{Period prevalence} = \frac{(\text{\# of outcomes at the beginning of the follow-up period}) + (\text{\# of incident cases that developed during the follow-up period})}{\text{Total population size at the beginning of the follow-up period}}$$

Although point prevalence is calculated using only data from a single point in time, period prevalence is calculated using data where participants have been observed during some follow-up period. An illustration of point prevalence and period prevalence is shown in **Figure 2.8**, where a population of 10 individuals has been followed for 1 year. At the beginning of the follow-up period, three of the individuals already had the outcome of interest. During the 1-year follow-up period, two people developed the outcome of interest. The period prevalence of the outcome can be calculated as follows:

$$\text{Period prevalence} = \frac{3 \text{ prevalent cases} + 2 \text{ incident cases}}{10 \text{ individuals in the population at the beginning of the period}}$$

$$= \frac{5}{10} = 0.5 = 50\%$$

## FIGURE 2.8 POINT PREVALENCE AND PERIOD PREVALENCE

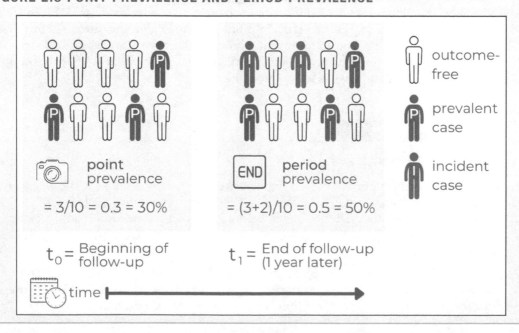

A summary of the definitions, calculations, and units for the measures of risk, rate, and prevalence are included in **Table M.1**, which appears in the middle of the textbook along with other tables that summarize key measures and concepts for easy reference.

---

### Highlights

### Measures of Frequency

- Measures of **incidence** describe the occurrence of *new* health outcomes in an *at-risk* population and require that the population be observed during a follow-up period.
  - **Risk** (cumulative incidence): The proportion of at-risk individuals who develop the outcome of interest during the follow-up period.
  - **Rate** (incidence density): A measure of how quickly new cases of a health outcome occur, where the number of new cases is divided by the amount of person-time contributed by at-risk individuals in the population.
- **Point prevalence:** Describes the proportion of the population with a health outcome at a single point in time and thus does not include a follow-up period.

---

## DESCRIBING OUTCOME FREQUENCY BY PERSON, PLACE, AND TIME (LEARNING OBJECTIVE 2.6)

Health-related outcomes are not randomly distributed throughout populations; some individuals are more likely to develop certain health outcomes, like cardiovascular disease or diabetes, than others. Measures of frequency can be used to describe the distribution of outcomes in different populations, including by person, place, and time characteristics.

### Person Characteristics

Health-related outcomes often differ by person characteristics such as age, biological sex, gender, race, ethnicity, and socioeconomic status (SES). Other factors that fall under the umbrella of person characteristics are health-related behaviors (e.g., diet, exercise, substance use) and biologic characteristics (e.g., blood type, immune status). Evaluating outcomes by person characteristics enables researchers to understand how outcomes vary across groups, consider different treatment or prevention needs for different groups, make policy decisions, and generate hypotheses about potential causes of these outcomes.

---

### Pause to Practice 2.4

### The Importance of Denominators

Age is almost always an important person characteristic to consider as most health-related outcomes vary by age. As shown in **Figure 2.9**, COVID-19 cases reported to the U.S. CDC in May 2020 varied by age.[13] Review these two panels carefully and answer the following questions.

1.  Review the axes in panels A and B of Figure 2.9. How are they similar? How are they different?

2.  According to these data, which age group had the highest number of COVID-19 cases? Which age group was proportionally most affected by COVID-19? Are these groups the same or different? If they are different, why might this be?

## FIGURE 2.9 COVID-19 CASES REPORTED TO THE U.S. CENTERS FOR DISEASE CONTROL AND PREVENTION BY AGE GROUP, MAY 2020

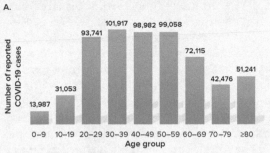
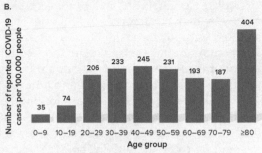

*Source:* Data from Boehmer TK, DeVies J, Caruso E, et al. Changing age distribution of the COVID-19 pandemic—United States, May-August 2020. *MMWR Morb Mortal Wkly Rep.* 2020;69(39):1404–1409. https://doi.org/10.15585/mmwr.mm6939e1

Biological sex is also an important person characteristic to consider as health-related outcomes may vary due to genetic, hormonal, or anatomical differences. For example, several autoimmune diseases occur more frequently in females than males, with some of this difference attributed to sex hormones.[14] While it is important to consider sex, which refers to biological differences between females and males, we must distinguish this from gender, which is socially constructed.[15] Consider the example of trachoma, a neglected tropical disease, which is the leading infectious cause of blindness worldwide. Among those with trachoma, permanent blindness is four times as common among women than among men. This difference is not driven by sex, meaning it is not driven by biologic differences between males and females. Rather, these differences have been explained by sociocultural factors. For example, in settings where trachoma is prevalent, women are responsible for the vast majority of childcare and thus spend more time in direct contact with children who may be repeatedly infected with trachoma.[16] This additional exposure due to socially prescribed gender roles puts women at an increased risk for permanent blindness.

The frequency of health-related outcomes may also vary by SES. SES is a complex measure comprised of factors like education, occupation, income, and housing—factors that may be relatively easy to measure—as well as concepts like social position and SES-related stigma, which are more difficult to measure. Many poor health outcomes are more common among those with lower SES and are often linked to limited access to material, human, and social capital needed to support health.[17–19]

## Using Proxies to Stand in for Factors That Are Difficult to Measure: The Case of Race

Researchers often describe health outcomes by person, place, or time characteristics that are **proxies**, or stand-ins, for the factor that actually affects the frequency of those outcomes. A common example is describing the frequency of health outcomes in the United States by racial groups. It is relatively uncommon for genetic or biological racial differences to affect the distribution of health outcomes; most often, race is a proxy for the effects of the experience of racism on health. Racism in the United States is a public health crisis occurring at individual, institutional, and structural levels and is the driver of many observed links between race and negative health outcomes.[20]

For example, the distribution of hypertension by race and ethnicity in U.S. adults is shown in **Figure 2.10** using data from the CDC's National Health and Nutrition Examination Survey (NHANES).[21] These data show a much higher prevalence of hypertension in non-Hispanic Black adults compared with other groups, even after accounting or "adjusting" for the effect of age (more on adjustment in **Chapter 9, "Error in Epidemiologic Research and Fundamentals of Confounding"**). Although some research has suggested that genetic differences may predispose Black individuals to have higher blood pressure than other groups,[22] genetic differences have *not* been shown to significantly account for the large observed inequity in hypertension. Rather, data indicate that this inequity is largely driven by racial differences in SES caused by racism and discrimination.[17,23] Low SES is associated with lower health literacy and limited access to preventive healthcare, treatments, and healthy living environments.[17-19] Though beyond the scope of this textbook, social and behavioral epidemiology provides a robust set of methods to study social determinants of health, including how to study and address racial health inequities.[24]

In short, it is always important for epidemiologists to consider the context in which people are living, including the societal and systemic factors that may influence health. Sometimes these factors can be difficult to measure, and epidemiologists may use proxy measures to stand in for them. In doing so, we must keep these societal and systemic factors in mind when interpreting our results.

## FIGURE 2.10 PREVALENCE OF HYPERTENSION IN ADULTS BY RACE AND ETHNICITY, UNITED STATES, 2015 TO 2016

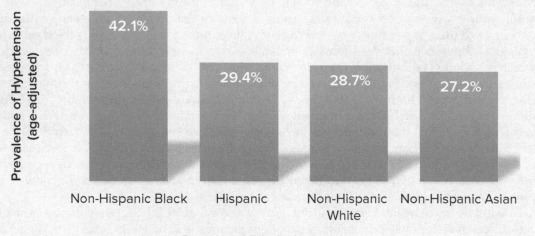

*Source:* Data from Centers for Disease Control and Prevention. National Health and Nutrition Examination Survey. 2021. https://www.cdc.gov/nchs/nhanes

## Place Characteristics

The frequency of health outcomes are often different by place, or *where* they occur. Place characteristics include any relevant geographic location, including country, state, city, or even neighborhood. Evaluating outcomes by place allows researchers to understand how patterns of a health outcome differ by geography, including whether certain areas have a higher frequency of the outcome than others. This information can also be used to make policy decisions related to treatment or prevention activities, as well as to generate hypotheses about what might be causing the outcomes. Such analyses are often visualized using heat maps or spot maps.

### Pause to Practice 2.5

#### Climate Change and Health: Malaria as an Example

Malaria is a mosquito-borne infectious disease caused by a parasite. Globally, the malaria "belt," where malaria risk is highest, is around the warmer, rainier, humid regions of the Equator (**Figure 2.11**). These regions are hospitable for the breeding of malaria-carrying mosquitos. Climate change is expected to have an impact on the global distribution of malaria, and the relationship between climate change and malaria is an area of active research. It is possible that malaria could become newly endemic in areas experiencing increasingly warmer weather.

1. How might climate change lead to an *increase* in the risk or rate of malaria in certain parts of the world?

2. How might climate change lead to a *decrease* in the risk or rate of malaria in certain parts of the world?

## FIGURE 2.11 GLOBAL DISTRIBUTION OF MALARIA AND CONTROL EFFORTS

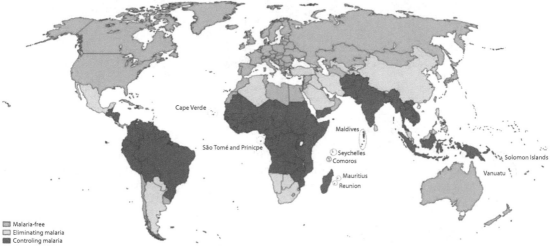

Malaria-free
Eliminating malaria
Controling malaria

*Source:* Feachem RG, Phillips AA, Hwang J, et al. Shrinking the malaria map: progress and prospects. *Lancet.* 2010;376(9752):1566-1578. https://doi.org/10.1016/S0140-6736(10)61270-6

## Time Characteristics

With the advent of new treatments and screening tools, along with the emergence of new pathogens, the temporal trends in health outcomes are constantly changing. Researchers often evaluate the frequency of health outcomes over time to generate hypotheses about potential causes, evaluate the success of treatment or prevention programs, make policy decisions related to treatment or prevention activities, and use trend data to predict future outcome occurrence.

Plots of the number of new health outcomes occurring during a particular time period are called **epidemic curves**. Epidemic curves are plots of the number of new cases on the *y*-axis and time on the *x*-axis (see **Figure 2.12** for an example epidemic curve for influenza in the United States). These plots are particularly useful when investigating an outbreak as they provide a visual representation of the occurrence of the health outcome and can provide some clues as to how the outbreak may have spread (see the CDC training lesson on epidemic curves at www.cdc.gov/training/quicklearns/epimode).

The time scale on the *x*-axis of an epidemic curve may vary, for example from hours to years, depending on the length of time we want to observe trends in the outcome. Graphing outcomes over long periods of time, often many years, can show **secular trends**, or changes in the frequency of an outcome over a longer period of time. There are many determinants that can influence secular trends, such as environmental changes, improved diagnostic technologies, treatment or prevention measures, and changes in population characteristics (e.g., behavioral changes, changing age distributions). In addition to considering secular trends, there may be some outcomes for which an examination of hourly or daily trends may be informative. For example, for foodborne outbreaks, the appropriate time scale may be days or hours. Some outcomes, like influenza, follow regular, seasonal trends and can be graphed by week or month over the course of a year or more to show their seasonal pattern (see **Figure 2.12**). For seasonal health outcomes, health officials coordinate prevention and treatment measures in advance—for example, planning for fall/winter influenza vaccination campaigns.

## FIGURE 2.12 TOTAL CASES OF INFLUENZA-POSITIVE SPECIMENS REPORTED BY PUBLIC HEALTH LABORATORIES, UNITED STATES, 2007 TO 2020

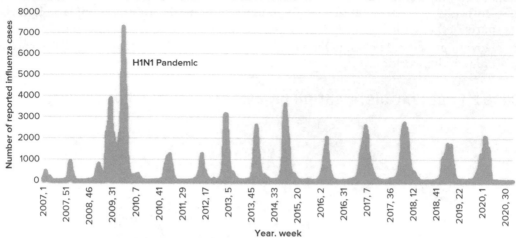

*Source:* FLUVIEW Interactive. https://gis.cdc.gov/grasp/fluview/flu_by_age_virus.html

While useful, these curves typically do not incorporate information about the size of the at-risk population (i.e., a denominator or the *contextualizing* information discussed previously). In lieu of presenting counts over time, researchers can also plot measures of frequency (i.e., risk, rate, or prevalence; see **Figure 2.7**).

### Pause to Practice 2.6

### Seasonal Variations in Influenza

Influenza virus is a communicable respiratory disease that typically follows a seasonal pattern and is monitored by surveillance systems in the U.S. The highest frequency of influenza cases is observed in winter months (typically between October and March in the northern hemisphere and April and August in the southern hemisphere) (see **Figure 2.12** for trends in reported influenza cases in the United States). Influenza outbreaks may be caused by many different influenza virus subtypes; for example, H1N1 ("swine flu") led to a global pandemic in 2009. Most cases of seasonal influenza are preventable by annual influenza vaccination and hand hygiene.

1. Why do you think that the frequency of influenza is typically higher in winter months?

### Digging Deeper

### The Epidemiologic Triangle

Although it is not broadly applicable to noninfectious causes of health outcomes, the epidemiologic triangle is a common framework to think about infectious disease epidemiology. It exemplifies the interconnection between person; place; and, though not explicitly stated, time by considering the interplay between:

- **A susceptible host:** This is the person who is at-risk of harboring the infectious disease.
- **The agent:** This is the pathogen (e.g., virus, bacteria) that causes the disease.
- **The environment:** These are situational characteristics that influence the likelihood of disease transmission (e.g., seasons, climate, crowding).
- **A vector:** This is a living organism that transmits the infectious agent between species, such as a mosquito transmitting the malaria parasite to humans. Not all infectious diseases are vector-borne.

## FIGURE 2.13 EPIDEMIOLOGIC TRIANGLE FOR LYME DISEASE

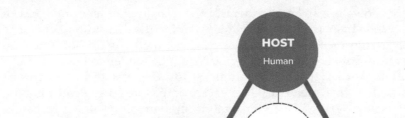

The epidemiologic triangle for Lyme disease, the most common vector-borne disease in the United States, is shown in **Figure 2.13**. The bacterium *Borrelia burgdorferi* (agent) is transmitted to humans (host) by infected deer ticks (vector). Although Lyme disease can occur at any time, cases are more likely to be reported during the summer months and after spending time in wooded areas (environment).

## Where Do Epidemiologic Data Come From?

It is useful to think about where the epidemiologic data we have been describing may come from. A (non-exhaustive) list of common epidemiologic data sources is shown in **Box 2.1.**

There are several sources of routinely collected data that can be used to describe health outcomes and answer research questions. We have already discussed the use of surveillance systems to systematically capture descriptive health-related data; if publicly available, these data may also be accessed for use by researchers to answer many different public health questions. Other common existing sources of epidemiologic data include national death indices (useful if you want to collect data on death, though these indices are not available in all countries and quality may vary), birth certificates (useful if you are interested in births or population dynamics), reportable disease databases, national registries, and medical records. Existing data sources may not be sufficient to describe a specific health outcome or to answer a specific research question, and data collection processes are often designed de novo, or from scratch. Researchers may design surveys or questionnaires in which participants may be asked to self-report health data or ask participants to complete medical exams, laboratory tests, or diagnostic tests to generate needed data.

Different data sources will have different strengths and limitations, particularly pertaining to the quality of the data (i.e., Is all of the information that was supposed to be recorded actually available? When data are available, is the information correct?). These are important questions to consider, and data quality issues will be explored in **Chapter 11, "Information Bias and Screening and Diagnostic Tests."**

### BOX 2.1. Common Sources of Epidemiologic Data

| | |
|---|---|
| Surveillance systems | Surveys/questionnaires (self-reported data) |
| National death indices | Medical exams |
| Birth certificates | Laboratory tests |
| Reportable disease databases | Diagnostic tests |
| Medical record abstraction | |

## WHERE WE'VE BEEN AND WHAT'S UP NEXT

Descriptive epidemiology allows researchers to identify the *who, what, where,* and *when* of health-related outcomes. While there is great utility in describing the distribution of health outcomes in a population using measures of frequency, these methods do not allow researchers to identify *why* health-related outcomes occur. Analytic epidemiology, the focus of **Chapter 3, "Introduction to Analytic Epidemiologic Study Designs and Measures of Association,"** allows researchers to evaluate whether certain exposures (i.e., determinants) cause certain health outcomes. As you will learn, in analytic epidemiology allows researchers to test hypotheses about the association between an exposure and an outcome by *comparing* measures of frequency across two or more groups. Often, analytic epidemiologic studies are required to justify healthcare, policy, or behavior changes that will ultimately improve public health. For example, as we will soon see, it was an analytic epidemiologic study that identified the cause of the water crisis in Flint, Michigan in 2015.

---

## END OF CHAPTER PROBLEM SET

1. Which of the following statements about chronic kidney disease[25] are examples of descriptive epidemiology? *Select all that apply.*
   a. The prevalence of chronic kidney disease increased from 11.8% in 1988 to 14.23% in 2016 among adults in the United States.
   b. Chronic kidney disease is most common among individuals in the United States age 70 years and older, with a prevalence of 44%.
   c. One in four adults in the United States with advanced chronic kidney disease is food insecure.
   d. High blood pressure causes chronic kidney disease in some older adults in the United States.
   e. The rates of chronic kidney disease are highest in the southeastern United States.

2. "Autism, or autism spectrum disorder (ASD), refers to a broad range of conditions characterized by challenges with social skills, repetitive behaviors, speech and nonverbal communication" (para. 1).[26] The term *infantile autism* was first coined in 1943 in a case series written by Leo Kanner[27] and first appeared in the second edition of the American Psychiatric Association's *Diagnostic and Statistical Manual of Mental Disorders* (*DSM-2*) in 1952, where it was defined as a psychiatric condition—specifically, a form of childhood schizophrenia. Over time, new editions of the *DSM* have been released, with each revision further expanding the definition of autism. Initially, children were required to be diagnosed before age 30 months; however, this restriction was lifted in 1987. In 1994, the definition was expanded to categorize autism as a spectrum of disorders.
   a. What impact do you think the evolving case definition for ASD has had on the estimates of the prevalence of ASD over time?
   b. In the United States, White children had been more likely to be identified as having ASD than Black or Hispanic children.[28] This difference was not driven by true differences in the *occurrence* of ASD, but rather by an inequity in the *detection* of ASD in Black and Hispanic children. It is important to close the gap in the detection of ASD because children with an ASD diagnosis are entitled to specialized support services. Inequities in health will persist if Black and Hispanic children with ASD are unable to access these support services because they do not have an ASD diagnosis. Fortunately, this gap in ASD detection has narrowed over time. What are some possible reasons that the frequency of ASD detection increased in Black and Hispanic children?

3. Dengue is a mosquito-borne viral infection which is found in both tropical and subtropical climates across the globe.[29] While most dengue infections result in nonlethal illness, a small subset cause severe dengue, which can be lethal. The incidence of dengue has increased globally in recent years, with an estimated 100 to 400 million new infections each year. Early detection of dengue infection, mosquito control, and active surveillance of both mosquitoes and disease are essential to controlling this public health problem.

Answer the following questions, which relate to Figure 2.14 which shows trends in dengue incidence in Singapore from 2018 to 2023:

   a. Why is it important to compare trends in dengue cases across multiple years?

   b. Do you see any concerning trends in dengue cases across years in Singapore?

   c. Hypothesize some reasons why the number of cases of dengue may have increased in 2020 over what would be expected.

   d. How could these data be used to improve public health?

**FIGURE 2.14 DENGUE CASES REPORTED WEEKLY FROM 2018 TO 2023 IN SINGAPORE (EXPECTED PEAK TRANSMISSION IS DURING THE MID-YEAR RAINY SEASON)**

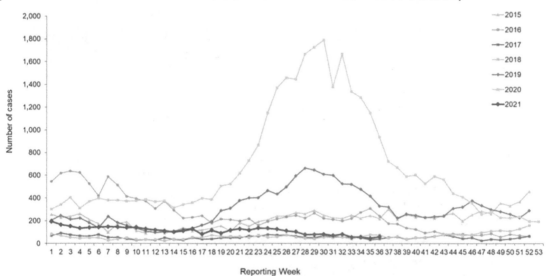

*Source:* World Health Organization. Update on the Dengue situation in the Western Pacific region. July 20, 2023. https://www.who.int/docs/default-source/wpro---documents/emergency/surveillance/dengue/dengue-20210923.pdf

4. Figure 2.15 shows hypothetical study data. All individuals entered the study on January 1, 2020, with the goal of estimating the 5-year risk of a particular health outcome. However, we see that individuals 4 and 5 were lost to follow-up before January 1, 2025. The purpose of the questions that follow is to help underscore the importance of having complete data on all study participants when calculating risk. Having complete data means that participants either were followed for the entire study period or developed the outcome of interest during the study.

   a. Calculate the *true* 5-year risk of the outcome, *if* the investigators had been able to observe all of the outcomes that occurred among everyone who was at-risk on January 1, 2020.

   b. Calculate the 5-year risk of the outcome that the investigators would obtain if they (incorrectly!) assumed that those who were lost to follow-up did *not* develop the outcome during the 5-year period.

  c. Calculate the 5-year risk of the outcome that the investigators would obtain if they (incorrectly!) restricted their analysis to those for whom they had complete data.

  d. Compare your answers to the three previous questions. What is the true 5-year risk of the outcome in this group? What impact did different assumptions have on this calculation?

## FIGURE 2.15 HYPOTHETICAL STUDY ENTRY, FOLLOW-UP, AND EXIT DATA FOR FIVE STUDY PARTICIPANTS: CHALLENGES WHEN CALCULATING RISK

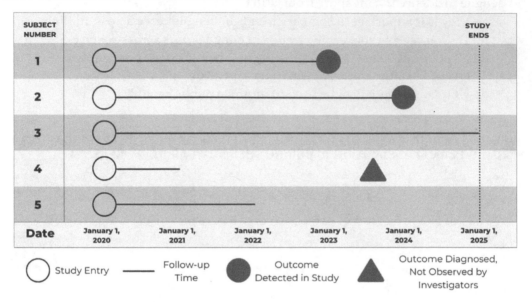

5. Revisit Figure 2.5, which illustrates an example of an epidemiologic study in which individuals contributed varying amounts of person-time to the study. Calculate and interpret the rate of the health outcome in this study population between January 1, 2020, and January 1, 2024, and report your answer per …

   a. 100 person-years
   b. 1,000 person-months
   c. 10,000 person-days

6. Electronic cigarettes (e-cigarettes) were introduced in the United States in the mid-2000s,[30] and by 2018 an estimated 5.4% of United States adults reported current e-cigarette use.[31] In 2019, the United States experienced a nationwide outbreak of lung injuries, called e-cigarette, or vaping, product use–associated lung injury (EVALI). The data in **Table 2.2** describe a population of individuals with EVALI who were included in an outbreak investigation.

   Sometimes investigators aren't able to collect all of the information that they would like for all individuals in a study. As shown in **Table 2.2**, a total of 1,378 EVALI patients were evaluated ($N = 1,378$); however, not everyone had available data for all of the characteristics of interest. The number of people who provided data for each of the characteristics in **Table 2.2** is denoted with a lowercase $n$ next to the characteristic description. *NOTE: A capital* N *is typically used to denote the size of the total study population, while a lowercase* n *is typically used to denote the size of a* subset *of the total study population.*

   a. Name and calculate the measure of frequency that describes the proportion of individuals with EVALI with any use of tetrahydrocannabinol (THC, the main psychoactive ingredient in cannabis)-containing products.

b. Using the data shown in **Table 2.2**, calculate the distribution of EVALI cases within each of the four person characteristics listed. For example, how are EVALI cases proportionally distributed across the six age groups?

c. What hypotheses might these descriptive data generate?

d. What additional information would you like to have in order to better understand and ultimately respond to this outbreak?

**TABLE 2.2 CHARACTERISTICS OF REPORTED CASES OF ELECTRONIC CIGARETTE (E-CIGARETTE), OR VAPING, PRODUCT USE-ASSOCIATED LUNG INJURY (EVALI), UNITED STATES, 2019**

| Characteristic | Number of Individuals with EVALI |
|---|---|
| **Sex ($n = 1,378$)** | |
| Male | 964 |
| Female | 414 |
| **Age Group** (Years; $n = 1,364$) | |
| 13–17 | 196 |
| 18–24 | 541 |
| 25–34 | 344 |
| 35–44 | 172 |
| 45–64 | 87 |
| 65–75 | 24 |
| **Race/Ethnicity ($n = 383$)** | |
| White | 298 |
| Black or African American | 9 |
| American Indian or Alaska Native | 4 |
| Asian, Native Hawaiian, or other Pacific Islander | 5 |
| Other | 5 |
| Hispanic | 62 |
| **Substances Used in E-Cigarette, or Vaping, Products ($n = 867$)** | |
| THC-containing products, any use | 749 |
| Nicotine-containing products, any use | 552 |
| Both THC- and nicotine-containing products, any use | 455 |
| THC-containing products, exclusive use | 294 |
| Nicotine-containing products, exclusive use | 97 |
| No THC- or nicotine-containing products reported | 21 |

*Source:* Data from Moritz ED, Zapata LB, Lekiachvili A, et al. Update: characteristics of patients in a national outbreak of e-cigarette, or vaping, product use-associated lung injuries—United States, October 2019. *Morb Mortal Wkly Rep.* 2019;68(43):985–989. https://www.cdc.gov/mmwr/volumes/68/wr/pdfs/mm6843e1-H.pdf

7. Revisit **Figure 2.6**, which illustrates factors that lead to an increase or a decrease in the number of prevalent cases of an outcome in a population. Recall that the number of individuals in the classroom represents the number of prevalent cases of a health outcome in a population. We can think of this group of prevalent cases as the numerator of the prevalence calculation. Of course, a classroom doesn't exist in isolation; it is part of a school, which we can think of as representing the *total* population, and thus the denominator of the prevalence calculation.

If all else stays the same, what impact would the following changes have on the prevalence of the health outcome in this population?

a. The school expands to include another grade level none of whom have the outcome.

b. A new drug is developed that shortens the duration of the outcome.

c. The health outcome is an infectious disease, and unfortunately many students are exposed during a school-wide celebration and become sick.

8. Herpes zoster, commonly called shingles, is caused by the varicella zoster virus (VZV), which is the same virus that causes chicken pox. VZV remains dormant in those who have had chicken pox and can reactivate many years later as shingles.

   To prevent this reactivation, investigators tested a new shingles vaccine, where 7,344 individuals received two doses of the new vaccine. Of these individuals, six developed shingles during the 3-year study period.[32]

   a. Given these data, name, calculate, and interpret the appropriate measure of frequency for the occurrence of shingles.

   b. The goal of this study was to understand the effectiveness of the new vaccine. What additional information is needed in order to answer this question?

## REFERENCES

1. Schultz MG, Bloch AB. Memoriam: Sandy Ford (1950–2015). *Emerg Infect Dis*. 2016;22(4):764–765. https://doi.org/10.3201/eid2204.151336

2. Fowler JR, Jack BW. *Cervical Cancer*. StatPearls Publishing; 2020.

3. Centers for Disease Control and Prevention. Gonorrhea (*Neisseria gonorrhoeae* infection) 2023 case definition. 2023. https://ndc.services.cdc.gov/case-definitions/gonorrhea-neisseria-gonorrhoeae

4. The Lancet. ICD-11. *The Lancet*. 2019;393(10188):2275. https://doi.org/10.1016/S0140-6736(19)31205-X

5. Centers for Disease Control. *Pneumocystis* pneumonia—Los Angeles. *MMWR Morb Mortal Wkly Rep*. 1981;30(21):250–252. https://www.cdc.gov/mmwr/preview/mmwrhtml/lmrk077.htm

6. Thacker SB, Berkelman RL. Public health surveillance in the United States. *Epidemiol Rev*. 1988;10:164–190. https://doi.org/10.1093/oxfordjournals.epirev.a036021

7. Centers for Disease Control. Surveillance and data analytics: the latest in COVID-19 data and surveillance. March 26, 2021. https://www.cdc.gov/coronavirus/2019-ncov/php/surveillance-data-analytics.html

8. Lee LM, Teutsch SM, Thacker SB, St. Louis ME. *Principles and Practice of Public Health Surveillance*. 3rd ed. Oxford University Press; 2010.

9. Centers for Disease Control and Prevention. Introduction to public health surveillance. 2018. https://www.cdc.gov/training/publichealth101/surveillance.html

10. Amorim LDAF, Cai J. Modelling recurrent events: a tutorial for analysis in epidemiology. *Int J Epidemiol*. 2015;44(1):324–333. https://doi.org/10.1093/ije/dyu222

11. Rothman K, Lash T. Measures of occurrence. In: Lash TL, VanderWeele TJ, Haneuse S, Rotjman KJ, eds. *Modern Epidemiology*. 4th ed. Wolters Kluwer; 2021:69.

12. Forsythe SS, McGreevey W, Whiteside A, et al. Twenty years of antiretroviral therapy for people living with HIV: global costs, health achievements, economic benefits. *Health Aff*. 2019;38(7):1163–1172. https://doi.org/10.1377/hlthaff.2018.05391

13. Boehmer TK, DeVies J, Caruso E, et al. Changing age distribution of the COVID-19 pandemic—United States, May-August 2020. *MMWR Morb Mortal Wkly Rep*. 2020;69(39):1404–1409. https://doi.org/10.15585/mmwr.mm6939e1

14. Ngo ST, Steyn FJ, McCombe PA. Gender differences in autoimmune disease. *Front Neuroendocrinol*. 2014;35(3):347–369. https://doi.org/10.1016/j.yfrne.2014.04.004

15. Tseng J. Sex, gender, and why the differences matter. *Virtual Mentor*. 2008;10(7):427–428. https://doi.org/10.1001/virtualmentor.2008.10.7.fred1-0807

16. Burki T. Gender disparities in neglected tropical diseases. *Lancet Infect Dis*. 2020;20(2):175–176. https://doi.org/10.1016/S1473-3099(20)30013-X

17. Fiscella K, Williams DR. Health disparities based on socioeconomic inequities: implications for urban health care. *Acad Med.* 2004;79(12):1139–1147. https://doi.org/10.1097/00001888-200412000-00004

18. McMaughan DJ, Oloruntoba O, Smith ML. Socioeconomic status and access to healthcare: interrelated drivers for healthy aging. *Front Public Health.* 2020;8:231. https://doi.org/10.3389/fpubh.2020.00231

19. Institute of Medicine. Socioeconomic disparities: food insecurity and obesity. In: Troy LM, Miller EA, Olson S, eds. *Hunger and Obesity: Understanding a Food Insecurity Paradigm: Workshop Summary.* National Academies Press (US); 2011:33–50. https://doi.org/10.17226/13102

20. Devakumar D, Selvarajah S, Shannon G, et al. Racism, the public health crisis we can no longer ignore. *Lancet.* 2020;395(10242):e112–e113. https://doi.org/10.1016/S0140-6736(20)31371-4

21. Centers for Disease Control and Prevention. National Health and Nutrition Examination Survey. 2021. https://www.cdc.gov/nchs/nhanes

22. Graham G. Disparities in cardiovascular disease risk in the United States. *Curr Cardiol Rev.* 2015;11(3):238–245. https://doi.org/10.2174/1573403x11666141122220003

23. Forde AT, Sims M, Muntner P, et al. Discrimination and hypertension risk among African Americans in the Jackson Heart Study. *Hypertension.* 2020;76(3):715–723. https://doi.org/10.1161/HYPERTENSIONAHA.119.14492

24. Boyd RW, Lindo EG, Weeks LD, McLemore MR. On racism: a new standard for publishing on racial health inequities. *Health Affairs Blog.* July 2, 2020. https://www.healthaffairs.org/content/forefront/racism-new-standard-publishing-racial-health-inequities

25. Centers for Disease Control and Prevention. Kidney disease surveillance system. https://nccd.cdc.gov/CKD/detail.aspx?Qnum=Q8#refreshPosition

26. Autism Speaks. What is autism? https://www.autismspeaks.org/what-autism

27. Kanner L. Autistic disturbances of affective contact. *Nervous Child.* 1943;2:217–250. http://simonsfoundation.s3.amazonaws.com/share/071207-leo-kanner-autistic-affective-contact.pdf

28. Centers for Disease Control and Prevention. Spotlight on: racial and ethnic differences in children identified with autism spectrum disorder (ASD). https://www.cdc.gov/ncbddd/autism/addm-community-report/differences-in-children.html

29. World Health Organization. Dengue and severe dengue. March 17, 2023. https://www.who.int/news-room/fact-sheets/detail/dengue-and-severe-dengue

30. Centers for Disease Control and Prevention. *2016 Surgeon General's Report: E-Cigarette Use Among Youth and Young Adults.* U.S. Department of Health and Human Services; 2016:1–24. https://www.cdc.gov/tobacco/data_statistics/sgr/e-cigarettes/pdfs/2016_SGR_Chap_1_508.pdf

31. Obisesan OH, Osei AD, Uddin SMI, et al. Trends in e-cigarette use in adults in the United States, 2016–2018. *JAMA Intern Med.* 2020;180(10):1394–1398. https://doi.org/10.1001/jamainternmed.2020.2817

32. Maltz F, Fidler B. Shingrix: a new herpes zoster vaccine. *PT.* 2019;44(7):406–409, 433. https://www.ncbi.nlm.nih.gov/pmc/articles/PMC6590925

# CHAPTER 3

## INTRODUCTION TO ANALYTIC EPIDEMIOLOGIC STUDY DESIGNS AND MEASURES OF ASSOCIATION

### KEY TERMS

analytic epidemiology

experimental studies

hypothesis

measures of association

observational studies

### LEARNING OBJECTIVES

3.1 Distinguish between descriptive and analytic epidemiologic study designs.

3.2 Identify the important components of an epidemiologic study hypothesis.

3.3 Differentiate between experimental and observational research.

3.4 Describe the basic design features of randomized controlled trial, cohort, case-control, cross-sectional, and ecological designs.

3.5 Distinguish between association and causation.

3.6 Understand how epidemiologic data are presented in an R×C table.

3.7 Identify the null value for a given measure of association.

3.8 Construct an R×C table given a description of epidemiologic study data.

### DR. MONA HANNA-ATTISHA: PEDIATRIC PUBLIC HEALTH WHISTLEBLOWER

Dr. Hanna-Attisha is considered one of the key public health "whistleblowers" who brought the Flint, Michigan, water crisis to light. In 2014, when the water supply in Flint, Michigan, was changed from Lake Huron to the Flint River, residents began to voice concerns about the color, taste, and smell of the water. Reports of skin rashes also increased. Dr. Mona Hanna-Attisha, a first-generation Iraqi immigrant and pediatrician in Flint, began observing elevated blood lead levels in her patients. Lead is a neurotoxin that can affect behavior and cognition, and there are no safe levels of lead.[1] Dr. Hanna-Attisha hypothesized that blood lead levels were higher in children who used water from the Flint River. She conducted an analytic epidemiologic study that found much higher blood lead levels in children after Flint changed its water supply source. Like John Snow, Dr. Hanna-Attisha's findings were initially met with skepticism. When she presented her data,[2] the state of Michigan initially discredited her and accused her of causing panic. However, she continued publicizing her work, and the state ultimately acknowledged the water lead crisis and began to take public health action.

## WHAT IS ANALYTIC EPIDEMIOLOGY? (LEARNING OBJECTIVE 3.1)

Recall that in descriptive epidemiology, investigators describe the **distribution** of health-related outcomes using **measures of frequency**. Descriptive studies help answer the questions of *who* is affected, along with *where* and *when* health outcomes occur, which can lead to hypotheses about potential determinants (see **Figure 2.1**). For example, as previously described, Dr. Hanna-Attisha noticed elevated blood levels among her patients and hypothesized that this was due to the transition from sourcing water from Lake Huron to the Flint River.

In **analytic epidemiology**, the focus of this chapter, investigators still describe health outcomes using measures of frequency. However, they additionally ask *why* outcomes occur by making quantitative *comparisons* of measures of frequency across two or more groups. Most often, analytic epidemiologic studies are designed to test hypotheses about associations between **determinants** (often called **exposures**) and health-related outcomes. Exposures may be any number of factors potentially associated with an outcome, including the person, place, and time characteristics described in **Chapter 2, "Descriptive Epidemiology, Surveillance, and Measures of Frequency."** Dr. Hanna-Attisha used an analytic study to explore whether blood levels in her patients (the health outcome) were associated with drinking water source (the determinant, or exposure). She answered this question by comparing the blood levels among children in Flint, Michigan, before and after the transition to the new water source.

As another example, suppose an investigator hypothesized that rates of cervical cancer are lower among women who receive the human papillomavirus (HPV) vaccine compared with those who do not. The hypothesized exposure potentially leading to a reduction in cervical cancer is HPV vaccination status. Additional examples of different types of exposures, classified as person, place, and time characteristics, are shown in **Table 3.1**.

TABLE 3.1 **EXAMPLES OF EXPOSURES\* IN EPIDEMIOLOGIC RESEARCH**

| Person Characteristics (WHO?) | Place Characteristics (WHERE?) | Time Characteristics (WHEN?) |
|---|---|---|
| Age | Country of residence | Time trends over decades |
| Occupation | Neighborhood of residence | Before and after a policy change |
| Health conditions | Urban vs. rural locations | Seasons |
| Behaviors (e.g., condom use, physical activity) | Environmental (e.g., air pollution, pesticides) | Time of day |

\*Like health outcomes, exposures (i.e., determinants) should be well-defined, including a description of what constitutes both **exposure** and **non-exposure**.

## THE CYCLE OF ANALYTIC EPIDEMIOLOGY

The steps involved in conducting an analytic epidemiologic study are shown in **Figure 3.1**, which highlights the cyclic nature of this process. Descriptive studies often generate hypotheses that lead to analytic studies. While an analytic epidemiologic study may address one (or more) study hypotheses, it may also generate new hypotheses that can lead to new studies.

In this chapter, we focus on the three elements of this cycle that are noted with a blue star in **Figure 3.1**: how to develop a strong epidemiologic study hypothesis; a brief overview of the main analytic study designs (described in detail in upcoming chapters); and defining, calculating, and interpreting common measures of association within those studies.

## FIGURE 3.1 THE CYCLE OF ANALYTIC EPIDEMIOLOGY

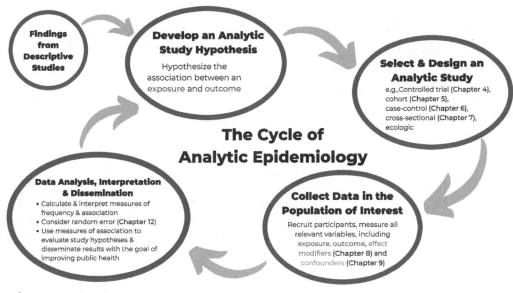

⚠ Recognize that error can happen at any stage along the way - we will discuss how to minimize these errors throughout the text

# DEVELOPING EPIDEMIOLOGIC STUDY HYPOTHESES
## (LEARNING OBJECTIVE 3.2)

Developing an epidemiologic study hypothesis is foundational for an analytic epidemiologic study. An epidemiologic study **hypothesis** is a statement that posits that an exposure of interest is associated with an outcome of interest. Hypotheses may be structured in several different ways; an example of one such structure is as follows:

> In a **population**, those who are **exposed** have a **<different/higher/lower/not different> frequency** of the outcome compared to those who are **unexposed**.

We've already explored two hypotheses in this chapter related to two different exposure-outcome relationships: water sourcing and blood lead levels, and HPV vaccination and cervical cancer. **Table 3.2** shows how we can frame these hypotheses using the above structure.

To develop a strong hypothesis, investigators should think through the following five basic components which are shown in bold in the hypothesis above:

1. **What is the health outcome of interest and how is it defined?** We have already discussed applying rigorous case definitions to define health-related outcomes of interest in **Chapter 2, "Descriptive Epidemiology, Surveillance, and Measures of Frequency."** It is equally important to define the group of individuals *without* the outcome of interest.

    As an example, in Flint, Michigan, there was an interest in learning whether children were experiencing elevated blood lead levels after transitioning to the new water source. Blood lead levels are measured in micrograms of lead per deciliter of blood (mcg/dL), and children are often classified as having an elevated

**TABLE 3.2 IDENTIFYING THE BASIC COMPONENTS OF AN EPIDEMIOLOGIC STUDY HYPOTHESIS**

| Hypothesis | Population of interest | Outcome | Direction of association | Measure of frequency | Exposed group | Unexposed group |
|---|---|---|---|---|---|---|
| Children in Flint, Michigan had a higher prevalence of high blood lead levels when water was sourced from the Flint River compared to when water was sourced from Lake Huron. | Children in Flint, Michigan | Blood lead levels (high vs. low) | Positive | Prevalence | Time period when water was supplied by the Flint River | Time period when water was supplied by Lake Huron |
| Among women in the United States, those who received HPV vaccines have a lower rate of cervical cancer compared to those who did not receive HPV vaccines. | Women in the United States | Cervical cancer (yes vs. no) | Negative | Rate | Received HPV vaccines | Did not receive HPV vaccines |

HPV, human papillomavirus.

blood lead level if this value is greater than 5 mcg/dL.[1] When investigating Flint's water crisis, Dr. Hanna-Attisha and her colleagues defined those *with* the outcome as children whose blood lead levels were greater than 5 mcg/dL, and those *without* the outcome as those with blood lead levels of 5 mcg/dL or less.

2. **What is the exposure of interest and how is it defined?** Investigators must also rigorously define the exposure of interest. As is the case when defining the outcome, investigators must define both the exposed *and* the unexposed (often called the **referent, reference,** or **comparison**) groups. Exposed and unexposed groups are often defined not just by whether an exposure occurred but also account for the exposure's dose (i.e., how much) and duration (i.e., for how long).

When investigating the Flint water crisis, Dr. Hanna-Attisha and her colleagues considered two different exposures, as shown in **Table 3.3**. They began by comparing the distribution of elevated blood lead levels by *time*: before (unexposed) versus after (exposed) the water source transition. They also compared the distribution of elevated blood lead levels in children by *place*: comparing municipalities and wards in and around Flint, Michigan, to determine whether one or more areas had an increased frequency of elevated blood lead levels compared to others.

Returning to the HPV vaccination example, we can use the United States Centers for Disease Control and Prevention's (CDC's) recommended doses and timing as shown in **Table 3.3** to define our exposed group as those who received both doses of the HPV vaccine between 11 and 12 years of age, spaced 6 to 12 months apart. However, the unexposed group could be defined in multiple ways. For example, the unexposed group could comprise those who received no doses of the HPV vaccine by age 13. Alternatively, the unexposed group could be defined as those who received either zero or one dose of the HPV vaccine by age 13.

Ultimately, the decision about how to define your exposed and unexposed groups is dependent on the research question you are trying to answer. For example, if you wanted to understand whether the HPV vaccine is effective at preventing cervical cancer relative to no vaccination at all, then you would select those who received no doses of the HPV vaccine by age 13 as your unexposed group. However, if you wanted to understand the benefits of the full recommended

**TABLE 3.3 DEFINING EXPOSURE GROUPS: FLINT WATER CRISIS AND HPV VACCINATION EXAMPLES**

| Exposure (Determinant) | Type of Comparison | Possible Ways to Define the Exposed Group | Possible Ways to Define the Unexposed Group |
|---|---|---|---|
| Water Source in Flint, Michigan | Comparison across **time** | Time when Flint River water was used (**after** the water source transition) | Time when Lake Huron water was used (**before** the water source transition) |
| | Comparison across **place** | Municipalities with **high** water lead levels | Municipalities with **low** water lead levels |
| HPV Vaccination | Comparison across **personal characteristics** (i.e., vaccination status) | U.S. CDC Recommendation:<br>• Receipt of HPV vaccine dose #1 at ages 11–12<br>• Receipt of HPV vaccine dose #2 6–12 months after dose #1 | **No HPV vaccination:** Neither dose #1 nor dose #2 by age 13<br>-OR-<br>**Incomplete HPV vaccination:** No HPV vaccination or dose #1 only by age 13 |

CDC, Centers for Disease Control and Prevention; HPV, human papillomavirus.
*Source*: U.S. Centers for Disease Control and Prevention. *HPV Vaccine*. https://www.cdc.gov/hpv/parents/vaccine.html

course of the HPV vaccine relative to incomplete vaccination, then you would choose the second definition for your unexposed group.

When considering how exposure status is defined, the key point is to always ask "*compared to what*?" It is important that the study hypothesis specify not just who is considered to be exposed, but also who is considered to be unexposed.

3. **What measures of frequency are being compared?** We often test hypotheses by quantitatively comparing the experience of one group to that of another. For example, we may compare the prevalence of elevated blood lead levels in children before versus after a change in water source. **Measures of association**, described in detail later in this chapter, are derived from the comparison of measures of frequency (**Chapter 2, "Descriptive Epidemiology, Surveillance, and Measures of Frequency"**). During our discussion of the main epidemiologic study designs, you will learn how the study hypothesis determines which of these designs is most appropriate, which then determines what measures can be calculated (Figure 3.2).

4. **What is the direction of the hypothesized association?** Investigators may hypothesize that the difference in the frequency of health outcomes between exposure groups is higher, lower, the same or different.

5. **What is the population?** When constructing a hypothesis, it is important to specify the population that we want to learn about. This helps inform who you will sample for your study.

## FIGURE 3.2 RELATIONSHIP AMONG HYPOTHESES, STUDY DESIGN, AND MEASURES OF FREQUENCY AND ASSOCIATION

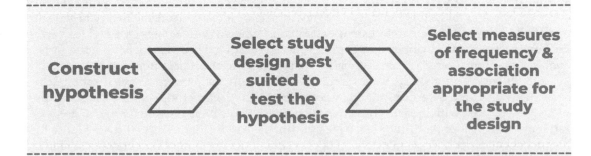

**Pause to Practice 3.1**

### Hypothesis Formulation

Hypotheses are designed to explore meaningful public health questions. Before developing a study hypothesis, it is important to thoroughly read the peer-reviewed literature on the topic area of interest. This review of the literature helps investigators to:

- Identify potential causes of a health-related outcome.
- Learn how exposures and outcomes have previously been defined.
- Learn which populations were studied and why.
- Get a sense of the possible direction of the hypothesized association.
- Identify gaps in the literature that could be answered using an analytic epidemiologic study.

The three hypotheses that follow aim to evaluate the association among three different exposure–outcome pairings; however, each of these is lacking the specificity that is required for constructing a robust hypothesis. For each hypothesis, identify what additional information could be useful to include.

1.   Hypothesis 1: Red meat intake is associated with coronary heart disease (CHD).
2.   Hypothesis 2: Physical activity is associated with a decreased risk of depression in young adults.
3.   Hypothesis 3: Air quality is associated with the prevalence of asthma in children.

## A NOTE ABOUT EXPLORATORY ANALYTIC EPIDEMIOLOGIC STUDIES

There are times when researchers are interested in evaluating the associations between several different exposures and outcomes. This research is often classified as exploratory, and can be helpful (a) when little is known about the etiology of an outcome and/or (b) to generate hypotheses for future studies. For example, an exploratory study sought to identify many potential factors associated with two health outcomes in the United States: breastfeeding initiation (ever versus never breastfed) and exclusive breastfeeding (only breastfeeding versus any amount of formula feeding).[3] Researchers were interested in learning whether several characteristics of the breastfeeding parent (e.g., age, education), child (e.g., birth weight), and home environment (e.g., family structure, presence of a smoker in the home) were associated with whether a child was ever or exclusively breastfed. They found that, for example, maternal age was associated with exclusive breastfeeding, but not breastfeeding initiation; while children with birth weights lower than 1,500 g were more likely to have *ever* been breastfed, they were the least likely to have been *exclusively* breastfed.

When conducting exploratory research, it is important to carefully select the exposures and health outcomes of interest such that there is some rationale for why these factors have been chosen; the best way to accomplish this is by reviewing the relevant literature. We caution against choosing any and all factors that might be measurable or already available in a data set—this approach is often referred to as a "fishing expedition," whereby researchers cast a wide net with the hope of turning up an interesting finding. This is considered bad science since these sorts of analyses are more likely to raise false alarms and are not grounded in a hypothesis.

In the breastfeeding study, it was important for the investigators to have a rationale for selecting each of the exposures that they considered. The factors they selected had been previously associated with breastfeeding initiation or exclusive breastfeeding or had a biological rationale for consideration, and thus were appropriate to consider in this study. Suppose that the investigators had access to a data set that included hundreds of other variables, including maternal blood type. In theory, they could conduct an analysis to investigate the relationship between maternal blood type and breastfeeding initiation, even though there is no biological rationale to support this hypothesis. We caution readers to be judicious in selecting which exposures to study and to avoid exploring all possible exposure-outcome relationships, even if they have access to the data to do so.

## CLASSIFICATION OF EPIDEMIOLOGIC STUDIES

We have already noted that analytic epidemiologic studies differ from descriptive epidemiologic studies in that they make quantitative comparisons across two or more groups, most often with the goal of testing a hypothesis. Epidemiologic studies can also be classified as being either experimental or observational (Learning Objective 3.3). The hallmark of an **experimental study** is that the study investigator *assigns* the exposure status to participants. This assignment is often, but not always, achieved by random assignment, or **randomization** (discussed further in **Chapter 4, "Randomized Controlled Trial Designs"**). Although you will learn that experimental studies have some great advantages, often the exposures that we are interested in studying (e.g., smoking, air pollution, diet) cannot easily (or ethically!) be assigned to study participants. In these cases, investigators rely on **observational studies**, where the exposure is not assigned; rather, the investigators observe the exposure status that has occurred or will occur anyway.

Returning to our cervical cancer example, suppose an investigator hypothesizes that rates of cervical cancer are lower among U.S. women who receive the HPV vaccine compared to those who do not. To test this hypothesis in an experimental study, researchers could compare the rate of cervical cancer in those who were assigned to receive the HPV vaccine to the rate of cervical cancer in those who were assigned to receive an inert injection (i.e., a placebo). If vaccination could not be assigned by the investigator, this hypothesis could be tested in an observational study by comparing rates of cervical cancer among those who either received or did not receive HPV vaccination by their own choosing.

One way to classify different types of epidemiologic studies is shown in **Figure** 3.3. This classification system begins by differentiating how analytic designs, in contrast to descriptive designs, make a quantitative comparison between at least two groups. We then further differentiate between the two types of analytic epidemiologic study designs defined above: experimental and observational.

## FIGURE 3.3 CLASSIFICATION OF EPIDEMIOLOGIC STUDY DESIGNS

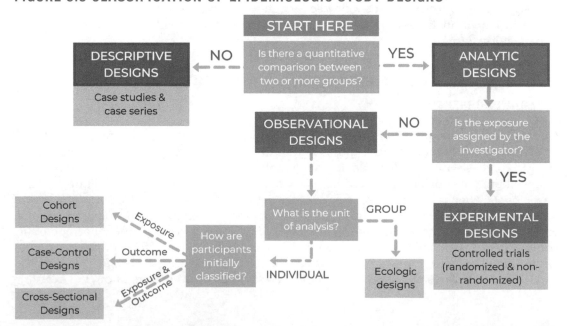

As also shown in **Figure 3.3**, the observational designs can be differentiated by their **unit of analysis**. The unit of analysis is the "level" at which study data are analyzed and is typically either at the individual- or group-level.[4] If we have detailed information that includes the exposure and outcome status for each individual in our study, then the unit of analysis is the individual. However, if we only have aggregate (group-level) data—meaning that we know the average frequency of exposure and/or outcome across different groups, but we don't know the specific exposure and outcome status for each individual—then the unit of analysis is the group (**Figure 3.4**). To study whether HPV vaccination is associated with a reduction in cervical cancer using an individual-level analysis, we would need to know the vaccination *and* cervical cancer statuses of everyone in the study. If we didn't have access to this individual-level information, and instead only knew the proportion of people who were vaccinated and the proportion of people who had cervical cancer, we would conduct our study using a group-level analysis. The unit of analysis in epidemiologic studies is determined by the available data. The unit of analysis informs how the study results are interpreted, as we will soon discuss.

## FIGURE 3.4 UNITS OF ANALYSIS FOR EPIDEMIOLOGIC STUDY DESIGNS

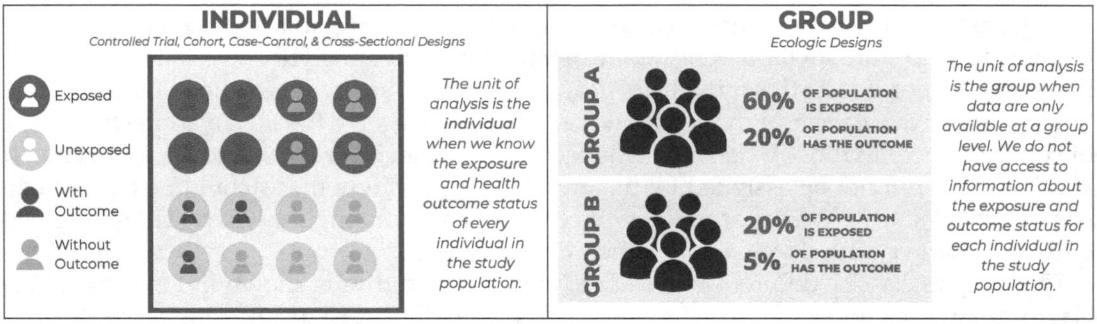

Now that we know about how to construct hypotheses and have an idea of the different levels at which an analysis can occur, we are ready for a broad overview of the analytic study designs shown in **Figure 3.3**: controlled trial, cohort, case-control, cross-sectional, and ecologic designs. This overview will be followed by a description of common measures of association, which quantify the association between an exposure and a health outcome, that are used in each study design.

## OVERVIEW OF ANALYTIC EPIDEMIOLOGIC STUDY DESIGNS
### (LEARNING OBJECTIVE 3.4)

**Controlled trial.** A controlled trial (also called a clinical trial) is an experimental study design in which the investigator *assigns* exposure status to the study participants. After developing a study hypothesis, investigators identify and enroll a sample from a population that is at-risk of developing the outcome of interest. Investigators then *assign* the exposure status to study participants, often randomly. A schematic of the design features of a controlled trial is shown in **Figure 3.5**. Simple random assignment, a type of randomization, is equivalent to assigning an exposure by tossing a fair coin (e.g., one side of the coin = exposed; the other side of the coin = nonexposed) and is not based on patients' or study investigators' preferences. After exposure assignment, study participants are followed forward for a specified time period to measure new cases of the outcome(s) of interest. Since investigators know the exposure

## FIGURE 3.5 SCHEMATIC OF A CONTROLLED TRIAL DESIGN

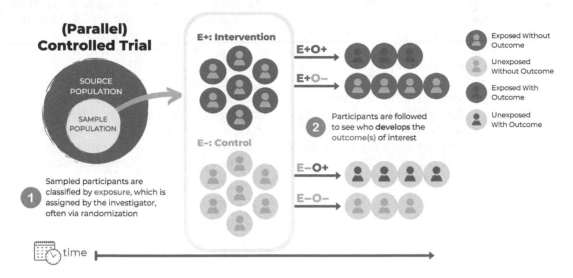

and outcome status for everyone in the study, the unit of analysis for a controlled trial is the individual. Given that at-risk individuals are followed for *new* cases of the outcome in this design, investigators may describe the frequency of the outcome using a risk or rate. Consequently, the association between exposure and outcome may be quantified using risk- and rate-based measures of association, described later in this chapter. Controlled trials, including the rationale for exposure assignment and randomization, are discussed in detail in **Chapter 4, "Randomized Controlled Trial Designs."**

## Pause to Practice 3.2

### An Example of a Controlled Trial

The safety and effectiveness of vaccines for prevention of SARS-CoV-2 have been evaluated in controlled trials. One study was conducted with participants from Argentina, Brazil, Germany, South Africa, Turkey, and the United States.[5] Participants were assigned to receive either two injections of a candidate mRNA vaccine (mRNA vaccines use messenger RNA to instruct our cells to create proteins that can trigger a protective immune response) or two placebo (meaning dummy or sham) injections. Participants were followed for a median of 2 months for incident COVID-19 diagnoses occurring at least 7 days after the second injection. Relatively few participants were lost to follow-up.

1.   What is the exposure of interest?
2.   What is the outcome of interest?
3.   Who is the study population?
4.   The investigators were interested in identifying new COVID-19 diagnoses during the follow-up period. Given this goal, what measures of frequency might be calculated?
5.   Formulate a possible study hypothesis.
6.   What features described above indicate that this is a controlled trial?

**Cohort Design.** The cohort design is an observational design, which means that the study investigator does not assign exposure status to participants; rather, they observe what occur anyway. After developing a study hypothesis, investigators identify and enroll a sample from an at-risk population. Then, investigators collect information about participants' exposure status and classify them as exposed or unexposed. Finally, participants are followed for a specified period of time to measure new cases of the outcome of interest. A schematic of the features of the cohort design is shown in **Figure 3.6**. Since investigators know the exposure and outcome status for everyone in the study, the unit of analysis for a cohort design is the individual. Given that at-risk individuals are followed for *new* cases of the outcome, investigators can describe the frequency of the outcome using a risk or rate. Consequently, the association between exposure and outcome is quantified using risk- and rate-based measures of association, described later in this chapter. Cohort designs are discussed in detail in **Chapter 5, "Cohort Designs."**

## FIGURE 3.6 SCHEMATIC OF A COHORT DESIGN

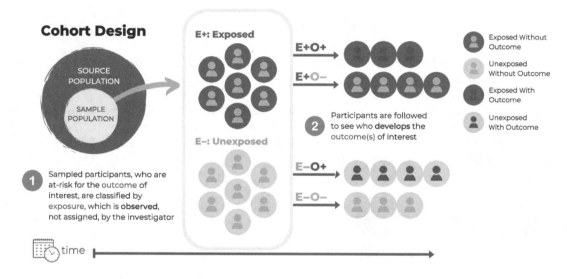

### An Example of a Cohort Design

Many studies have evaluated the effect of red meat consumption on various health outcomes, including coronary heart disease (CHD). In one study, 43,272 men in the United States who did not have CHD were recruited, and their level of red meat intake was measured. These men were then followed for 30 years to identify newly diagnosed cases of CHD.[6]

1.  What is the exposure of interest?
2.  What is the outcome of interest?
3.  Who is the study population?
4.  The investigators were interested in studying new cases of CHD during the 30-year follow-up period. Given this goal, what measures of frequency might be calculated?
5.  Formulate a possible study hypothesis.
6.  What features described above indicate that this is a cohort design?

**Case-Control Design.** The case-control design is also an observational design. After developing a study hypothesis, investigators identify and enroll a group of individuals with the outcome (the cases) and a suitable comparison group without the outcome (the controls). Next, investigators use tools like questionnaires or medical records to ascertain the exposure history of the study participants. Note that, in contrast to trials and cohort designs, there is no follow-up of participants enrolled in a case-control study. A schematic of these design features is shown in **Figure 3.7.** Since investigators know the exposure and outcome status for everyone in the study, the unit of analysis for a case-control design is the individual.

Importantly, no measure of outcome frequency can be directly calculated in a case-control design. Since investigators using a case-control design select participants based on outcome status, the investigators "fix" the proportion of those with the outcome by design. For example, if researchers enrolled one control for every case, a common strategy, and inappropriately calculated a measure of outcome frequency, they would find that 50% of the study participants had the outcome of interest. This is not a measure of outcome frequency, but rather a proportion determined by the relative number of cases to controls that the investigator selected. Even though no measure of outcome frequency can be directly calculated for a case-control design, epidemiologists have derived a meaningful measure of association called the exposure odds ratio (EOR), which is described later in this chapter. Case-control designs are discussed in detail in **Chapter 6, "Case-Control Designs."**

## FIGURE 3.7 SCHEMATIC OF A CASE-CONTROL DESIGN

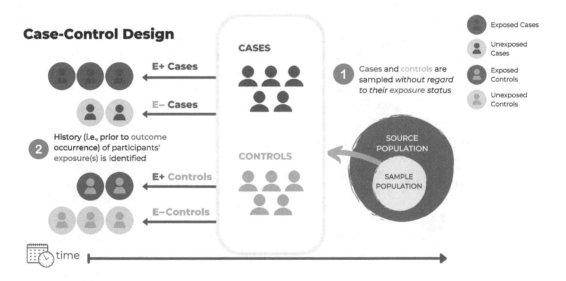

## Pause to Practice 3.4

### An Example of a Case-Control Design

Although stillbirths (defined in the United States as pregnancy losses occurring at 20 weeks' gestation or later) account for over half of the deaths that occur between 20 weeks' gestation and the first year of life, little is known about their causes.[7] To help address this gap, one study in the United States recruited and enrolled a group of individuals who experienced a stillbirth and a separate group whose babies were born alive. Investigators then reviewed the study participants' medical records and administered questionnaires to see whether there were any factors (e.g., age at conception, obesity/overweight, smoking prior to pregnancy) that were associated with stillbirth.[8]

Note that this is an example of an **exploratory study** where the investigators did not have a particular exposure of interest in mind. Rather, they explored whether a range of factors were associated with stillbirth, which means that they evaluated several different study hypotheses. Importantly, each of these hypotheses considered factors that were plausibly related to stillbirth based on what was already known.

1. What is the exposure of interest?
2. What is the outcome of interest?
3. Who is the study population?
4. What measures of outcome frequency might be calculated given this study design?
5. Formulate a possible study hypothesis for one of the exposures noted previously.
6. What features described above indicate that this is a case-control design?

**Cross-Sectional Design.** The cross-sectional design is also an observational design. First, after developing a study hypothesis, researchers must identify a population that is at-risk of the outcome of interest, and select study participants from this group. Then, researchers use tools like questionnaires or medical records to simultaneously collect information about their exposure and outcome statuses. A schematic of these design features is shown in **Figure 3.8**. There is no follow-up of study participants in the cross-sectional design; rather, their exposure and outcome are measured at a single point (a "snapshot") in time. Given that the exposure and outcome status are known for everyone in the study, the unit of analysis for a cross-sectional design is the individual. Since investigators measure existing cases of an outcome at one point in time, the outcome frequency is described using prevalence, and the association between exposure and outcome is quantified using prevalence-based measures of association, described later in this chapter.

A key feature of the cross-sectional design is that the investigator may not be able to differentiate which came first, the exposure or the outcome. This lack of temporality between the exposure and the outcome is a limitation for supporting causality. Cross-sectional designs are discussed in detail in **Chapter 7, "Cross-Sectional Designs."**

## FIGURE 3.8 SCHEMATIC OF A CROSS-SECTIONAL DESIGN

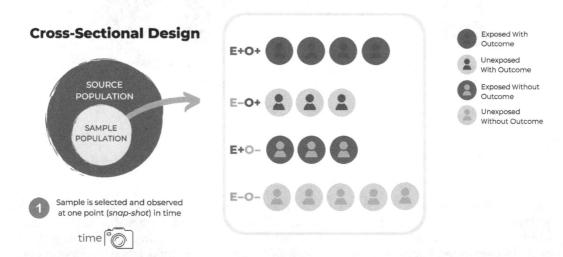

## Causality and Temporality in Analytic Study Designs

When conducting an analytic epidemiologic study, our goal is often to understand causality; that is, we want to know whether a particular exposure causes a particular health outcome. A cause is defined in *Modern Epidemiology* as "an antecedent event, condition, or characteristic that was necessary for the occurrence of the disease at the moment it occurred, given that other conditions are fixed".[9]

The word *antecedent* means something that came before in time, and it relates to the concept of temporality, which is one critical component in causal thinking: *If an exposure caused an outcome, the exposure must have occurred first.* We know that an exposure cannot possibly have been the cause of an outcome if it happened after the outcome occurred. We discuss how analytic epidemiologic studies attempt to (or fail to) establish temporality between exposures and outcomes in **Chapter 4 "Randomized Controlled Trial Design"; Chapter 5, "Cohort Designs"; Chapter 6, "Case-Control Designs"**; and **Chapter 7, "Cross-Sectional Designs."**

## Pause to Practice 3.5

### An Example of a Cross-Sectional Design

The U.S. CDC has conducted the National Health Interview Survey (NHIS) since 1957.[10] This survey has been used to monitor and compare the frequency of autism spectrum disorder (ASD) diagnoses among children in the United States at sequential cross-sectional time points and across demographic groups.[11] In 2016, researchers found a higher frequency of ASD in biological men than in biological women.

1.  What is the exposure of interest?
2.  What is the outcome of interest?
3.  Who is the study population?
4.  The investigators were interested in understanding how common ASD was in 2016. Given this goal, what measures of frequency might be calculated?
5.  Formulate a possible study hypothesis.
6.  What features described above indicate that this is a cross-sectional design?

The key aspects of the four common analytic epidemiologic study designs discussed previously are summarized for reference in **Table M.2**.

**Ecologic Design.** An ecologic design is another observational design; however, it differs from those previously discussed because the unit of analysis is a group of people defined in a meaningful way (e.g., by country or state) rather than individuals (see **Figure 3.4**).[12] The exposure and outcome data are aggregated, or combined, across these defined groups, and then used for analysis. This means that we do not know both the exposure and the outcome data for each individual in the study. For example, a study examining the association between a country's aggregate prevalence of cigarette smoking and aggregate prevalence of poverty would be an ecologic study. In such a study, we would not know whether those who smoke are the same people who are living in poverty, or vice versa.

Since ecologic studies use groups as the unit of analysis, the interpretation of these study findings is sometimes prone to the **ecologic fallacy**. This fallacy occurs when findings from an ecologic study are presumed to apply to individuals.[13] For example, while there may be an association between smoking and poverty at the country level, we don't have enough information to say whether this relationship holds for individuals. Even if this association were to appear at the country level, it is possible that *no* individual in the country experienced both smoking and poverty, meaning that there would be no causal association between smoking and poverty in individuals.

Findings from ecologic studies cannot support causal relationships in individuals, which is the primary focus of most public health questions. Despite this limitation, ecologic studies have generated important public health data, and their uses include:

- Exploration of existing, publicly available aggregate data on outcomes and exposures to generate data more quickly and inexpensively than de novo individual-level data collection. For example, an ecologic study of smoking and poverty may be able to quickly and inexpensively generate data to support funding for a more robust analytic study at the individual level.
- Evaluation of associations for which exposures can only be measured at the population level, such as broad-reaching policy changes. For example, exploring the effect of U.S. state-level cigarette smoking ban policies on state lung cancer prevalence would be an ecologic study, as it would be difficult to measure exposure to statewide smoking ban policies at the individual level.

## Pause to Practice 3.6

### Ecologic Studies and the Ecologic Fallacy

Consider Figure 3.9, which shows country-level gender inequality (using an index rank, in which a lower rank represents less inequality) on the *y*-axis and country-level life expectancy at birth in years on the *x*-axis. These data come from publicly available World Health Organization Key Indicator data for 195 countries around the world.[14] This figure shows that, on average, lower gender inequality appears to be associated with increased life expectancy at the country level.

1. What is the exposure of interest?
2. What is the outcome of interest?
3. What is the study population?
4. Formulate a possible study hypothesis.
5. What features define this study as an ecologic design?
6. Can it be assumed that experiencing less gender inequity leads an individual to live longer?

### FIGURE 3.9 COUNTRY-LEVEL GENDER INEQUALITY AND LIFE EXPECTANCY (*N* = 195 COUNTRIES)

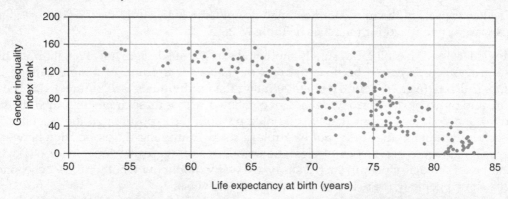

*Source:* Data from World Health Organization. Key country indicators. 2020. https://apps.who.int/gho/data/node.cco.latest?lang=en

### Proving Causality: The Unachievable Goal of Analytic Epidemiologic Studies
(LEARNING OBJECTIVE 3.5)

Though epidemiologic hypotheses posit an *association* between an exposure and a health outcome, epidemiologists are ultimately interested in whether the exposure *causes* the outcome. Unfortunately, proving a causal relationship between an exposure and an outcome is impossible in an epidemiologic study. We can conduct a useful thought experiment to conceptualize a situation that would definitively establish causality. Ideally, we would like to know the health outcome for an exposed individual as well as the health outcome for that *exact same* individual *had they been unexposed* (i.e., in an alternate universe where the only difference was their exposure status). We could "prove" causality if the individual experienced different outcomes in these alternate universes would be able to say that the exposure had a causal (i.e., etiologic) effect on the outcome in that individual. Of course, we can't observe the exposed and unexposed conditions for the exact same individual, all else remaining the same. We only observe an individual under one exposure condition. The other unobservable condition is called the **counterfactual**, meaning that, counter to fact, it did not occur.

As an example, suppose a woman received an HPV vaccination and did not develop cervical cancer. Further, suppose that we were able to observe what happened to her in an alternate universe where she did *not* receive an HPV vaccination (and everything else in her life otherwise stayed the same). Unfortunately, in this alternate universe, she *did* develop cervical cancer. In this hypothetical scenario, we have proven that the HPV vaccination had a *causal*, in this case preventive, effect on cervical cancer.

Although we can never prove causality between an exposure and an outcome, we use analytic study designs to estimate their *association* while attempting to control for as many sources of error as possible. It is important to keep in mind that an association (what we measure in a study) does not imply causation (which is unobservable). Fortunately, as you will learn throughout this text, epidemiologists have access to many tools that help us gather evidence to support or refute hypotheses, such as selecting suitable comparison groups to help us get as close to the counterfactual ideal as possible.

## Which Design Is Best?

No matter how robust a given study is, scientific knowledge on the determinants of health-related outcomes is advanced through multiple studies and an accumulation of evidence. Students of epidemiology are often taught that there is a hierarchy to study designs and that randomized controlled trials are the gold standard study design, with cross-sectional and ecologic studies generating the least robust evidence of the analytic designs (**Figure 3.10**). While it is true that trials have unique design attributes that attempt to reduce error and approximate the counterfactual ideal (namely, randomization of the exposure, as you will learn in **Chapter 4, "Randomized Controlled Trial Designs"**), the reality is that any well-conducted study of any design can provide robust evidence. The answer to the question "What is the best study design?" is dependent on the research question at hand, as well as ethical and practical considerations. These issues are explored in **Chapter 4, "Randomized Controlled Trial Designs"; Chapter 5, "Cohort Designs"; Chapter 6, "Case-Control Designs"; and Chapter 7, "Cross-Sectional Designs."**

## FIGURE 3.10 RETHINKING THE HIERARCHY OF STUDY DESIGNS

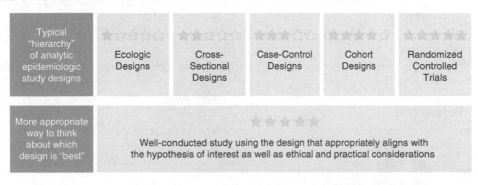

## CALCULATING AND INTERPRETING MEASURES OF ASSOCIATION

In the first part of this chapter, we described the importance of a well-constructed hypothesis and introduced the main analytic epidemiologic study designs. We can now turn our attention to learning about the measures that can be calculated using data from each of these designs with the goal of evaluating whether there is an association between an exposure and a health outcome. These **measures of association** make use of the measures of frequency described in **Chapter 2, "Descriptive Epidemiology, Surveillance, and Measures of Frequency."** Before moving on, we suggest that readers review the summary of measures of frequency shown in **Table M.1.**

To calculate and interpret measures of association, we must first orient ourselves to the "R×C" (row × column) tables (sometimes called contingency tables) commonly used to present exposure and outcome data. Epidemiologists typically create 2×2 tables since we often consider dichotomous, meaning binary, exposures and outcomes (i.e., there are only two categories, like vitamin use and no vitamin use or cancer and no cancer). An example 2×2 table is shown in **Figure 3.11** (Learning Objective 3.6).

### FIGURE 3.11 EXAMPLE 2×2 TABLE USED TO ORIENT COUNT DATA (USED FOR CALCULATION OF RISK-, PREVALENCE-, AND ODDS-BASED MEASURES)

|  | Exposed (E+) | Unexposed (E−) | TOTAL |
|---|---|---|---|
| **Outcome (O+)** | A | B | $M_1$ (=A+B) |
| **No Outcome (O−)** | C | D | $M_0$ (=C+D) |
| **TOTAL** | $N_1$ (=A+C) | $N_0$ (=B+D) | N |

- $N$ is the total number of individuals in the study population.
- The letters A, B, C, and D represent count data for each of four groups:
  - A is the number of people who are categorized as **exposed** *and* **who have the outcome.**
  - B is the number of people who are categorized as **unexposed** *and* **who have the outcome.**
  - C is the number of people who are categorized as **exposed** *and* **who do** *not* **have the outcome.**
  - D is the number of people who are categorized as **unexposed** *and* **who do** *not* **have the outcome.**
- $N_1$ and $N_0$ represent the total number of exposed and unexposed individuals, respectively.
- $M_1$ and $M_0$ represent the total number of individuals with and without the outcome, respectively.

## Notation Notice

The values $N_1$, $N_0$, $M_1$, and $M_0$ are often referred to as *marginal totals*. The subscript 1 is traditionally used to note that a group *has* a particular characteristic of interest ($N_1$ = exposed [E+], $M_1$ = outcome [O+]), whereas the subscript 0 is traditionally used to note that a group *does not have* a particular characteristic of interest ($N_0$ = unexposed [E–], $M_0$ = no outcome [O–]).

## 2×2 Table Thoughts

Notice that the 2x2 table in **Figure 3.11** includes individuals in four different categories:

- Exposed with the outcome
- Unexposed with the outcome
- Exposed without the outcome
- Unexposed without the outcome

An analytic epidemiologic study usually provides information from individuals belonging to all four of these groups. When thinking about a relationship between an exposure and an outcome, those new to the field of epidemiology sometimes mistakenly assume that everyone who is exposed has the outcome of interest, and that everyone who is unexposed does not have the outcome of interest. While this scenario would provide strong evidence of a link between the exposure and the outcome, it is highly unlikely to occur.

For example, consider the association between smoking tobacco and lung cancer. It is well-established that smoking is associated with lung cancer, meaning lung cancer is more common among smokers than among nonsmokers. However, there are some individuals who have smoked for decades and never develop lung cancer (belonging to cell C in **Figure 3.11**); additionally, there are some who never smoked a day in their life but develop lung cancer (belonging to cell B in **Figure 3.11**). These three things can be true simultaneously: smoking is strongly associated with lung cancer, some smokers will never develop lung cancer, and some non-smokers will develop lung cancer.

## R×C Table Orientation (LEARNING OBJECTIVE 3.6)

There is variation in how individuals or organizations prefer to orient their R×C tables. For this reason, we must always examine the orientation of the table when analyzing data. Throughout this text, we will orient our 2×2 table with exposure data in the columns and outcome data in the rows, as shown in **Figure 3.11**.

**TABLE 3.4 R×C TABLE ORIENTATION**

| | Outcome (O+) | No Outcome (O–) | TOTAL |
|---|---|---|---|
| Exposed (E+) | A | C | $M_1$ |
| Unexposed (E–) | B | D | $M_0$ |
| TOTAL | $N_1$ | $N_0$ | N |

However, others may orient 2×2 tables with the outcome presented in the columns and the exposure in the rows, as shown in **Table 3.4**. Note that to make the letter notation shown in **Figure 3.11** equivalent to **Table 3.4**, the letters B (the number of unexposed with the outcome) and C (the number of exposed without the outcome) must switch places.

It is important for readers to know that the orientation of the R×C table does not matter. What is important is to be able to navigate a 2×2 table so that you know what information you must use to calculate the measure(s) of interest. We'll discuss this further throughout the text.

In the text that follows, we provide a description of each main measures of association, their formulae, and their key features: null value, units, the range of possible values, interpretation, and application. The **null value** is the value that a measure of association takes on when there is no association between the exposure and outcome (i.e., the exposure does not affect the outcome of interest; Learning Objective 3.7). We provide generic sentences for interpreting the measures of association, but note it is important to always substitute the specific exposure and outcome of interest when generating your own interpretations. As you will see, the choice of which measure to calculate depends on which study design has been used; there are some measures of associations that are unique to a given study design, and there are some that are appropriate for more than one. For reference, the measures of association and their key features are summarized in **Table M.4**.

## Risk-Based Measures of Association

The **risk ratio** (often abbreviated RR) is a measure of association that divides the risk of the outcome in the exposed group by the risk of the outcome in the unexposed group. Using the notation from **Figure 3.11**, the formula for calculating the risk ratio is shown in **Equation 3.1**.

$$\text{Risk ratio (RR)} = \frac{\text{Risk in the exposed}}{\text{Risk in the unexposed}} = \frac{A/N_1}{B/N_0} \tag{3.1}$$

### INTERPRETATION OF THE RISK RATIO

The interpretation of the risk ratio is: *the risk of the outcome among those who are exposed is [insert value of RR] times the risk of the outcome among those who are unexposed over the study follow-up period.*

Recall that risks are always presented with the length of the follow-up period over which participants were observed (e.g., the *5-year* risk of death among breast cancer survivors is 10%). Similarly, it is important that an interpretation of the risk ratio also incorporates information about the length of the follow-up period.

### NULL VALUE OF THE RISK RATIO (LEARNING OBJECTIVE 3.7)

When the risks in both the exposed and the unexposed group are the same, there is no association between the exposure and the outcome. Thus, taking the ratio of these risks yields a risk ratio of 1. The null value for all ratio measures of association is 1.

### UNITS OF THE RISK RATIO

Although risks can be reported as a percentage, there are no units associated with the risk ratio because they cancel upon division.

### RANGE OF POSSIBLE VALUES FOR THE RISK RATIO

Since risks are bound between 0 and 1, a risk ratio can never be negative; however, there is no upper limit for the values that the risk ratio can take. If no one in the unexposed group gets the outcome of interest, the risk ratio will be *undefined* due to division by zero.

### APPLICATION OF THE RISK RATIO

The risk ratio can be calculated in any study that includes a follow-up period (e.g., a trial or cohort study). Recall that it may not be possible to calculate risk if not everyone in a population is followed until they either get the outcome or complete the same study follow-up time.

The **risk difference** (often abbreviated RD) is a measure of association that subtracts risk of the outcome in the unexposed group from the risk of the outcome in the exposed group. Using the notation in **Figure 3.11**, the formula for calculating the risk difference is shown in **Equation 3.2**.

$$\text{Risk difference } (RD) = \text{Risk in exposed} - \text{Risk in unexposed} = \frac{A}{N_1} - \frac{B}{N_0} \qquad (3.2)$$

### INTERPRETATION OF THE RISK DIFFERENCE

The interpretation of the risk difference is: *the difference between the risk of the outcome in the exposed and the unexposed is [insert value of RD] during the study follow-up period.*

When the risk difference is positive, it is often interpreted as the additional (or excess) risk of an outcome in a population due to exposure, as shown visually in **Figure 3.12**. When the risk difference is negative, it is sometimes interpreted as the *reduction* in risk of an outcome in a population due to exposure. As with the risk ratio, the interpretation of a risk difference must also include the length of time that the study participants were followed.

### NULL VALUE OF THE RISK DIFFERENCE (LEARNING OBJECTIVE 3.7)

Again, when there is no association between the exposure and the outcome, the risk in the exposed and unexposed groups will be the same. Taking the difference between these risks yields a risk difference of 0. The null value for all difference measures of association is 0.

### FIGURE 3.12 INTERPRETING POSITIVE AND NEGATIVE RISK DIFFERENCES

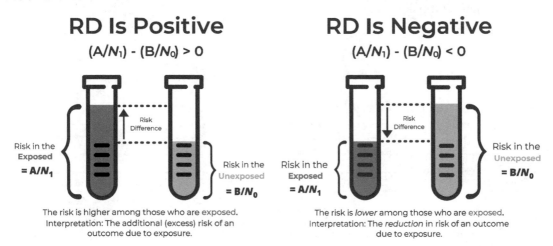

**RD Is Positive**
$(A/N_1) - (B/N_0) > 0$

Risk in the **Exposed** $= A/N_1$

Risk Difference

Risk in the Unexposed $= B/N_0$

The risk is higher among those who are exposed.
Interpretation: The additional (excess) risk of an outcome due to exposure.

**RD Is Negative**
$(A/N_1) - (B/N_0) < 0$

Risk Difference

Risk in the **Exposed** $= A/N_1$

Risk in the Unexposed $= B/N_0$

The risk is *lower* among those who are exposed.
Interpretation: The *reduction* in risk of an outcome due to exposure.

### UNITS OF THE RISK DIFFERENCE

When subtracting one risk from another, the units do not cancel as they do for the risk ratio. For this reason, the risk difference is expressed as a decimal or a percentage.

### RANGE OF POSSIBLE VALUES FOR THE RISK DIFFERENCE

When a risk difference is expressed as a decimal, its possible values can range from −1 to 1; when the risk difference is expressed as a percentage, its possible values range from −100% to 100%.

### APPLICATION OF THE RISK DIFFERENCE

The risk difference can be calculated in any study that includes a follow-up period (e.g., a trial or cohort study). However, recall that it may not be possible to calculate risk if not everyone in a population is followed until they either get the outcome or complete the same study follow-up time.

## Pause to Practice 3.7

### Calculating and Interpreting Risk Ratios and Risk Differences

COVID-19 became a major threat to global public health in 2020, and a race to develop effective vaccines began right away. Recall the randomized trial from **Pause to Practice 3.2**. This was a multinational, randomized controlled trial where researchers sought to evaluate whether the candidate COVID-19 vaccine was associated with a lower risk of COVID-19 diagnosis among the multinational study participants compared to a placebo injection.[5] Participants were followed for a median of 2 months. Among participants without baseline COVID-19 infection:

- A total of 18,198 participants received injections with the candidate COVID-19 vaccine.

- A total of 18,325 participants received injections with a saline placebo.

- Eight cases of COVID-19 occurred in participants assigned to receive the candidate COVID-19 vaccine at least 7 days after the second injection.

- A total of 162 cases of COVID-19 occurred in participants assigned to receive the placebo at least 7 days after the second injection.

The study data have been organized into **Table 3.5**. Practice creating this table using the study description yourself (Learning Objective 3.8).

1. Calculate the risk ratio.
2. Interpret the risk ratio.
3. Calculate the risk difference.
4. Interpret the risk difference.

TABLE 3.5 **CANDIDATE COVID-19 VACCINE TRIAL DATA**

|  | Candidate Vaccine (E+) | Placebo (E−) | TOTAL |
|---|---|---|---|
| COVID-19 diagnosis (O+) | 8 | 162 | 170 |
| No COVID-19 diagnosis (O−) | (18,198 − 8) = 18,190 | (18,325 − 162) = 18,163 | 36,353 |
| TOTAL | 18,198 | 18,325 | 36,523 |

*Source*: Data from Polack FP, Thomas SJ, Kitchin N, et al. Safety and efficacy of the BNT162b2 mRNA Covid-19 vaccine. N Engl J Med. 2020;383(27):2603-2615. https://doi.org/10.1056/NEJMoa2034577

### Comparing Ratio and Difference Measures of Association

The risk ratio is a measure of the strength of the *relative* risk of an outcome between an exposed and an unexposed group. The risk difference is a measure of the *absolute* difference in risk of an outcome between an exposed and unexposed group.

Taking the previous example:

Though the *relative* risk is quite large, the *absolute* difference in the risks remains small. Compare the candidate vaccine (our exposed group) to the placebo (our unexposed group):

- risk ratio = 0.05
- risk difference = −0.80%

Equivalently, we can "flip" the comparison group to present these data in a more intuitive way by taking the inverse of the risk ratio or 1 (or 100%) minus the risk difference.

- risk ratio = $1/0.05 = 20$
- risk difference = $100\% - (-0.80\%) = 100.80\%$

To see the impact that the risk in the unexposed can have on the magnitude of the risk difference, we can consider an example where the risk in the exposed group is 0.6 and the risk in the unexposed group is 0.03. In this case, the risk ratio (0.6/0.03) equals 20, just as in the example with the COVID-19 vaccine. However, the risk difference (0.6 − 0.03 = 0.57) is much larger.

Since ratio and difference measures of association provide different information, both may be calculated in a given study.

## Rate-Based Measures of Association

The **rate ratio** (also called the **incidence density ratio**, and abbreviated IDR, thus avoiding the confusion of having the same abbreviation as the risk ratio [RR]) is a measure of association that divides the rate of the outcome in the exposed group by the rate of the outcome in the unexposed group. Since rates are calculated using person-time as the denominator, a slightly different 2×2 table is needed to accommodate rate data, as shown in **Figure 3.13**.

Just like in the 2×2 table shown in **Figure 3.11**, **Figure 3.13** presents count data for those who have the outcome of interest and are either exposed or unexposed in one row. However, instead of presenting *count data* for those without the outcome, investigators record the *person-time* accumulated by all individuals in each exposure group.

### FIGURE 3.13 EXAMPLE 2×2 TABLE USED TO ORIENT COUNT AND PERSON-TIME DATA (USED FOR CALCULATION OF RATE-BASED MEASURES OF ASSOCIATION)

|  | Exposed (E+) | Unexposed (E−) | TOTAL |
|---|---|---|---|
| **Outcome (O+)** | A | B | $M_1$ (A+B) |
| **Person-Time\*** | $PT_1$ | $PT_0$ | $PT_{Total}$ ($PT_1 + PT_0$) |

*Person-time included in a 2×2 table for rate-based data corresponds to the time that all individuals who were exposed or unexposed contributed to the study. This includes person-time for people who did and did not get the outcome of interest during the follow-up period.

### A Note About the 2×2 Table for Rate-Based Data

There is a common misconception among those first learning about rates that the person-time presented in a rate-based 2×2 table only corresponds to the time contributed by those who eventually got the outcome of interest. It is important to have denominator information about those who do and do not get the outcome—and thus, these tables incorporate the person-time for both groups.

Using the notation in **Figure 3.13**, the formula for calculating the rate ratio is shown in **Equation 3.3**.

$$\text{Rate ratio (IDR)} = \frac{\text{Rate in the exposed}}{\text{Rate in the unexposed}} = \frac{A/PT_1}{B/PT_0} \tag{3.3}$$

## INTERPRETATION OF THE RATE RATIO

The interpretation of the rate ratio is: *the rate of the outcome among those who are exposed is [insert value of IDR] times rate of the outcome among those who are unexposed.*

## NULL VALUE OF THE RATE RATIO

When the rates in both the exposed and the unexposed group are the same, there is no association between the exposure and the outcome. If we were to take the ratio of these rates, we would yield a rate ratio of 1. The null value for all ratio measures of association is 1.

## UNITS OF THE RATE RATIO

Although rates are reported using person-time denominators (e.g., 35 cases *per 10,000 person-years*), these units cancel upon division, and thus the rate ratio is unitless. For this reason, it is imperative to calculate the rate of the outcome among the exposed and unexposed groups using the same units; a rate ratio that is calculated by dividing a rate in the exposed group expressed per 10,000 person-years by a rate in the unexposed group expressed per 100,000 person-years will yield an incorrect answer.

## RANGE OF POSSIBLE VALUES FOR THE RATE RATIO

Since rates can never be negative, neither can the rate ratio. However, there is no upper limit for the values that the rate ratio can take. If no one in the unexposed group gets the outcome of interest, the rate ratio will be *undefined* due to division by zero (the rate in the unexposed).

## APPLICATION OF THE RATE RATIO

A rate ratio can be calculated in any study that includes a follow-up period and the length of follow-up time is known for all study participants (e.g., a trial or cohort study). The rate ratio is particularly useful when there is loss to follow-up or if everyone isn't followed for the same length of time.

The **rate difference** (also called **incidence density difference**, and abbreviated IDD) is a measure of association that subtracts the rate of the outcome in the unexposed group from the rate of the outcome in the exposed group. Using the notation in **Figure 3.13**, the formula for calculating the rate difference is shown in **Equation 3.4**.

Rate difference (IDD)

$$= \text{Rate in exposed} - \text{Rate in unexposed} = \frac{A}{PT_1} - \frac{B}{PT_0} \tag{3.4}$$

## INTERPRETATION OF THE RATE DIFFERENCE

The interpretation of the risk difference is: *the difference between the rate of the outcome in the exposed and the unexposed is [insert value of IDD].*

## NULL VALUE OF THE RATE DIFFERENCE (LEARNING OBJECTIVE 3.7)

As before, when there is no association between the exposure and the outcome, the rate in the exposed and unexposed groups will be the same. Thus, if we were to take the difference between these rates, this would yield a rate difference of 0. The null value for all difference measures of association is 0.

## UNITS OF THE RATE DIFFERENCE

When subtracting one risk from another, the units do not cancel as they do for the rate ratio. For this reason, rate differences must retain the units that describe the context in which the rates were observed (e.g., IDD = 15 cases per 10,000 person-years). As with the rate ratio, it's important to ensure that the rates in the exposed and unexposed groups have been calculated using the same units to avoid errors.

### RANGE OF POSSIBLE VALUES FOR THE RATE DIFFERENCE

Since there is no upper limit on a rate, there is no limit on the range of values that the rate difference can assume. Similarly, there is also no lower limit.

### APPLICATION OF THE RATE DIFFERENCE

A rate difference can be calculated in any study that includes a follow-up period and the length of follow-up time is known for all study participants (e.g., a trial or cohort study). Although we provide details on the calculation and interpretation of rate differences, they are not commonly calculated in epidemiologic studies.

## Pause to Practice 3.8

### Calculating and Interpreting Rate Ratios

Recall from **Chapter 1, "Introduction to Public Health and the Fundamentals of Epidemiology,"** that ischemic heart disease, also called coronary heart disease (CHD), is the leading cause of mortality worldwide. In **Pause to Practice 3.3**, we presented a cohort study designed to evaluate whether men in the U.S. with higher red meat consumption had higher rates of CHD compared to those with lower red meat consumption.[6] Understanding more about dietary risk factors for CHD could help to inform prevention interventions to reduce CHD mortality.

In this cohort study, meat consumption was categorized into quintiles (i.e., five evenly distributed, mutually exclusive categories). To organize the study data in a 2x2 table, we can compare the highest quintile of meat consumers (exposed) to the lowest four quintiles of red meat consumers (unexposed).

During the study:

- A total of 204,079 person-years of follow-up were contributed by men in the highest quintile of red meat consumption.

- A total of 819,792 person-years of follow-up were contributed by men in the lowest four quintiles of red meat consumption.

- A total of 1,087 CHD outcomes occurred in men in the highest quintile of red meat consumption.

- A total of 3,368 CHD outcomes occurred in men in the lowest four quintiles of red meat consumption.

The study data have been organized into **Table 3.6** for rate-based data. Practice creating this table using the study description yourself (Learning Objective 3.8).

1. Calculate the rate ratio.
2. Interpret the rate ratio.
3. Think about how we can calculate measures of association using a different definition for the unexposed group. This is important because different definitions for the exposed and/or unexposed groups may yield different values for the measures of association and be interpreted differently.

**TABLE 3.6 DATA FROM A COHORT STUDY DESIGNED TO EVALUATE WHETHER HIGHER RED MEAT CONSUMPTION WAS ASSOCIATED WITH A HIGHER RATE OF CHD AMONG MEN IN THE UNITED STATES**

| | High Red Meat Consumption Highest Quintile (E+) | Low Red Meat Consumption Lowest 4 Quintiles Combined (E−) | TOTAL |
|---|---|---|---|
| CHD Diagnosis (O+) | 1,087 | 3,368 | 4,455 |
| Person-Years (PY) | 204,079 | 819,792 | 1,023,871 |

CHD, coronary heart disease.
*Source:* Data from Al-Shaar L, Satija A, Wang DD, et al. Red meat intake and risk of coronary heart disease among US men: prospective cohort study. *BMJ.* 2020;371:m4141. https://doi.org/10.1136/bmj.m4141

Assume that investigators continue to define the exposed group as men in the highest quintile of red meat consumption. However, they now define the unexposed group as men in the single lowest quintile of red meat consumption (instead of the lowest four quintiles combined). The new study data are shown in **Table 3.7**.

**TABLE 3.7 STUDY DATA DEFINING THE UNEXPOSED GROUP AS MEN IN THE SINGLE LOWEST QUINTILE OF RED MEAT CONSUMPTION**

| | High Red Meat Consumption Highest Quintile (E+) | Low Red Meat Consumption Lowest Quintile (E−) | TOTAL |
|---|---|---|---|
| CHD Diagnosis (O+) | 1,087 | 811 | 1,898 |
| Person-Years (PY) | 204,079 | 203,879 | 407,958 |

CHD, coronary heart disease.
*Source:* Data from Al-Shaar L, Satija A, Wang DD, et al. Red meat intake and risk of coronary heart disease among US men: prospective cohort study. *BMJ.* 2020;371:m4141. https://doi.org/10.1136/bmj.m4141

Practice calculating the new rate ratio, which you should find is equal to 1.34. This measure of association is slightly stronger (i.e., further from the null value of 1) than the rate ratio calculated previously, which is expected given the change in our definition of the unexposed group. Why might this be?

## Prevalence-Based Measures of Association

The **prevalence ratio** (often abbreviated PR) is a measure of association that divides the prevalence of the outcome in the exposed group by the prevalence of the outcome in the unexposed group. Using the notation in **Figure 3.11**, the formula for the prevalence ratio is shown in **Equation 3.5**.

$$\text{Prevalence ratio } (PR) = \frac{\text{Prevalence in the exposed}}{\text{Prevalence in the unexposed}} = \frac{A/N_1}{B/N_0} \tag{3.5}$$

If you look closely, you will notice that the formulae for the risk ratio and the prevalence ratio are identical. The difference between these is in whether the observed outcomes are *newly occurring* (i.e., incident cases—and thus yielding a risk ratio) or if they are *existing* outcomes (i.e., prevalent cases—thus yielding a prevalence ratio). As we'll continue to discuss throughout this text, it is important to be familiar with your data in order to calculate and interpret the measures appropriately.

### INTERPRETATION OF THE PREVALENCE RATIO

The interpretation of the prevalence ratio is: *the prevalence of the outcome among those who are exposed is [insert value of PR] times the prevalence of the outcome among those who are unexposed.*

## NULL VALUE OF THE PREVALENCE RATIO (LEARNING OBJECTIVE 3.7)

When there is no association between an exposure and a health outcome, this means that the prevalence in both the exposed and the unexposed group is the same. Thus, dividing the prevalence in the exposed by the prevalence in the unexposed yields a prevalence ratio of 1. The null value for all ratio measures of association is 1.

## UNITS OF THE PREVALENCE RATIO

Although prevalence can be reported as a percentage, there are no units associated with the prevalence ratio because they cancel upon division.

## RANGE OF POSSIBLE VALUES FOR THE PREVALENCE RATIO

Since the prevalence is bound between 0 and 1, a prevalence ratio can never be negative; however, there is no upper limit for the values that the prevalence ratio can take. If no one in the unexposed group has the outcome of interest, the prevalence ratio will be *undefined* due to division by zero (the prevalence in the unexposed).

## APPLICATION OF THE PREVALENCE RATIO

A prevalence ratio is an appropriate measure to calculate for cross-sectional designs.

The **prevalence difference** (often abbreviated PD) is a measure of association that subtracts the prevalence of the outcome in the unexposed group from the prevalence of the outcome in the exposed group. Using the notation in **Figure 3.11**, the formula for calculating the prevalence difference is shown in **Equation 3.6**.

$$\text{Prevalence difference (PD)} =$$

$$(\text{Prevalence in exposed}) - (\text{Prevalence in unexposed}) = \frac{A}{N_1} - \frac{B}{N_0} \tag{3.6}$$

As with the prevalence ratio, you will notice that the formula for the prevalence difference is identical to that of risk difference. Again, it's important to know whether you are considering incident or prevalent cases of an outcome in order to determine whether to interpret the measure as a risk difference or a prevalence difference.

## INTERPRETATION OF THE PREVALENCE DIFFERENCE

The interpretation of the prevalence difference is: *the difference between the prevalence of the outcome in the exposed and the unexposed is [insert value of PD].*

Like the risk difference, the prevalence difference can also use the "excess" or "additional" prevalence interpretation (replacing the word *risk* with *prevalence*).

## NULL VALUE OF THE PREVALENCE DIFFERENCE (LEARNING OBJECTIVE 3.7)

As before, when there is no association between the exposure and the outcome, the prevalence in the exposed and unexposed groups will be the same. Thus, taking their difference yields a prevalence difference of 0. The null value for all difference measures of association is 0.

## UNITS OF THE PREVALENCE DIFFERENCE

When subtracting one prevalence from another, the units do not cancel as they do for the prevalence ratio. For this reason, the prevalence difference is expressed as a decimal or a percentage.

## RANGE OF POSSIBLE VALUES FOR THE PREVALENCE DIFFERENCE

When a prevalence difference is expressed as a decimal, its possible values can range from −1 to 1; when the prevalence difference is expressed as a percentage, the possible values range from −100% to 100%.

## APPLICATION OF THE PREVALENCE DIFFERENCE

A prevalence difference is an appropriate measure to calculate for cross-sectional designs.

## Pause to Practice 3.9

### Calculating and Interpreting Prevalence-Based Measures of Association

An improved understanding of factors associated with Autism Spectrum Disorder (ASD) may shed light on ASD etiology and improve screening. Recall the study described in **Pause to Practice 3.5**, which considered a cross-sectional study comparing ASD diagnoses among males and females. One hypothesis that could be evaluated using these data is whether male (versus female) biological sex was associated with a higher prevalence of ASD diagnoses among children in the United States.[12] Investigators hypothesized that biological sex may be associated with ASD diagnoses due to exposure to sex hormones from an early age.

During the study:

- A total of 15,727 biological males were surveyed.

- A total of 14,775 biological females were surveyed.

- A total of 545 biological males were diagnosed with ASD.

- A total of 166 biological females were diagnosed with ASD.

The study data have been organized into **Table 3.8**. Practice creating this table using the study description yourself (Learning Objective 3.8).

1. Calculate the prevalence ratio.
2. Interpret the prevalence ratio.
3. Calculate the prevalence difference.
4. Interpret the prevalence difference.

**TABLE 3.8 DATA FROM A SURVEY USED TO COMPARE THE FREQUENCY OF ASD DIAGNOSES AMONG CHILDREN IN THE UNITED STATES**

|  | Biologically Male (E+) | Biologically Female (E−) | TOTAL |
|---|---|---|---|
| ASD Diagnosis (O+) | 545 | 166 | 711 |
| No ASD Diagnosis (O−) | 15,182 | 14,609 | 29,791 |
| TOTAL | 15,727 | 14,775 | 30,502 |

ASD, autism spectrum disorder.
*Source:* Xu G, Strathearn L, Liu B, Bao W. Prevalence of autism spectrum disorder among US children and adolescents, 2014–2016. *JAMA.* 2018;319(1):81–82. https://doi.org/10.1001/jama.2017.17812

## The Exposure Odds Ratio

For completeness, we conclude our discussion of measures of association with the **exposure odds ratio** (often abbreviated EOR), which is the appropriate measure of association for case-control designs. This measure differs from those discussed previously in that it is derived from a measure called the **odds** (as opposed to a risk, rate, or prevalence). The utility and derivation of this measure are described in detail in **Chapter 6, "Case-Control Designs."**

For now, all you should know is that the exposure odds ratio is a measure of association that divides the odds of the exposure in those with the outcome by the odds of the exposure in those without the outcome. The formula for the exposure odds ratio using the notation in **Figure 3.11** is shown in **Equation 3.7**. This formula is sometimes called the "cross-product" because it is calculated by multiplying the values in opposite corners of the 2×2 table.

$$\text{Exposure odds ratio (EOR)} = \frac{A \times D}{B \times C} \tag{3.7}$$

### INTERPRETATION OF THE EXPOSURE ODDS RATIO

The interpretation of the exposure odds ratio is: *the odds of exposure among the cases is [insert value of EOR] the odds of exposure among the controls*.

### NULL VALUE OF THE EXPOSURE ODDS RATIO (LEARNING OBJECTIVE 3.7)

As with all ratio measures of association, the null value for the exposure odds ratio is equal to one.

### UNITS OF THE EXPOSURE ODDS RATIO

Like the other ratio measures of association, the exposure odds ratio is unitless.

### RANGE OF POSSIBLE VALUES FOR THE EXPOSURE ODDS RATIO

Odds, which will be formally defined in **Chapter 6, "Case-Control Designs"** are always greater than 0, so the exposure odds ratio cannot take on negative values. There is no upper limit on the value for an exposure odds ratio. If there are no individuals in cells B or C in the 2×2 table, the exposure odds ratio will be undefined due to division by zero.

### APPLICATION OF THE EXPOSURE ODDS RATIO

The exposure odds ratio is the only measure of association that is calculated for case-control designs. However, as you will learn, there are times when an odds ratio is calculated in other designs. Therefore, if you see an odds ratio, you can't automatically assume the data come from a case-control study.

## Pause to Practice 3.10

### Calculating and Interpreting the Exposure Odds Ratio

Recall the study described in **Pause to Practice 3.4**, which was a case-control study evaluated whether certain prior exposures were more common among study participants who experienced a stillbirth than among those whose babies were born alive.[8] This is an important research question since, even today, much less is known about the etiology or risk factors for stillbirth relative to other pregnancy outcomes. One of the risk factors considered was the age of the birthing person at the time of delivery. Below is a summary of key data required to evaluate the association between age of the birthing parent at delivery and stillbirth.

- Investigators enrolled 614 individuals who experienced a stillbirth.
- Investigators enrolled 1,354 individuals whose babies were born alive.
- Among those who had a stillbirth, 28 participants were aged 40 years or older.
- Among those whose babies were born alive, 28 participants were aged 40 years or older.

The study data have been organized into **Table 3.9**. Practice creating this table using the study description yourself (Learning Objective 3.8).

1. Calculate the exposure odds ratio.
2. Interpret the exposure odds ratio.

**TABLE 3.9 STUDY DATA EVALUATING THE ASSOCIATION BETWEEN STILLBIRTH AND AGE OF THE BIRTHING PARENT AT DELIVERY**

| | Age at Delivery ≥ 40 Years (E+) | Age at Delivery < 40 Years (E−) | TOTAL |
|---|---|---|---|
| Stillbirth (O+) | 28 | 586 | 614 |
| Livebirth (O−) | 28 | 1,326 | 1,354 |
| TOTAL | 56 | 1,912 | 1,968 |

*Source:* Stillbirth Collaborative Research Network Writing Group. Association between stillbirth and risk factors known at pregnancy confirmation. *JAMA.* 2011;306(22):2469–2479. https://doi.org/10.1001/jama.2011.1798

# USING MEASURES OF ASSOCIATION TO EVALUATE STUDY HYPOTHESES

## Magnitude and Direction of Measures of Association

The concepts of magnitude and direction of measures of association are shown in Figure 3.14.

### FIGURE 3.14 MAGNITUDE AND DIRECTION OF MEASURES OF ASSOCIATION

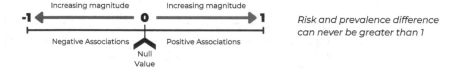

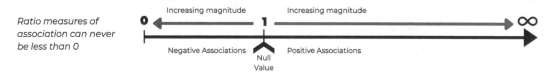

### WHAT IS THE DIRECTION OF A MEASURE OF ASSOCIATION?

The direction of a measure of association refers to *where* it lies relative to its null value, above (sometimes called a positive association) or below (sometimes called a negative association).

When there is a **negative association** between an exposure and a health outcome, being exposed is associated with a *decrease* in the occurrence of the health outcome, and thus the measure of association falls *below* the null value. When an association is negative, the difference measures of association range from [−1, 0), and the ratio measures of association range from [0, 1). In these situations, the exposure is often described as being "protective" for the outcome. While intuitive, this terminology is only appropriate when the presence of the outcome is defined as something that is harmful. For example, while we could say that not using illicit drugs was protective for death in a given study, we would not say that illicit drug use was protective for survival.

When there is a **positive association** between an exposure and a health outcome, that means being exposed is associated with an *increase* in the health outcome, and thus the measure of association falls *above* the null value. When an association is positive, the difference measures of association can range from (0, 1], while the ratio measures of association range from (1, ∞).

## WHAT IS THE MAGNITUDE OF A MEASURE OF ASSOCIATION?

The magnitude (or "strength") of a measure of association can be thought of as *how far* the measure is from its null value. The closer the difference measures are to −1, and the ratio measures to 0, the stronger the negative association. Conversely, the closer the difference measures are to 1, and the further the ratio measures are from 1, the stronger the positive association.

**Figure 3.14** shows the symmetry in the range of possible values for the difference measures of association. This means that the strength of possible difference measures of association is equivalent, regardless of whether they are positive or negative in direction (e.g., a risk difference of −0.3 has the same strength as a risk difference of 0.3).

This is not true, however, for the ratio measures of association. All possible values for a negative association are bound between 0 and 1, while positive associations can take on any value greater than 1. The magnitude of the range of ratio measures of association that fall between [0, 1) is the same as for (1, ∞). For this reason, understanding the strength of a negative ratio measure of association can be misleading. For example, a risk ratio of 0.3 might not seem to be a very strong measure of association. To get a sense for the strength of a ratio measure of association that falls on the left side of the null, we can take its inverse to get the corresponding measure of association that falls on the right side of the null. In our example, the inverse of the risk ratio of 0.3 is 3.33—meaning that the risk in the *unexposed* group is 3.33 times the risk in the *exposed* group.

The strength of a measure of association depends on the research question under study, and there are no global cutoffs for determining what are considered strong or weak measures of association.

# Causality and Interpretation of Measures of Association
## (LEARNING OBJECTIVE 3.5)

We've already discussed how association does not imply causation. We must remember that although an association may be observed between two variables, this does not necessarily mean that one of these variables causes the other. For some unexpected and funny examples of spurious correlations, check out http://www.tylervigen.com. Investigators must be careful to interpret measures of association as *associations* between exposures and outcomes, rather than causal relationships.

For example, we previously considered the following study hypothesis: consuming higher (versus lower) amounts of red meat is associated with increased rates of CHD among men in the United States. It would be incorrect to interpret the previously calculated rate ratio of 1.30 to mean that higher red meat consumption *caused* the study participants to have a higher rate of CHD. However, it is appropriate to say that an rate ratio of 1.30 supports the study hypothesis.

In many introductory epidemiology courses, students learn about the guidelines proposed by a statistician named Sir Austin Bradford Hill in 1965 to establish whether a relationship is likely to be causal.[16] (**Table 3.10**). While Hill's intention was for these guidelines to be items for consideration when thinking about causal relationships, they are routinely mischaracterized as a checklist of elements that are required to establish causality. Notably, all of these guidelines need not be met to 'prove' causality (which as we've discussed, is impossible). Each of Hill's guidelines is described in **Table 3.10** along with some considerations for why these guidelines may not hold in all cases.

## TABLE 3.10 BRADFORD HILL'S GUIDELINES FOR CAUSALITY

| Guideline | Concept | Considerations for When the Guideline Might Not Hold |
|---|---|---|
| Strength | Stronger associations (i.e., those with larger magnitude) between an exposure and outcome are more likely to be causal than weak ones. | The strength of an association may depend upon the scale on which it was measured (i.e., ratio vs. difference measures) and may also be invalid due to errors in the study design. |
| Consistency | The same association is observed in different study populations. | Unfortunately, errors can be repeated across multiple studies leading to consistent yet invalid conclusions. |
| Specificity | A given health outcome is caused by one exposure. | Specificity seeks to link one exposure with a health outcome. However, we now know that many exposures can lead to multiple health outcomes and that most health outcomes are multifactorial. |
| Temporality | The exposure must precede the health outcome in time. | This is the only guideline on this list which is an absolute requirement for causality. An exposure can only cause a health outcome if it occurs prior to it. |
| Biological Gradient / Dose Response | Higher levels of exposure lead to an increased frequency of the health outcome. | Not all exposure levels have a linear relationship with the frequency of a health outcome. As an example, there is a U-shaped relationship between maternal age and stillbirth where the risk of stillbirth is highest among the youngest and oldest pregnant persons. |
| Biological Plausibility | Is the association between the exposure and outcome supported by what is known about the biological mechanisms causing that health outcome? | This will not hold if the current knowledge of the biological mechanisms of a health outcome is limited or incorrect. |
| Coherence | Similar to biological plausibility, coherence requires that the association between the exposure and health outcome align with what is already known. | Coherence will not hold if current knowledge is limited or incorrect. |
| Experiment | Evidence drawn from experimental studies provides strong support of a causal relationship. | Experimental studies are not always ethical or feasible in epidemiologic research. |
| Analogy | When one causal relationship has been presumed, other similar relationships are more likely to also be causal. | As before, the existing knowledge that we draw upon may be limited or incorrect. |

*Source:* Data from Hill AB. The environment and disease: association or causation? *J R Soc Med.* 2015;108(1):32–37. https://doi.org/10.1177/0141076814562718

# WHERE WE'VE BEEN AND WHAT'S UP NEXT

Now that you have learned about epidemiologic study hypotheses and been introduced to the main analytic epidemiologic designs, it may be helpful to revisit the cycle of analytic epidemiology summarized in **Figure 3.1**. Our overarching goal when designing an analytic epidemiologic study is to test the study hypothesis using the best and most appropriate methods available. While we have noted that the study hypothesis informs the choice of study design, there are other practical considerations (e.g., time, resources, ethics, exposure[s] or outcome[s] of interest); we will discuss these in **Chapter 4, "Randomized Controlled Trial Designs"; Chapter 5, "Cohort Designs"; Chapter 6, "Case-Control Designs";** and **Chapter 7, "Cross-Sectional Designs,"** where we explore both the strengths and the limitations of each study design in detail.

TABLE 3.11 **DESCRIPTIVE OR ANALYTIC EPIDEMIOLOGIC STUDIES?**

|  | Descriptive Epidemiology | Analytic Epidemiology |
|---|---|---|
| Calculate measures of frequency |  |  |
| Make a quantitative comparison between at least two groups |  |  |
| Calculate measures of association |  |  |
| Generate hypotheses |  |  |
| Test hypotheses |  |  |

## END OF CHAPTER PROBLEM SET

1. Fill in **Table 3.11** to note whether each of the statements applies to descriptive or analytic epidemiologic studies.
2. Do the following statements describe descriptive or analytic epidemiologic study results? For any statements that reflect a descriptive result, describe what could be added to calculate an analytic result.
   a. Data show that individuals who previously experienced homelessness were three times more likely to contract HIV than those who did not previously experience homelessness.
   b. A quarter of cardiovascular disease diagnoses occur among persons with diabetes.
   c. Though gaps are closing, Black men and women in the United States experience higher cancer-related death rates than White men and women.
   d. Pregnant persons who smoke tobacco are 2 to 3 times more likely to have a stillbirth than those who do not smoke tobacco.
   e. Approximately 6% of children in India have been diagnosed with asthma.
3. You have been tasked with conducting a study to determine whether energy drink consumption leads to poor sleep among college students.
   a. What is the exposure? How might you define the exposed and unexposed groups?
   b. What is the outcome? How might you define those with and without the outcome?
   c. Develop a hypothesis for this study using the structure shown in this chapter.
4. Smoking is sometimes an exposure of interest in analytic epidemiologic studies as it is known to have a negative impact on health. One challenge of studying smoking as an exposure is that there are a number of ways that exposed and unexposed groups could be defined. Brainstorm at least two possible ways to define exposed and unexposed smoking groups; keep both the dose and the duration of exposure in mind as you consider different definitions.

5. Identify the study design that corresponds to each study description that follows. For each study description, answer the following questions:

- What defining features helped you identify the study design?
- What is (are) the exposure(s) and what is (are) the health outcome(s)?
- Are there any measures of frequency reported for the study?
- What is (are) the appropriate measure(s) of association for the study?
  a. Investigators analyzed data from the U.S. CDC to identify factors associated with inadequate sleep.[16] Participants were randomly selected to answer questions about their sleep habits and demographic characteristics. Overall, 65% of the study population reported meeting the recommended healthy sleep duration of at least 7 hours each night. Respondents who were aged 65 years or older were more likely to report sleeping at least 7 hours relative to younger respondents.
  b. An innovation in HIV prevention was the discovery that individuals who were at risk for HIV acquisition could benefit from taking antiretroviral drugs (which are also used to treat those *with* HIV) *before* being exposed to HIV, and thus prevent infection. This approach, called pre-exposure prophylaxis (PrEP), was discovered through a series of studies, one of which enrolled a group of men who have sex with men who did not have HIV but were at a high risk of HIV acquisition.[17] Participants were randomly assigned to begin PrEP immediately or after a 1-year delay. Of the 523 individuals enrolled, 23 were diagnosed with HIV during the 48-week study period. The rate of HIV among those who deferred PrEP initiation for 1 year was 7.5 times the corresponding rate among those who initiated PrEP immediately.
  c. Researchers began investigating the source of an outbreak of *Salmonella* (a bacterium that infects the intestinal tract) Havana in South Australia by identifying individuals with a laboratory-confirmed case of *S.* Havana reported to the Communicable Disease Control Branch.[18] The recent food and drink consumption of these individuals with *S.* Havana was compared to the recent food and drink consumption of a selection of individuals identified using a randomly generated list from a population health survey in South Australia. Investigators determined that the outbreak was caused by alfalfa sprouts, since those with a *S.* Havana infection were more likely to have recently eaten alfalfa sprouts than were those without such an infection.
  d. Chinese health officials investigated an outbreak of COVID-19 among a group of 300 individuals who attended a 150-minute worship event.[19] Two groups of attendees traveled to the event by bus, the second of which carried an individual who had a SARS-CoV-2 infection (Bus 1, $n = 60$; Bus 2, $n = 68$). The at-risk individuals who rode Bus 2 were more likely to later be diagnosed with COVID-19 than those who rode Bus 1. COVID-19 diagnoses were also more common among those who rode Bus 2 than among all of those who attended the worship event but did not arrive by bus.

6. Using Figure 3.15, write the letter indicator of the measure of association that corresponds to each description that follows.
  a. No association between the exposure and the outcome on the difference scale
  b. The strongest negative association on the difference scale
  c. The weakest positive association on the ratio scale
  d. The weakest negative association on the ratio scale
  e. Write the descriptions of the other measures of association that appear in Figure 3.15, but were not answers to parts a to d.

## FIGURE 3.15 COMPARING MAGNITUDE AND DIRECTION OF MEASURES OF ASSOCIATION

**Difference Measures of Association: Risk & Prevalence Difference**

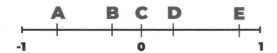

*Risk and prevalence difference can never be greater than 1*

**Ratio Measures of Association: Risk, Rate, Prevalence, and Odds Ratio**

*Ratio measures of association can never be less than 0*

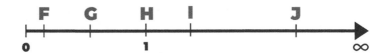

7. Although there is little debate in the scientific community about the effectiveness of masks to prevent transmission of SARS-CoV-2, the virus that causes COVID-19,[20] there has been much public discourse in the United States about the utility of masks. To support the position that masks should not be required, some individuals cited a pre-print (meaning not yet peer reviewed or published in the peer-reviewed literature) article that concluded that there was not an association between mask mandates or mask use and reduced COVID-19 spread in the continental United States.[21]

This study compared rates of COVID-19 in states with mask mandates to rates of COVID-19 in states without mask mandates. Additionally, they explored whether COVID-19 rates were associated with the percent of the population that always wears masks in public settings.

   a. What study design is this?

   b. Supposing that their results are valid (i.e., correct), hypothesize how it might be true that...

     – Mask mandates and population-level mask use are not associated with reductions in the rates of COVID-19 at the population-level, AND

     – Masks do prevent the spread of COVID-19.

## REFERENCES

1. Centers for Disease Control and Prevention. Blood lead levels in children. 2020. https://www.cdc.gov/nceh/lead/prevention/blood-lead-levels.htm

2. Hanna-Attisha M, LaChance J, Sadler RC, Champney Schnepp A. Elevated blood lead levels in children associated with the Flint drinking water crisis: a spatial analysis of risk and public health response. *Am J Public Health*. 2015;106(2):283–290. https://doi.org/10.2105/AJPH.2015.303003

3. Jones JR, Kogan MD, Singh GK, Dee DL, Grummer-Strawn LM. Factors associated with exclusive breastfeeding in the United States. *Pediatrics*. 2011;128(6):1117–1125. https://doi.org/10.1542/peds.2011-0841

4. Sedgwick P. Unit of observation versus unit of analysis. *BMJ*. 2014;348:g3840. https://doi.org/10.1136/bmj.g3840

5. Polack FP, Thomas SJ, Kitchin N, et al. Safety and efficacy of the BNT162b2 mRNA COVID-19 vaccine. *N Engl J Med*. 2020;383(27):2603–2615. https://doi.org/10.1056/NEJMoa2034577

6.  Al-Shaar L, Satija A, Wang DD, et al. Red meat intake and risk of coronary heart disease among US men: prospective cohort study. *BMJ*. 2020;371:m4141. https://doi.org/10.1136/bmj.m4141

7.  Macdorman MF, Kirmeyer S. The challenge of fetal mortality. *NCHS Data Brief*. 2009;(16):1–8. https://www.cdc.gov/nchs/products/databriefs/db16.htm

8.  Stillbirth Collaborative Research Network Writing Group. Association between stillbirth and risk factors known at pregnancy confirmation. *JAMA*. 2011;306(22):2469–2479. https://doi.org/10.1001/jama.2011.1798

9.  Rothman KJ, Greenland S, Lash TL. *Modern Epidemiology*. Vol. 3. Wolters Kluwer Health/Lippincott Williams & Wilkins; 2008.

10. Parsons VL, Moriarity C, Jonas K, Moore TF, Davis KE, Tompkins L. Design and estimation for the National Health Interview Survey, 2006–2015. *Vital Health Stat*. 2014;2(165):1–53. https://www.cdc.gov/nchs/data/series/sr_02/sr02_165.pdf

11. Xu G, Strathearn L, Liu B, Bao W. Prevalence of autism spectrum disorder among US children and adolescents, 2014–2016. *JAMA*. 2018;319(1):81–82. https://doi.org/10.1001/jama.2017.17812

12. Sedgwick P. Ecological studies: advantages and disadvantages. *BMJ*. 2014;348:g2979. https://doi.org/10.1136/bmj.g2979

13. Sedgwick P. Understanding the ecological fallacy. *BMJ*. 2015;351:h4773. https://doi.org/10.1136/bmj.h4773

14. World Health Organization. Key country indicators. 2020. https://apps.who.int/gho/data/node.cco.latest?lang=en

15. Hill AB. The environment and disease: association or causation? (First published in *JRSM*. 1965;58(5)). *J R Soc Med*. 2015;108(1):32–37. https://doi.org/10.1177/0141076814562718

16. Liu Y, Wheaton AG, Chapman DP, et al. Prevalence of healthy sleep duration among adults—United States, 2014. *Morb Mor Wkly Rep*. 2016;65(6):137–141. https://www.cdc.gov/mmwr/volumes/65/wr/mm6506a1.htm

17. McCormack S, Dunn DT, Desai M, et al. Pre-exposure prophylaxis to prevent the acquisition of HIV-1 infection (PROUD): effectiveness results from the pilot phase of a pragmatic open-label randomised trial. *Lancet*. 2016;387:P53–P60. https://doi.org/10.1016/S0140-6736(15)00056-2

18. Harfield S, Beazley R, Denehy E, et al. An outbreak and case-control study of *Salmonella* Havana linked to alfalfa sprouts in South Australia, 2018. *Commun Dis Intell (2018)*. 2019;43:10.33321/cdi.2019.43.45. https://doi.org/10.33321/cdi.2019.43.45

19. Shen Y, Li C, Dong H, et al. Community outbreak investigation of SARS-CoV-2 transmission among bus riders in Eastern China. *JAMA Intern Med*. 2020;180(12):1665–1671. https://doi.org/10.1001/jamainternmed.2020.5225

20. Howard J, Huang A, Li Z, et al. An evidence review of face masks against COVID-19. *Proc Natl Acad Sci USA*. 2021;118(4):e2014564118. https://doi.org/10.1073/pnas.2014564118

21. Guerra DD, Guerra DJ. Mask mandate and use efficacy for COVID-19 containment in US states. *medRXiv*. https://doi.org/10.1101/2021.05.18.21257385

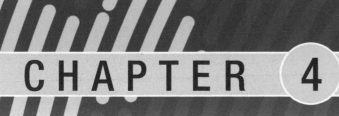

# CHAPTER 4

# RANDOMIZED CONTROLLED TRIAL DESIGNS

## KEY TERMS

allocation concealment

controlled trials

effectiveness

efficacy

equipoise

intention-to-treat analysis

masking

per-protocol analysis

placebo

randomization

## LEARNING OBJECTIVES

4.1 Understand the difference between preventive and therapeutic exposures in a controlled trial.

4.2 Discuss why a control group is critical in controlled trials and when use of a placebo control group is appropriate.

4.3 Differentiate between trials that hypothesize intervention superiority, non-inferiority, or equivalence.

4.4 Describe the rationale for randomization in a controlled trial.

4.5 Define simple and stratified randomization techniques.

4.6 Differentiate between individual and cluster level randomization, and describe when each unit of randomization would be appropriate.

4.7 Differentiate between the basic features of three common controlled trial designs: parallel, crossover, and factorial.

4.8 Understand what masking and allocation concealment are and how they differ.

4.9 Distinguish between intervention efficacy and effectiveness, and the analyses associated with each.

4.10 Describe the phases of U.S. Food and Drug Administration pharmaceutical trials.

4.11 Discuss ethical considerations that are important for controlled trials.

4.12 Describe the strengths and limitations of controlled trials.

## PERSISTENCE PAYS OFF: MESSENGER RNA VACCINE DEVELOPMENT

Scientist Dr. Katalin Karikó left Hungary for the United States in the mid-1980s in search of better scientific infrastructure to continue her research on messenger RNA (mRNA) vaccines. During her career, Dr. Karikó struggled to garner support for her research, which was viewed for many years as not particularly promising. This led to frequent rejection by funding agencies and scientific journals. Finally in 2005, after years of persistence, she and collaborator Dr. Drew Weissman discovered how to allow synthetic RNA to circumvent the immune system. This work helped develop the underpinnings of using synthetic mRNA to create proteins that convinced the immune system to mount an immune response. Today, Dr. Karikó's decades-long work is the basis for the mRNA vaccines that have a high effectiveness in preventing hospitalization and death due to the novel coronavirus COVID-19. mRNA vaccines also hold promise to tackle other diseases such as HIV, cancer, influenza, and malaria. Drs. Karikó and Weissman were honored with the 2023 Nobel Prize in Physiology or Medicine for this groundbreaking work.

## CONTROLLED TRIAL DESIGN BASICS

**Controlled trials** (sometimes simply called trials) belong to the experimental branch of epidemiologic research (you can revisit the classification of epidemiologic studies in **Figure 3.3**). As noted in **Chapter 3, "Introduction to Analytic Epidemiologic Study Designs and Measures of Association,"** the defining feature that distinguishes experimental from observational designs is that experimental research involves the allocation, or assignment of the exposure(s) of interest by the investigators. As you will see throughout this chapter, there is a lot of terminology that is unique to controlled trials, and this begins with terms that are used to describe those with and without the exposure(s) of interest. The exposed group in a trial is often referred to as the **intervention** or **treatment** group, and a trial's unexposed group is often referred to as the **control** group. The different exposure groups in a trial are often referred to as the trial's **arms**.

A schematic of the most basic randomized controlled trial, called a **parallel controlled trial**, is shown in **Figure 4.1**. In this design, investigators sample participants from a source population that is at-risk of developing the outcome of interest into a sample population. As with all

### FIGURE 4.1 SCHEMATIC OF A PARALLEL RANDOMIZED CONTROLLED TRIAL

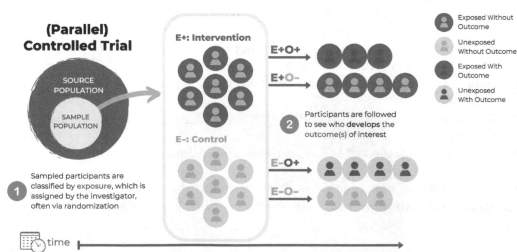

study designs, it is imperative that investigators carefully define their **source population** (the group of people from which study participants will be selected) and then thoughtfully select participants to be included in the **sample population** (the people who are actually selected from the source population to participate in the study). You will learn more about defining the source population and sampling strategies in later chapters.

After participants are sampled, investigators then assign participants to the exposure or control arms, often via randomization. After exposure assignment, study participants are followed forward in time to measure new (i.e., incident) cases of the outcome(s) of interest. Throughout this chapter, you will learn about other common variations of randomized controlled trials.

The basic steps involved in designing and conducting a randomized controlled trial are shown in **Table 4.1**. The steps fall into four broad categories, which are relevant for all study designs: formulating a research question, designing the study, conducting the study, and analyzing and reporting the data. As you navigate through **Chapter 4, "Randomized Controlled Trial Designs"; Chapter 5, "Cohort Designs"; Chapter 6, "Case-Control Designs";** and **Chapter 7, "Cross-Sectional Designs,"** you will see that although there is consistency in these three categories, the specific details differ for each study design. Each of the blue terms in **Table 4.1** is discussed in detail in the text that follows. The topics are listed in order in **Table 4.1** as you would approach designing a trial; however, since formulating hypotheses can be complicated, we begin with a discussion about defining the exposure.

**TABLE 4.1 BASIC STEPS IN DESIGNING AND CONDUCTING A RANDOMIZED CONTROLLED TRIAL**

| State the Research Question |
| --- |
| State the trial objective and study hypothesis. |
| Define the exposure and define outcome(s) with case definitions. |
| **Design the Trial** |
| Determine the randomization strategy, select the type of trial, and decide whether there will be masking. |
| **Conduct the Trial** |
| Select subjects from an at-risk source population and obtain informed consent. |
| Allocate subjects to exposure groups with concealment. |
| Follow subjects and collect data on incident outcomes as well as key covariates. |
| **Analyze and Report Data** |
| Calculate measures of frequency and association from an intention-to-treat analysis and/or a per-protocol analysis. |
| Report findings using the CONSORT reporting guidance. |
| Consider the strengths and limitations of the study. |

## DEFINING THE EXPOSURE IN A CONTROLLED TRIAL

As discussed in earlier chapters, defining the exposure, which includes defining both the exposed *and* the unexposed status, is critical for all analytic epidemiologic studies.

In controlled trials, exposures are often categorized as either preventive or therapeutic (**Learning Objective 4.1**). A **preventive exposure** is administered to individuals *without* the health outcome of interest to assess whether the intervention can *prevent* negative health outcomes relative to a control. A **therapeutic exposure** is given to individuals *with* a particular health condition to assess whether the intervention can *improve* their health status relative to a control.

As in all analytic epidemiologic studies, trials must include a comparison group (**Learning Objective 4.2**); as previously noted, this is often called the control group in a controlled trial, which is equivalent to the unexposed group in other analytic epidemiologic studies. Individuals included in the control arm often receive either a **placebo** or the **standard of care** preventive or therapeutic option.

A placebo is an inert or "fake" treatment, such as a sugar pill or sham procedure. The purpose of conducting a placebo-controlled trial is to account for a phenomenon called the **placebo effect**, where individuals report benefits derived from the act of simply *receiving* an intervention, even if that intervention does not have any clinical benefit. An interesting example of the placebo effect comes from a randomized controlled trial of patients with irritable bowel syndrome (IBS) who were assigned to receive placebo or no intervention at all.[1] Participants in the trial were aware of their group assignment, and those who received the placebo were told that they were taking "placebo pills made of an inert substance, like sugar pills, that have been shown in clinical studies to produce significant improvement in IBS symptoms through mind-body self-healing processes." Despite knowing they received a pill with no active ingredient, those in the placebo arm reported significant improvement in their IBS symptoms relative to the arm that received no intervention at all. While the mechanism for the placebo effect is unclear, as is the magnitude of its effect,[2] the use of a placebo control arm allows investigators to estimate the effect of an intervention above and beyond any benefits derived from the act of simply *receiving* an intervention.

A placebo control may be appropriate when studying health outcomes that have no existing treatment or preventive option (such as with some newly emerging diseases). However, when an effective standard of care exists, many investigators argue that it is not ethical to use a placebo control.[3] The rationale is that participants in a trial should not be denied an existing and effective option; rather, they should be offered the best available standard of care to prevent or treat the health outcome of interest. This rationale may seem obvious today, but this wasn't always the case. For example, a 1985 randomized controlled trial of ivermectin to treat onchocerciasis, also known as river blindness, used a placebo control arm even though the drug diethylcarbamazine had been used as standard of care for several decades.[4] Another trial in 1992 evaluated the antidepressant drug paroxetine in a sample of patients who all had severe depression.[5] Half of these participants were given a placebo despite the availability of effective antidepressants. In 1996, the Declaration of Helsinki was revised to specify that control groups in clinical research should be offered the best standard of care, if one exists.[6] Still, some regulatory authorities allow the use of placebo controls under certain conditions, even if an effective standard of care exists.[7]

When effective standards of care exist, the use of a placebo control not only has ethical and health implications for study participants, but also affects the resulting measure(s) of association calculated using the trial data. The effect of a new drug compared to placebo may be very different (and typically stronger) compared to the best available standard of care. As Bradford Hill described in 1963: "Is it [*sic*] Ethical to Use a Placebo, or Dummy Treatment? The answer to this question will depend, I suggest, upon whether there is already available an orthodox treatment of proved or accepted value. If there is such an orthodox treatment the question hardly arises, for the doctor will wish to know whether a new treatment is more, or less, effective than the old, not that it is more effective than nothing"(p. 1048).[8]

## STATING THE TRIAL OBJECTIVES AND HYPOTHESES
### (LEARNING OBJECTIVE 4.3)

Depending on the researcher's objective, trials may be defined as **superiority**, **non-inferiority**, or **equivalence trials**. A schematic that differentiates these three trial objectives and their relationships to the null value is shown in **Figure 4.2**.

**Superiority trials.** A superiority trial is likely what comes to mind when thinking about a controlled trial. A superiority trial is designed to evaluate whether or not an intervention is *superior* (i.e., better) at reducing negative health outcomes relative to the control group. If an intervention is superior to the control at reducing a negative health outcome, that implies that

## FIGURE 4.2 TYPES OF CONTROLLED TRIAL OBJECTIVES AND THEIR HYPOTHESES

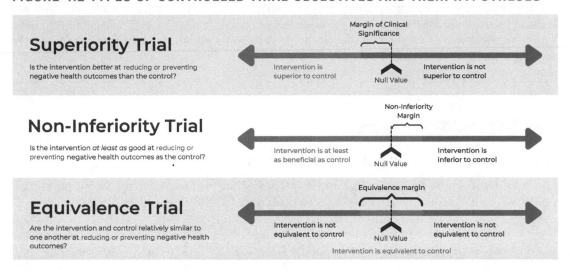

there would be a negative relationship between the intervention and outcome, thus yielding an association that is less than the null value.

An example of a superiority trial would be one designed to determine whether a new antidepressant drug is better at reducing depressive symptoms compared to an existing drug regimen. If an intervention is only *slightly* better at reducing depressive symptoms, it may not be worthwhile to pursue. Suppose physicians conducted a randomized superiority trial and screened for depression using the Patient Health Questionnaire-9 (PHQ-9), which is a nine-item questionnaire with possible scores ranging from 0 (no evidence of depression) to 27 (severe depression).[9] Suppose the new drug improves PHQ-9 scores by one point. Although the new drug *does* perform better than the existing treatment, this difference may not be clinically meaningful and thus wouldn't warrant consideration as a *superior* treatment to the existing regimen. In a superiority trial, researchers identify a margin beyond which the intervention would be classified as being superior to the control in a way that truly makes a difference in clinical practice; this is called the **margin of clinical significance**.[10]

**Non-inferiority trials.** Non-inferiority trials are designed to evaluate whether an intervention is *at least* as good at reducing the frequency of negative health outcomes when compared to a control. Non-inferiority trials are particularly useful for evaluating interventions that have greater availability, have reduced cost, are less invasive, have fewer side effects, or are easier to administer compared to the current standard of care. Like superiority trials, non-inferiority trials include a margin within which the intervention would still be considered at least as clinically beneficial as the control, even if the measure of association falls above the null value. This is called the **non-inferiority margin**—an interval in which the control condition outperforms the intervention, but which is seen as an acceptable tradeoff given the benefits of the new intervention such as greater availability or reduced cost. Keeping with our example of an antidepressant drug trial, a non-inferiority trial might be designed to determine whether use of a new, inexpensive antidepressant drug reduces depressive symptoms with at least the same frequency as a commonly used, very expensive drug regimen.

**Equivalence trials.** Equivalence trials are designed to evaluate whether the intervention is relatively similar to the control in terms of its effect on the frequency of health outcomes. Equivalence trials may be conducted for similar reasons as non-inferiority trials, but instead of demonstrating that an intervention is at least as beneficial as the control, investigators seek to demonstrate that the intervention is equivalent to the control. Investigators must specify what is meant by *not too different* using an **equivalence margin**, which is an interval centered around the null value within which the intervention and control would be considered to have a similar effect. For example, a trial designed to determine whether use of a new, inexpensive antidepressant drug reduces depressive symptoms with similar frequency as a more expensive existing drug regimen would be an equivalence trial.

## Pause to Practice 4.1

### COVID-19 Vaccine Trial: Exposures, Objectives, and Hypotheses

You may recall **Pause to Practice 3.2** and **3.7**, which discussed a randomized controlled trial, published by Polack et al.,[11] that evaluated a candidate COVID-19 vaccine. In December 2020, the U.S. Food and Drug Administration (FDA) issued an Emergency Use Authorization allowing the vaccine to be administered to individuals aged 16 years and older;[12] the vaccine was subsequently distributed throughout the United States and in other countries.

In this trial, participants aged 16 years or older who were at risk of a COVID-19 infection were randomly assigned to receive two doses of either the candidate vaccine or a placebo control, with each dose spaced 21 days apart. One of the main trial objectives was to assess whether the frequency of incident, laboratory-confirmed COVID-19 infections that occurred at least 7 days after the second dose was lower in individuals who received the candidate vaccine compared to the placebo. At the time of the trial, there were no approved vaccines or other pharmaceutical preventive options for COVID-19.

1. Is the intervention evaluated in this trial a preventive or therapeutic exposure?
2. Was use of a placebo control appropriate? Why or why not?
3. Was this a superiority, non-inferiority, or equivalence trial?

## Highlights

### Controlled Trial Basics: Defining Exposures, Trial Objectives, and Hypotheses

- **Controlled trials** belong to the **experimental** branch of epidemiologic research in which the investigator assigns participants to one of the exposure groups, often via randomization.
- The different exposure groups in a trial are often referred to as trial **arms**.
  - The **exposed** group in a trial is sometimes referred to as the **intervention** or **treatment** group.
  - The **unexposed** group is sometimes referred to as the **control** group.
    - The control condition is often either a placebo or the standard of care.
- Exposures may be either **preventive** or **therapeutic**.
  - A **preventive exposure** is administered to individuals *without* the health outcome of interest to assess whether the intervention can reduce negative health outcomes relative to the control.
  - A **therapeutic exposure** is given to individuals *with* a particular health condition to assess whether the intervention can improve their health status relative to the control.

- Depending on the objective, trials may be defined as either superiority, non-inferiority, or equivalence trials.
  - **Superiority trials** are designed to evaluate whether an intervention is *better* at reducing the frequency of negative health outcomes when compared to a control group.
  - **Non-inferiority trials** are designed to evaluate whether an intervention is *at least as beneficial* at reducing the frequency of negative health outcomes when compared to a control group.
  - **Equivalence trials** are designed to evaluate whether the intervention is *similar* to the control in terms of their effect on the frequency of health outcomes.

Now that we have discussed defining our exposure groups and formulating hypotheses based on the objective of the research, we will discuss four key controlled trial design elements: randomization, trial types, masking, and allocation concealment.

# RANDOMIZATION

As discussed previously, allocation (i.e., assignment) of the exposure by the study investigator is the hallmark that distinguishes experimental from observational analytic epidemiologic designs. Typically, this assignment is achieved via **randomization**, a process by which every individual has an equal chance of being assigned to each exposure condition. Importantly, when the exposure is assigned randomly, that assignment is independent of patients' or study investigators' preferences.

## Rationale for Randomization (LEARNING OBJECTIVE 4.4)

The primary benefit of randomization is that, on average, random assignment of the exposure should yield exposed and unexposed groups that are comparable on all factors *except* for the exposure status, thus isolating the effect of the exposure. If investigators observe an association between the exposure and the health outcome in a randomized controlled trial, it increases their confidence relative to observational study designs that the association is due to the effect of the exposure and not any other factors. Randomization attempts to control for all factors that could introduce error (i.e., bias) study results if they were imbalanced across the study arms.

The bias that occurs when one or more external factors can explain the observed association between an exposure and a health outcome is called confounding, which will be discussed in detail in **Chapter 9, "Error in Epidemiologic Research and Fundamentals of Confounding."** Randomized controlled trials present a perfect opportunity to introduce confounding. Let's consider a hypothetical example.

Suppose you conducted an *observational* study to examine whether a hypertension drug is associated with reduced mortality using a cohort design. You identified a group of individuals who are alive (and thus at-risk for the outcome of interest: death), and you observe who among this group is currently taking the hypertension drug. You then follow them over time to see who dies during the course of follow-up. Given the known correlation between age and death (i.e., as individuals get older, their probability of dying increases), you would expect that those who are older might be more likely to die during your study follow-up compared to those who are younger. This only becomes a problem if those who are older are more (or less) likely to be taking the hypertension drug compared to their younger counterparts. If it turns out that, as might be expected, older individuals are more likely to be taking this drug than younger individuals, it might appear that the hypertension drug is actually associated with an *increased* risk of death among the study participants, even if the drug truly reduces mortality. In this example, we can say that the association between the hypertension drug and mortality is *confounded* by age: the hypertension drug does not truly lead to increased mortality, and the observed association can be explained by age. Confounding by age occurred because those who were older were more likely to be taking the hypertension drug *and* they were also more likely to die during the follow-up period.

If instead we conducted a randomized controlled trial where the hypertension drug is randomly allocated to study participants, there should be no difference in the age distribution between the intervention and control arms of the study. For example, if 30% of the study population is aged 65 years or older, we would expect that roughly 30% of participants in the intervention group and 30% of participants in the control group would be aged 65 years or older. It would still be the case that those who are older would be more likely to die during the follow-up period; however, this cannot introduce bias in our study results if the distribution of age is balanced across the exposure groups. By allocating the hypertension drug via randomization, we are able to remove the potential confounding effect of age.

It is important to note that we could choose to simply control for confounders during data analysis if they were accurately measured during the study (more on such analytic techniques appears in **Chapter 9, "Error in Epidemiologic Research and Fundamentals of Confounding"**). However, one of the main advantages of randomization is that we should also achieve balance on factors that were unmeasured. This makes randomization one of the strongest tools for estimating the causal effect of exposures on health outcomes.

## Randomization Attempts to Approximate the Counterfactual

In **Chapter 3, "Introduction to Analytic Epidemiologic Study Designs and Measures of Association,"** we discussed causality, and described a cause as something that must have occurred in order for some outcome to have happened when it did, assuming that all other conditions are unchanged. Causality is a concept that we strive to understand with an analytic epidemiologic study; however, we are unable to know with certainty whether an intervention has a causal (i.e., true) effect on the outcome because we cannot observe outcomes for individuals under both the intervention and control exposures, while holding all other conditions constant. An individual's **counterfactual** exposure status is the one that they did not actually experience. Randomization is one of the strongest tools in our epidemiologic toolbox that allows us to approximate the counterfactual by creating comparison groups that should be identical on all factors except for the exposure.

## Randomization Techniques (LEARNING OBJECTIVE 4.5)

There are several techniques that can be used to achieve randomization. Here we discuss two common randomization techniques that are represented schematically in **Figure 4.3 (panels A and B)**: **simple randomization** and **stratified randomization**.

**Simple randomization.** In simple randomization, each study participant is randomly assigned to one of the exposure conditions. Computer-generated random numbers can be used for simple randomization. For example, in a trial with two arms, participants who receive an odd number could be assigned to the intervention arm and those who receive an even number could be assigned to the control arm. Simple randomization is often easy to implement relative to other techniques; however, when sample sizes are small (roughly less than 100), this approach may lead to imbalances between the trial arms by confounding factors. In **Figure 4.3A**, we see that randomization of this small sample

## FIGURE 4.3A SCHEMATIC ILLUSTRATING SIMPLE RANDOMIZATION FOR A CONTROLLED TRIAL

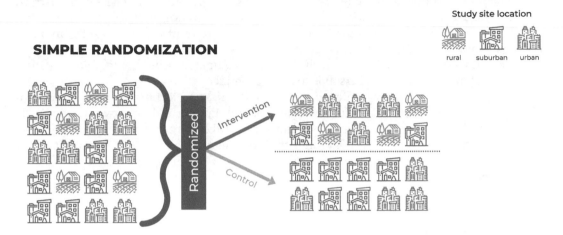

($N$ = 20) led to an imbalance in study site location, a potential confounder, across the two trial arms: only two of the eight suburban sites and all four of the rural sites were assigned to the intervention arm.

**Stratified randomization.** When investigators conduct stratified randomization, trial participants are first **stratified**, or separated, based on important characteristics (e.g., sex, age, study site). These stratification variables should be factors that could confound the association between the exposure and the health outcome if they happened to be imbalanced across the trial arms. Randomization then occurs in the same way as for simple randomization, except it happens *within* these strata. Stratified randomization ensures that the stratified factors are balanced across the trial arms. This is particularly useful when the overall sample is small or if there are small numbers of individuals belonging to a particular group that the investigators want to ensure are equally distributed across each of the trial arms. In **Figure 4.3B**, we

## FIGURE 4.3B SCHEMATIC ILLUSTRATING STRATIFIED RANDOMIZATION FOR A CONTROLLED TRIAL

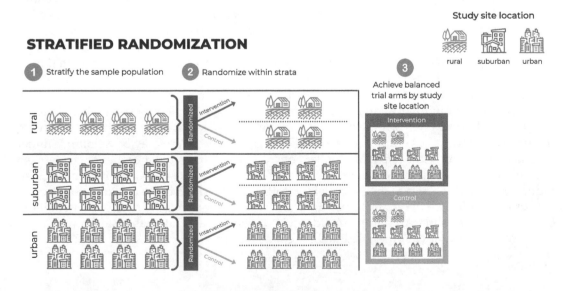

have stratified the study population by study site location, with one stratum each for rural, suburban, and urban sites. Randomization occurred within each of these strata, and we see that this has ensured that both the intervention and the control arms have an equal distribution of individuals by study site location. Note that stratified randomization is typically only conducted to achieve balance for one (or possibly two) important factors since the more we stratify our study population, the smaller the strata become. This could result in strata that have 0 or 1 individuals, which then precludes the investigators from being able to achieve balanced study arms if only one person is to be randomized.

It is important to note that regardless of which randomization technique you use, randomization may "fail," meaning not achieve a balance of both known and unknown factors in the study arms. Imbalances between exposure groups can still occur by chance, especially when randomizing smaller sample sizes. Consider the extreme example of randomizing just four people into two study arms, and the very low likelihood of balancing all possible factors that could bias the results.

## Units of Randomization (LEARNING OBJECTIVE 4.6)

The assignment of exposure conditions in a randomized controlled trial can occur at different **units**: individuals or clusters.

**Individual randomization.** As its name suggests, individual randomization allocates exposure status to each individual study participant, and the unit of randomization is the individual. This is the type of randomization that was used in the COVID-19 vaccine trial: the assignment of each participant to the intervention or control arm occurred on an individual basis.

**Cluster randomization.** Randomization can also occur among *groups* of individuals, called cluster randomization. In this case, the units of randomization are the groups, or clusters. A cluster should be a clearly defined group such as communities, families, hospitals, or schools. Cluster-randomized controlled trials are appropriate when the intervention must be delivered to an entire group for ethical or logistical reasons. Consider an intervention to promote healthy eating among students that includes promotional posters hung in the hallways of schools. There wouldn't be a way to randomize students attending the same school so that some saw the promotional posters while others did not. For this reason, schools, rather than individual children, would be randomized to receive the intervention or control. Another example is a trial exploring the effect of a package of household-based hygiene interventions (e.g., handwashing education, chlorine provision). It wouldn't be feasible to randomize individuals living in the same household to different arms of the trial and thus the randomization would need to happen at the household or even community level. Statistical techniques that are beyond the scope of this textbook are required to account for similarities that might exist among individuals within each cluster.

While cluster randomization allows for the possibility of a randomized controlled trial when individual randomization is not possible, it does have some important limitations. The first is that there is often a limited number of clusters from which to sample: even though there may be thousands of individuals living in each cluster, there may be a limited number of total clusters. As with simple randomization, randomizing a small number of clusters may not be sufficient to limit imbalances across the study arms. A second limitation of cluster randomized trials relates to the potential for **spillover**, in which exposure in an intervention cluster may influence the control cluster. For example, there may be concerns about spillover effects in the school-based intervention described earlier if a family has children who attend different schools that were assigned to different study arms.

## Pause to Practice 4.2

### Cluster Randomization: Sample Size and Spillover Effects

In the previous example, we considered the evaluation of a package of household-based hygiene interventions where cluster randomization was used. The following questions will help you think more about the relationship between two of the major limitations of cluster randomization: limited cluster size availability and spillover effects.

1. What are the benefits of conducting randomization at the household level versus the community level?

2. What are the drawbacks of conducting randomization at the household level versus the community level?

3. What are the benefits of conducting randomization at the community level versus the household level?

4. What are the drawbacks of conducting randomization at the community level versus the household level?

## TYPES OF TRIALS (LEARNING OBJECTIVE 4.7)

Now that we know about the different types of hypotheses and randomization techniques that can be considered in a controlled trial, we can think about three common controlled trial designs: **parallel**, **crossover**, and **factorial**.

**Parallel trials.** As indicated in **Figure 4.1**, each exposure group in a parallel trial receives a single exposure at the same time. A parallel trial design is probably what you envisioned when you first learned about controlled trials and is indeed the most common trial design.

## FIGURE 4.4 SCHEMATIC OF A RANDOMIZED CONTROLLED CROSSOVER TRIAL

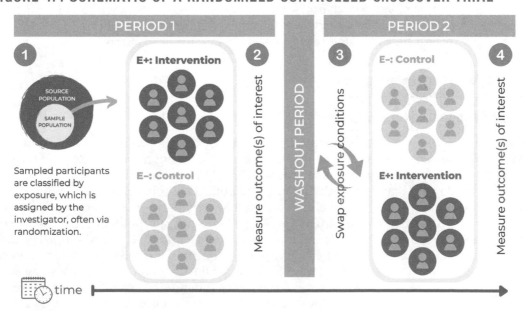

*Note*: Participants in a crossover trial are assigned to all exposure groups at some point during the study period.

**Crossover trials**. In a crossover trial, each subject receives both the intervention and the control exposure condition, one after the other (**Figure 4.4**). Some study participants receive the intervention condition first, followed by the control condition; other study participants receive the control condition first, followed by the intervention condition. The order is assigned via randomization. Subjects are followed under each exposure condition for a period of time during which the exposure could feasibly impact the outcome (e.g., if an antidepressant is expected to take 4 to 6 weeks to reach its maximum effectiveness, it wouldn't be appropriate for the follow-up period to only be 2 weeks long). Outcomes are measured during the first observation period. Then, before study participants are allocated to the other exposure condition (or "crossed over"), they enter a **washout period**, which is a time when individuals receive *neither* exposure condition. The goal of a washout period is to separate the effect of the first exposure condition from effect of the second exposure condition. This is particularly important for interventions that may continue to have an effect after the first observation period ends. For example, warfarin, a blood thinner, typically has an effect that lasts for 5 days after the last dose.[13] After the washout period, study participants receive the other exposure condition, and outcomes are measured during the second observation period.

The main advantage of a crossover trial design is that we observe outcomes in the same individuals under both exposure conditions allowing us to approximate the counterfactual, and thus the crossover design seeks to further minimize imbalances of confounding factors across the trial arms. Since each study participant essentially serves as their own control, the study arms should be balanced for factors that do not change systematically or meaningfully during the study. If, however, there are confounding factors that change during the course of the study period (for example, if study participants experience major weight fluctuations, begin to smoke, or start a new medication), this could inhibit our ability to approximate the counterfactual since more than just the exposure condition changed during the two study periods.

A crossover trial is not well suited for studying every exposure–outcome relationship. When an exposure has a long-term or even permanent effect on the outcome, we cannot measure the effect of each intervention separately. Any impact that an exposure might have that extends into the second observation period is called a **carryover effect**. For example, we might not be concerned about a potential carryover effect in a crossover design studying the effect of a drug that is eliminated from the body within a short, known amount of time; however, educational interventions may be more difficult to study in a crossover design since the effect of the first educational intervention will likely carry over into the second period. For this reason, crossover trial designs are best suited for studying exposures with short-term effects.

## Pause to Practice 4.3

### Cluster-Randomized Crossover Trials

Patient safety is a top priority for medical professionals, and efforts should be taken to eliminate medical errors. Medical residents often work shifts lasting more than 24 hours, which can lead to sleep deprivation and affect performance. In one study, investigators hypothesized that residents assigned to work shorter shifts would be less likely to make clinical errors compared to those working longer shifts. To test this hypothesis, investigators undertook a study among pediatric hospital resident physicians using a cluster-randomized crossover trial to determine whether shift length (i.e., number of hours worked) impacted serious medical errors. Participating hospitals were randomized to sequentially receive two different exposure conditions: shifts of 16 hours or less or shifts of 24 hours or more. Physicians' errors were observed over two 8-month observation periods, separated by a 4-month washout period. Contrary to the study hypothesis, the rate of serious medical errors was *higher* under the shortened shift schedule (97.1/1,000 patient days versus 79.0/1,000 patient days, rate ratio [IDR] = 1.23), although the findings varied by site.[14]

1.  Given the investigators' hypothesis, was this a superiority trial, a non-inferiority trial, or an equivalence trial?

2.  Why do you think the investigators chose cluster rather than individual randomization to answer this research question?

3.  Why was this research question well-suited for a crossover design?

4.  The study findings were *not* consistent with the investigators' hypotheses. Why do you think it might be the case that shorter shifts were associated with a higher rate of medical errors than longer shifts?

**Factorial trials.** As indicated in **Figure 4.5**, a factorial trial compares the effect of two (or more) interventions—both individually and jointly—to a control group. **Figure 4.5** shows a factorial design evaluating two interventions: A and B. A factorial trial is useful when the investigators are interested in how two interventions work both individually as well as when combined. This allows investigators to assess whether there is evidence of **interaction** between the interventions, which will be discussed in **Chapter 8, "Effect Measure Modification and Statistical Interaction."** As always, the particular research question at hand dictates whether a factorial design should be used.

For example, a factorial trial was used to evaluate whether individuals with alcohol dependence could achieve alcohol abstinence through pharmaceutical and/or behavioral interventions.[15] The investigators hypothesized that receiving both pharmaceutical and behavioral interventions in combination would be more beneficial than receiving either a pharmaceutical or a behavioral intervention on its own. Given that there are standard practices for managing alcohol dependence, all study participants received standard medical management, including the control group. One of the pharmacotherapies tested was naltrexone, a medication used to manage alcohol dependence by reducing alcohol cravings.

## FIGURE 4.5 SCHEMATIC OF A RANDOMIZED CONTROLLED FACTORIAL TRIAL WITH TWO INTERVENTIONS

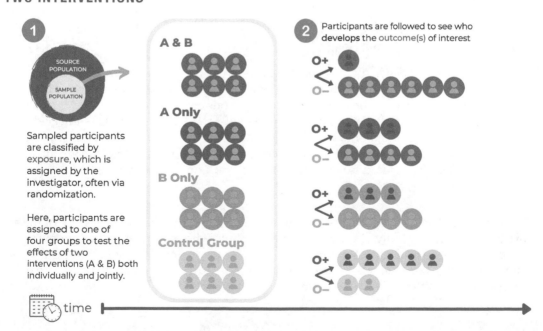

The investigators found that, compared to the control group, all three intervention groups experienced, on average, more days of alcohol abstinence: naltrexone alone (80.6% of study days with alcohol abstinence), behavioral intervention alone (79.2%), both naltrexone and behavioral intervention (77.1%), and placebo (75.1%). Interestingly, and contrary to the study hypothesis, the combined effect of the pharmaceutical and behavioral interventions did *not* exceed the effect of either intervention alone. The results indicated that either naltrexone or the behavioral intervention may be effective in helping individuals with alcohol dependence achieve abstinence.

## MASKING (LEARNING OBJECTIVE 4.8)

**Masking** (sometimes called blinding) is a term for withholding exposure status information from certain groups in a controlled trial, including study participants, investigators, and/or data analysts. By concealing the exposure status, masking prevents bias in how the study outcomes are ascertained or analyzed. The different types and reasons for masking in a controlled trial are described in the text that follows and are summarized in **Table 4.2**.

**TABLE 4.2 MASKING IN A CONTROLLED TRIAL**

| Masked Group | Masking Reduces the Likelihood of... |
|---|---|
| **Trial participants** | • Biased reporting of trial outcomes, symptoms, or other key data during the trial<br>• Differences between the intervention and control groups with respect to:<br>— Adherence to assigned exposure condition<br>— Loss to follow-up<br>— Use of supplementary interventions |
| **Investigators who have contact with trial participants (e.g., study physicians, interviewers)** | • Differences in engagement with participants that differ between the intervention and control groups, including:<br>— Withdrawing participants from the trial<br>— Adjusting intervention dosages or frequency<br>— Administering supplementary interventions<br>— Probing for side effects or asking additional questions |
| **Data analysts** | • Internal beliefs about the study hypothesis that could influence the data analysis |

### Evolving Terminology in Public Health

The use of the term *masking* instead of *blinding* represents an effort to remove ableist language from public health. Readers should also be aware that strides are being made in other areas, such as the use of more inclusive terminology around gender and race and the call to "put the person first" (e.g., saying "people living with HIV" instead of "HIV-infected people," or saying "people experiencing homelessness" instead of "homeless people"). Importantly, these changes should be driven by the preferences of the groups who are affected, and standards are different in different fields and will certainly continue to evolve.

A **single-masked** trial is one in which only one category of individuals is unaware of the exposure assignment. Typically, it is the study participants who are unaware of their exposure status in a single-masked trial. Masking participants can prevent bias stemming from how measures (outcomes or other covariates) are assessed. Additionally, masking makes participants less likely to differentially (meaning in a way that is different for each trial arm) adhere to study interventions, experience loss to follow-up, or use supplementary interventions due to knowing their exposure assignment. A study in which two groups of individuals are unaware of the exposure assignment is called a **double-masked** trial; typically, it is the investigator and the study participants who are unaware of the exposure status in a double-masked trial. Masked investigators are less likely to make decisions related to management of study participants that might be different by trial arm, such as withdrawing participants from the trial, adjusting the intervention dose or frequency, administering supplemental interventions, or asking questions to participants, such as probing for side effects. **Triple-masked** studies additionally mask the data analysts to prevent any internal beliefs about the intervention's effect from impacting the data analysis.

It is not always feasible or ethical to mask each of the groups involved in a controlled trial. To successfully mask participants and investigators, the control condition needs to resemble the intervention under study, which may not be possible. For example, it may be relatively easy to mask participants in a drug trial if the intervention drug can be made to look like and be administered similarly to placebo or standard of care drugs. On the other hand, surgical interventions may be more difficult to mask, and the ethics of conducting sham surgical procedures have been debated.[16] For example, investigators decided against masking participants in a trial of the effect of hormonal contraceptive methods on HIV acquisition,[17] in which masking participants would have required sham contraceptive implants and intrauterine device insertions. Of course, study physicians cannot be masked to certain exposures, such as surgical procedures that they conduct. It is generally possible to mask data collectors and is often recommended, especially in cases where the outcome of interest is measured in a more subjective manner such as with qualitative assessments of patient cognitive function.

Controlled trials in which participants are not masked are sometimes called **open-label trials**. An open-label trial may be used when masking is not feasible or ethical, or to mimic a real-world setting in which patients are aware of their exposures. Though study participants are not masked in open-label trials, it may be possible to mask some investigators and/or data analysts. For example, the trial studying the effect of hormonal contraceptive methods on HIV acquisition was an open-label study in which study staff who conducted outcome measurements were masked to patients' trial arm assignment.[17] Since participants in open-label trials are aware of their exposure status, it is best to use objective outcomes, such as laboratory results, to reduce bias. In the contraception and HIV trial, the outcome of incident HIV infection was assessed using a standardized HIV testing and confirmation algorithm.[17]

## ALLOCATION CONCEALMENT (LEARNING OBJECTIVE 4.8)

While it can be beneficial though not always possible to mask groups of individuals from knowing exposure assignment, it is always necessary to withhold information about the order in which participants will be assigned to trial arms. This process is called **allocation concealment**, whereby the order in which participants will be assigned to the trial arms is hidden until the moment of assignment. Allocation concealment is critical because it can prevent researchers from (consciously or unconsciously) influencing which participants are assigned to which trial arm, thereby forgoing the benefits of randomization. You may have encountered the medical-drama television show trope in which trial investigators break allocation concealment for personal reasons; for example, to ensure that a family member or friend is assigned to the treatment arm. Note that allocation concealment and masking are different and are performed for different purposes. While masking seeks to reduce biased *measurement of key variables*, allocation concealment seeks to prevent biased *allocation* and thus preserve randomization.

## A 2020 COVID-19 Vaccine Trial: Randomization, Trial Type, Masking, and Allocation Concealment

In the COVID-19 vaccine trial conducted in 2020 that we discussed earlier, 43,548 individuals were randomized to either the intervention (vaccine candidate) or the control (placebo saline injection) arms. Exposure assignment occurred in a 1:1 ratio, which means that an equal number of participants were assigned to each trial arm. The study protocol required that participants receive two injections of either the vaccine candidate or a placebo injection, spaced 21 days apart. After randomization, 43,448 study participants received injections with either the vaccine candidate or placebo.

Injections, both intervention and control, were 30 mcg each and administered in the deltoid muscle. Participants knew that they could receive either the candidate vaccine or placebo but were unaware of which one they received. Investigators, study coordinators, and other study site staff were also unaware of the exposure assignments. At the study sites, the staff involved in vaccine delivery, storage, dispensing, and administration were unmasked. Data analysts were also unmasked. To capture any immediate vaccine reactions, all participants were observed for 30 minutes after each injection.

1. What was the randomization technique: simple or stratified?
2. What was the unit of randomization?
3. Did the trial employ a parallel, crossover, or factorial design? Why?
4. Who was masked with respect to the trial participants' exposure status? What benefit may this masking provide in this trial?

## Randomization, Trial Types, Masking, and Allocation Concealment

- **Randomization** is a process by which every individual has an equal chance of being assigned to each exposure condition.
  - Randomization of exposure should yield exposed and unexposed groups that are comparable on all factors *except* for the exposure status, thus isolating the effect of the exposure.
  - Randomization attempts to remove confounding by both known and unknown confounders.
- Two common **randomization techniques**:
  - In **simple randomization**, each study participant is randomly assigned to one of the exposure conditions with no prior steps.
  - In **stratified randomization**, trial participants are first stratified based on important possible confounders (e.g., sex, age); randomization then occurs within each of these groups. This technique forces a balance in the stratified factors across study arms.
- The **unit of randomization** can be at the individual or cluster level.
  - **Individual randomization** allocates exposure status to each individual study participant.
  - **Cluster randomization** allocates exposure status to defined groups (i.e., clusters).
- Three common **trial types**:
  - In **parallel trials**, each exposure group receives a single exposure at the same time.
  - In **crossover trials**, each subject receives both the intervention and the control exposure condition, one after the other, often with a washout period in between.
  - In **factorial trials**, the effects of two (or more) interventions—both individually and jointly—are compared to a control group.

- **Masking** means withholding exposure status information from certain groups to prevent ascertainment bias.
  - In a **single-masked** trial, typically the study participants are masked.
  - In a **double-masked** trial, typically both the study participants and the investigators are masked.
  - In a **triple-masked** trial, typically the study participants, investigators, and data assessors are masked.
- **Allocation concealment** conceals the order in which participants will be assigned to the trial arms until the moment of assignment in order to maintain randomization.

## ANALYSIS OF RANDOMIZED CONTROLLED TRIAL DATA
### (LEARNING OBJECTIVE 4.9)

### Measures of Frequency and Association

Since investigators follow a group of at-risk participants for *new* cases of the outcome in a controlled trial, outcome frequencies can be reported using a risk or rate. Consequently, the association between the exposure and outcome can be quantified using risk- and rate-based measures of association (see **Table M.4**).

As discussed in the text that follows and shown in **Figure 4.6**, the analysis of trial data will require either a **per-protocol analysis** or an **intention-to-treat analysis**, and this decision hinges on whether the goal of the trial is to understand intervention **efficacy** or **effectiveness**, respectively.

### Intervention Efficacy and Per-Protocol Analyses

Intervention **efficacy** is defined as a measure of the ability of an intervention to prevent or treat a poor health outcome *among those who use the intervention according to the study protocol*. Efficacy is a measure of the etiologic, or causal, benefit of the intervention. To calculate a measure of association that reflects intervention efficacy, investigators conduct a **per-protocol analysis**,

## FIGURE 4.6 ESTIMATING EFFICACY AND EFFECTIVENESS IN A RANDOMIZED CONTROLLED TRIAL

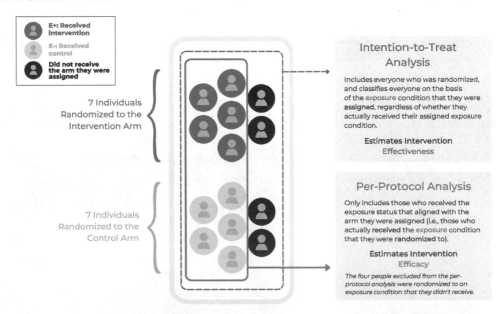

which only includes data from individuals with perfect adherence to their assigned trial arm. Anyone assigned to the intervention arm who did not actually take the intervention (e.g., participants assigned to take a drug but who did not), or anyone assigned to the control arm who ended up receiving an alternate treatment would be excluded from a per-protocol analysis.

## Intervention Effectiveness and Intention-to-Treat Analyses

In a controlled trial, the exposure *assignment* may differ from the exposure *received*. Intervention **effectiveness** is defined as a measure of the ability of an intervention to prevent or treat whatever health outcome it was designed for *among people who are randomized to the intervention, whether or not they actually receive the intervention*. Effectiveness provides a better estimate of the benefit of the intervention in a real-world setting where adherence is rarely perfect. To calculate a measure of association that reflects intervention effectiveness, investigators would conduct an **intention-to-treat analysis** (often described as "analyze what you randomize"), in which all study participants who underwent randomization are analyzed in their respective assigned arms, regardless of whether they adhered to their assigned arm. Although participants' exposure status may be misclassified (e.g., someone assigned to the intervention arm who never took the drug would still be included in the intervention group for analysis), this measure is still very useful.

Ultimately, controlled trials are conducted with the goal of rolling out effective interventions to individuals outside of a study setting. If investigators find that there is low adherence to the intervention during a trial, it will be important to investigate why this is to inform potential future expansion of the intervention. Reasons for non-adherence may include pain or discomfort associated with exposure administration, exposure side effects, or limited transportation to study visits. These barriers could be addressed by managing participants' expectations about potential side effects, providing pain relief as appropriate, or helping increase access to transportation.

## Comparing Intervention Effectiveness and Efficacy

Intervention efficacy, the estimate of the true etiologic benefit of an intervention, is a prerequisite for intervention effectiveness; an intervention that is not efficacious will not be meaningfully effective. Estimates of intervention effectiveness are generally closer to the null (i.e., more conservative) than estimates of intervention efficacy due to non-adherence but are a better reflection of what might be observed during a real-world rollout of an intervention. Note that in common vernacular, people (including researchers and the media) often use the term *effective* in a general sense to encompass both efficacy and effectiveness, although this usage to describe efficacy is not technically correct.

---

### Pause to Practice 4.5

#### A 2020 COVID-19 Vaccine Trial: Data Analysis

The primary analysis of the COVID-19 vaccine trial included data from participants age 16 years or older, without baseline infection, and who were randomized and actually received both injections. Data from this vaccine trial data are shown in **Table 4.3**.[11]

1. Calculate the rate ratio comparing the candidate vaccine to placebo.

2. Provide a one-sentence interpretation of this rate ratio.

Vaccine efficacy, which is a measure specific to vaccine studies, is expressed as a percent and is calculated as follows:

$$\text{Vaccine efficacy} = 100\% \times \left( \frac{\text{Risk}_{\text{Unvaccinated}} - \text{Risk}_{\text{Vaccinated}}}{\text{Risk}_{\text{Unvaccinated}}} \right) = 100\% \times (1 - \text{Risk ratio})$$

The same calculation can be performed using rates:

$$\text{Vaccine efficacy} = 100\% \times \left( \frac{\text{Rate}_{\text{Unvaccinated}} - \text{Rate}_{\text{Vaccinated}}}{\text{Rate}_{\text{Unvaccinated}}} \right) = 100\% \times (1 - \text{Rate ratio})$$

Vaccine efficacy is calculated among those who actually received their assigned exposure condition and is interpreted as the percentage reduction in disease among the vaccinated group compared to an unvaccinated group.

3.  Calculate the vaccine efficacy comparing the candidate vaccine to placebo.

4.  How would you interpret this vaccine efficacy?

5.  Does the previously noted summary provide a description of an intention-to-treat or a per-protocol analysis?

6.  Why might the effectiveness of the candidate vaccine be different from its efficacy?

**TABLE 4.3 COVID VACCINE TRIAL DATA FOR THOSE WHO RECEIVED BOTH INJECTIONS**

|  | Candidate Vaccine ($N = 17,411$) | Placebo ($N = 17,511$) |
|---|---|---|
| Number of confirmed incident COVID-19 cases at least 7 days after second injection | 8 | 162 |
| Person-time (years) | 2,214 | 2,222 |

*Source*: Data from Polack FP, Thomas SJ, Kitchin N, et al. Safety and efficacy of the BNT162b2 mRNA COVID-19 vaccine. *N Engl J Med.* 2020;383:2603–2615. https://doi.org/10.1056/NEJMoa2034577

**Digging Deeper**

## Effectiveness Measured in a Trial Versus Real-World Settings

Unlike the real-world, trial settings are typically rigorously controlled and structured. This means that participants are often closely followed, reminded of their study visits and study procedures, counseled about their health, and incentivized to participate and adhere to study procedures. Thus, a measure of association generated from a trial, even in an intention-to-treat analysis, is generally further from the null (i.e., a stronger effect) than what would be observed in a population that is not participating in a trial. For example, an observational study of the same COVID-19 vaccine discussed in this chapter was conducted among roughly 5.07 million U.S. individuals. Among fully vaccinated individuals in this observational study, effectiveness was 80% during the first month of full vaccination.[18]

# U.S. FOOD AND DRUG ADMINISTRATION (FDA) PHASES OF CONTROLLED DRUG TRIALS (LEARNING OBJECTIVE 4.10)

Though not all controlled trials evaluate drugs, a subset do. In the United States, the FDA regulates drugs, both those that require a prescription and those that do not.[19] Drugs that require FDA approval are tested over the course of several trials, which are defined by **study phase** as shown in **Figure 4.7** and discussed in the text that follows.

## FIGURE 4.7 PHASES OF U.S. FDA CONTROLLED DRUG TRIALS

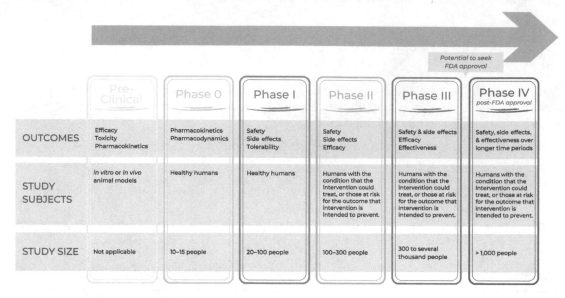

| | Pre-Clinical | Phase 0 | Phase I | Phase II | Phase III | Phase IV post-FDA approval |
|---|---|---|---|---|---|---|
| OUTCOMES | Efficacy Toxicity Pharmacokinetics | Pharmacokinetics Pharmacodynamics | Safety Side effects Tolerability | Safety Side effects Efficacy | Safety & side effects Efficacy Effectiveness | Safety, side effects, & effectiveness over longer time periods |
| STUDY SUBJECTS | *in vitro* or *in vivo* animal models | Healthy humans | Healthy humans | Humans with the condition that the intervention could treat, or those at risk for the outcome that intervention is intended to prevent. | Humans with the condition that the intervention could treat, or those at risk for the outcome that intervention is intended to prevent. | Humans with the condition that the intervention could treat, or those at risk for the outcome that intervention is intended to prevent. |
| STUDY SIZE | Not applicable | 10–15 people | 20–100 people | 100–300 people | 300 to several thousand people | > 1,000 people |

Potential to seek FDA approval

**Preclinical.** Before initiating studies with human subjects, investigators study new drugs using **preclinical studies**. In this phase, the efficacy, toxicity, and pharmacokinetics (the study of how drugs move within a body) of a new drug are studied in vitro or in vivo in animal models. Investigators may consider a range of drug doses, and the data from these studies may be used to obtain approval for testing in humans.

**Phase 0.** The first studies in humans occur during **Phase 0 trials**, which provide no data on drug safety or efficacy, but rather evaluate drug pharmacokinetics and pharmacodynamics (the study of the mechanism of drug action) in healthy humans. These studies often involve an exploratory assessment in a relatively small number of subjects using subtherapeutic dosages (e.g., micro-doses) of a drug.

**Phase I.** After drug pharmacokinetics and pharmacodynamics have been studied, investigators can enroll a larger number of healthy participants in **Phase I trials**, where drug safety, side effects, and tolerability are evaluated. Phase I studies may consider a range of drug doses.

**Phase II.** If the drug passes the safety and side-effect evaluations in a Phase I study, investigators may initiate a **Phase II trial** where they test the drug on individuals who actually have the condition that the drug is intended to treat, or are at-risk for the condition that the drug is intended to prevent. Phase II studies continue to assess drug safety and side effects; however, they are also used to evaluate drug efficacy. These trials enroll a larger number of participants, and therapeutic dosages are studied. Most drug trials do not make it past Phase II studies, typically because of limited efficacy and/or concerns related to toxicity.

**Phase III.** If Phase II trial data indicate that the intervention may be efficacious *and* any risks are deemed acceptable given the severity of the health outcome of interest, then a **Phase III trial** may be conducted to evaluate drug efficacy and possibly effectiveness. As with Phase II trials, Phase III trials continue to evaluate both safety and side effects. Phase III studies enroll a larger number of people, often across multiple sites and locations, and use therapeutic doses. As you might imagine, Phase III drug trials are very expensive, time-consuming, and challenging. With FDA approval, some drugs may be marketed to the public for a brief period while a Phase III trial is still under way. Successful Phase III trials may conclude with FDA approval and marketing of the intervention.

**Phase IV. Phase IV trials** are studies that occur *after* FDA approval that often enroll many thousands of people and assess longer-term outcomes and potentially find a new market for a drug (e.g., children who were excluded from earlier trials).

On average, it takes 7 to 15 years for a drug to move from preclinical testing to market, and it can cost hundreds of millions of dollars. Remarkably, several COVID-19 candidate vaccines moved from preclinical studies to Phase III studies and to market under an EUA in a matter of months without sacrificing rigor in scientific evaluation. As described at the beginning of this chapter, this accelerated process was due to decades of previous research on mRNA vaccines and was supported by the large-scale, organized, concerted efforts of multiple stakeholders.

## CONTROLLED TRIAL ETHICS (LEARNING OBJECTIVE 4.11)

Think back to our discussion of human subjects research ethics. As discussed in **Chapter 1, "Introduction to Public Health and the Fundamentals of Epidemiology,"** the ethics of human subjects research play an important role in all of epidemiologic research. Due to their experimental nature, there are additional considerations that are specific to controlled trials.

**Randomization.** It is not always ethical to randomize participants to receive exposures that are known to be harmful. For example, one could no longer randomize participants to cigarette smoking (although this might have not been considered unethical in the past before the deleterious effects of cigarettes were understood). Note that some exposures that have known harmful side effects (some chemotherapeutics, for example) might still be eligible for randomization if their benefits were thought to outweigh the risks in a given population.

**Equipoise.** For a trial to have **equipoise**, it means that none of the treatments should be already known to be inferior or superior prior to the trial. Once one treatment has been shown to be superior to another, investigators can no longer justify withholding it from patients in the control arm. The converse is also true: once an intervention has been found to be inferior, investigators can no longer justify assigning patients to receive it.

**Stopping rules.** The protocol for a controlled trial should include rules for when to stop the trial early. A trial may end early due to risks to participants that are judged to outweigh benefits, too few outcomes to evaluate the research question, and clear benefit or inferiority of the intervention (i.e., a lack of equipoise).

**Placebo control groups.** As discussed previously, many investigators argue that it is not ethical to use a placebo control when some other standard of care option exists,[3] and investigators typically only use placebo controls if there is no evidence-based standard of care.

**Standard of care control groups.** There is some debate about whether the standard of care control condition should be the best standard of care worldwide or the best standard of care that is locally available at the trial site.[20,21]

**Conducting trials in underserved populations.** Many trials enroll underserved populations due to higher healthcare needs. As with all studies involving human subjects, informed consent is crucial, and considerations such as literacy or coercion must be considered. Additionally, there is debate about whether trial participants should be guaranteed post-trial access to beneficial interventions, especially in countries where the intervention may not become widely available due to expense or feasibility.[22,23]

### Reporting Study Findings From Controlled Trials: The CONSORT Statement

All study designs, whether experimental or observational, have standard reporting guidance. Many journals require investigators to follow the CONSORT (CONsolidated Standards Of Reporting Trials) Statement when presenting results from a controlled trial. The CONSORT Statement is an evidence-based, minimum set of recommendations for reporting of randomized trials that provides a framework to support and maintain data integrity, validity, trial ethics, and transparency.[24] The statement consists of a 25-item checklist with items related to trial design, analysis, and interpretation along with a flow diagram that illustrates the progress of all participants throughout the trial.

## STRENGTHS AND LIMITATIONS OF CONTROLLED TRIALS
### (LEARNING OBJECTIVE 4.12)

### Strengths of Controlled Trials

**Temporality.** Given that investigators assign the exposure statuses in a trial and follow participants forward in time, the **temporality** between the exposure and the outcome (i.e., the exposure occurs and is recorded prior to when the outcome is observed) is established by the design. As we discussed in **Chapter 3, "Introduction to Analytic Epidemiologic Study Designs and Measures of Association,"** temporality is a core tenet of causality (i.e., for the exposure to have caused the outcome, The exposure must have occurred before the outcome). As you will later see, this contrasts with other study designs that do not establish temporality between the exposure and the outcome by design.

**Masking.** When feasible and ethical, masking is a key tool used to minimize bias due to personal beliefs.

**Randomization (with allocation concealment).** When feasible and ethical, randomization (with allocation concealment) is a key tool used to minimize confounding bias (i.e., imbalances in important factors across the study arms).

**Study of rare exposures.** Since the investigators assign the exposure conditions, trials are relatively well-suited for studying rare exposures, or exposures that would occur infrequently in an observational setting.

### Limitations of Controlled Trials

**Loss to follow-up.** As with all longitudinal designs, meaning those that involve tracking participants over time, there is the potential for loss to follow-up that may lead to selection bias, which will be discussed in detail in **Chapter 10, "Selection Bias."**

**Study of rare outcomes.** If the outcome of interest is rare, data from trials may not be able to detect differences in outcomes across the exposure groups.

**Study of outcomes with long induction or latency periods.** Longitudinal studies like trials may not be well-suited to study exposure-outcome relationships that have long **induction periods**, which is the time between when an exposure occurs and the outcome of interest occurs. Similarly, longitudinal studies like trials may not be well-suited to study exposure–outcome relationships that have long **latency periods**, which is the time between when an exposure occurs and the outcome of interest is detectable. If induction and/or latency periods are long, investigators would have to wait a long time to accrue enough outcomes to be able to draw conclusions, and the longer the follow-up period, the more likely it is that participants will be lost to follow-up. Induction and latency periods are discussed further in **Chapter 5, "Cohort Designs."**

**Logistics.** Trials are complicated and can be expensive, time-consuming, and resource intensive.

**Ethical considerations.** Investigators must always conduct research that stands up to current ethical guidelines, and controlled trials are no exception. Certain hallmark elements of controlled trials, such as randomization, may simply be unethical to pursue. Trials that could have been conducted ethically in the past may not meet current standards given what we know about certain exposures today.

**Generalizability.** Controlled trials often have strict eligibility criteria that can limit the **generalizability** (also called **external validity**) of trial findings. Generalizability refers to how well the study results can be applied to other populations or settings. For example, as mentioned earlier, pregnant people are often excluded from controlled trials, and findings from these trials may not be generalizable to pregnant populations. Similarly, given the highly controlled nature of these trials, the findings may not be generalizable to non-trial settings where there may be a lot of variation in how the interventions are used. We discuss generalizability further in **Chapter 10, "Selection Bias."**

## Pause to Practice 4.6

### A 2020 COVID-19 Vaccine Trial: Strengths and Limitations

The questions that follow ask you to explore some of the strengths and limitations related to the COVID-19 vaccine trial discussed in this chapter, and refer to **Table 4.4**, which presents data from the 2020 COVID-19 vaccine trial.

**TABLE 4.4 DEMOGRAPHICS OF THE 2020 COVID-19 VACCINE TRIAL PARTICIPANTS ($N$ = 37,706)**

| Variable | Candidate Vaccine Arm ($N$ = 18,860) % | Placebo Arm ($N$ = 18,846) % |
|---|---|---|
| **Biological sex** | | |
| Male | 51 | 50 |
| Female | 49 | 50 |
| **Self-reported race** | | |
| White | 83 | 83 |
| Black/African American | 9 | 9 |
| Asian | 4 | 4 |
| Other | 4 | 4 |

*Source:* Adapted from Polack FP, Thomas SJ, Kitchin N, et al. Safety and efficacy of the BNT162b2 mRNA COVID-19 vaccine. *N Engl J Med.* 2020;383:2603–2615. https://doi.org/10.1056/NEJMoa2034577

1.  Using the data in **Table 4.4**, is there evidence that randomization worked? How do you know? Is this what you would have expected given the sample size?

2.  What benefits would we expect from successful randomization?

3.  Of the 37,706 trial participants who underwent randomization and received either the candidate vaccine or the placebo and had a median of 2 months of follow-up, fewer than 200 were lost to follow-up. Do you think this would be considered meaningful loss to follow-up? Why or why not?

4.  Do you think there were any ethical concerns during the design and conduct of this trial?

5.  Consider the fact that only nonpregnant persons older than 16 years were enrolled in this trial, and look at the demographics presented in **Table 4.4**. Do you have any concerns about the generalizability of the trial results?

The strengths and limitations of controlled trials, along with all of the other analytic study designs discussed in this book, are presented in **Table M.3.** Some of these strengths and limitations are discussed in relation to the other designs, so reviewing them after you have read all the study design chapters (**Chapter 4, "Randomized Controlled Trial Designs"; Chapter 5, "Cohort Designs"; Chapter 6, "Case-Control Designs";** and **Chapter 7, "Cross-Sectional Designs"**) will be beneficial. Each of these study designs serves an important purpose, and we encourage readers to revisit these upon completion of **Chapter 7, "Cross-Sectional Designs."**

## Highlights

### Controlled Trial: Analyses, U.S. FDA Phases of Drug Trials, Ethics, Strengths, and Limitations

- In a controlled trial, the association between the exposure and the outcome can be quantified using **risk- and rate-based measures of association**.

- To calculate a measure of association that reflects intervention **efficacy**, investigators conduct a **per-protocol analysis** that only includes data from individuals with perfect adherence to the intervention in their assigned trial arm.

  - Efficacy is a measure of the etiologic (i.e., causal) benefit of an intervention.

- To calculate a measure of association that reflects intervention **effectiveness**, investigators conduct an **intention-to-treat analysis** that includes all study participants who underwent randomization, regardless of whether they adhered to their assigned intervention.

  - Effectiveness is a better measure of the real-world benefit of an intervention.

- Pharmaceuticals that require FDA approval are tested over the course of several trials, which are defined by **phases (preclinical to Phase IV)**.

- While all research with human subjects requires **ethical considerations**, there are additional considerations that are specific to controlled trials due to their experimental nature.

  - These include considerations related to randomization, equipoise, stopping rules, control conditions, and conducting trials in low- and middle-income countries.

- Common **strengths and limitations** of controlled trials:

  - **Strengths**: clear temporality between exposure and outcome; masking, allocation concealment, and randomization to prevent bias; and ability to study rare exposures.

  - **Limitations**: potential for loss to follow-up, difficult to study rare outcomes or outcomes with long latency periods, complicated logistics, additional ethical considerations, and limited generalizability.

## WHERE WE'VE BEEN AND WHAT'S UP NEXT

Controlled trials are often heralded as the best epidemiologic study design due to their experimental nature. While causality is most intuitively established when participants are randomized to their exposure conditions, controlled trials can only be used for exposures that can be ethically assigned *and* when there is a strong rationale to justify the resources required. Luckily, epidemiologists have another set of tools in their toolbox in the form of observational studies in which exposures are not assigned. **Chapter 5, "Cohort Designs"; Chapter 6, "Case-Control Designs";** and **Chapter 7, "Cross-Sectional Designs"** will provide an in-depth look at three of the most common observational study designs: cohort, case-control, and cross-sectional studies.

By the end of **Chapter 7, "Cross-Sectional Designs,"** you will see that each study design has its own strengths and limitations relative to the other designs, and that robust conclusions can be drawn from any study that is well-designed.

---

## END OF CHAPTER PROBLEM SET

1. Consider a cluster randomized trial of an intervention to provide postpartum family planning services. Healthcare providers in intervention facilities receive training on how to provide postpartum family planning methods. The outcome of interest is uptake of postpartum family planning methods. Name the phenomenon that might occur if providers from intervention facilities relocated to work at facilities randomized to the control arm, and describe the potential impact that this could have on the study results.

2. If conducting a crossover randomized trial, which of the following might inhibit our ability to approximate the counterfactual? *Select all that apply.*
   a. Factors changed during the course of the study period within individual participants, such as their employment status or living situation.
   b. A major global event, like a pandemic, occurred during the study period, which shifted individuals' stress levels and behaviors in a way that could influence the outcome of interest.
   c. The intervention being studied has no "wash-out" period, and its effects persist over a lifetime.

3. Describe the difference between masking and allocation concealment.

**Questions 4 to 12 are based on the study described in the text that follows.**

As described earlier and in **Chapter 3, "Introduction to Analytic Epidemiologic Study Designs and Measures of Association,"** new mRNA vaccines have been tested as *preventive* exposures, with the goal of keeping people from getting sick in the first place. Meanwhile, randomized trials of remdesivir, a drug that may shorten time of recovery, have been conducted in adults hospitalized with COVID-19 from across 60 trial sites. To evaluate the efficacy and safety of remdesivir, the investigators conducted a Phase III, randomized, double-blind, placebo-controlled trial.[25]

4. Is the intervention evaluated in this trial a preventive or a therapeutic exposure?

5. The investigators used a placebo control. Under what circumstances would use of a placebo control be appropriate?

6. Read the excerpt below from the study's publication[25] which pertains to masking. Who was masked with respect to the trial participants' exposure status? What benefit may this masking provide?

> *Remdesivir was administered intravenously as a 200-mg loading dose on day 1, followed by a 100-mg maintenance dose administered daily on days 2 through 10 or until hospital discharge or death. A matching placebo was administered according to the same schedule and in the same volume as the active drug. A normal saline placebo was used at the European sites and at some non-European sites owing to a shortage of matching placebo; for these sites, the remdesivir and placebo infusions were masked with an opaque bag and tubing covers to maintain blinding.*

7. Was this a superiority, non-inferiority, or equivalence trial?

8. Read the following excerpt from the study's publication,[25] which describes the main study findings. What do these data indicate in terms of the superiority of remdesivir versus placebo?

> *Those who received remdesivir had a median recovery time of 10 days (95% confidence interval [CI], 9 to 11), as compared with 15 days (95% CI, 13 to 18) among those who received placebo (rate ratio for recovery, 1.29; 95% CI, 1.12 to 1.49; P <0.001).*

9. As a secondary outcome, the investigators considered the association between remdesivir and mortality during a 14-day follow-up period. Using **Table 4.5**, name and calculate the appropriate measure of association.

**TABLE 4.5 REMDESIVIR AND MORTALITY DURING A 14-DAY FOLLOW-UP PERIOD DATA**

|  | Remdesivir (*N* = 541) | Placebo (*N* = 521) |
|---|---|---|
| Died during 14 days of follow-up | 35 | 61 |
| No death during 14 days of follow-up | 506 | 460 |

*Source:* Data from Beigel JH, Tomashek KM, Dodd LE, et al. Remdesivir for the treatment of COVID-19—final report. *N Engl J Med.* 2020;383:1813–1826. https://doi.org/10.1056/NEJMoa2007764

10. Interpret in words the measure of association calculated in Question 9.

11. Read the following excerpt from the study's publication,[25] which describes adverse events in the treatment and control arms. Do these data raise safety concerns about use of remdesivir? Why or why not?

> *Serious adverse events were reported in 131 of the 532 patients who received remdesivir (24.6%) and in 163 of the 516 patients who received placebo (31.6%).*

12. The remdesivir trial is an example of a Phase III trial. What are some characteristics of this trial that indicated it was a Phase III trial?

# REFERENCES

1. Kaptchuk TJ, Friedlander E, Kelley JM, et al. Placebos without deception: a randomized controlled trial in irritable bowel syndrome. *PLoS One.* 2010;5(12):e15591. https://doi.org/10.1371/journal.pone.0015591

2. Colloca L, Barsky AJ. Placebo and nocebo effects. *N Engl J Med.* 2020;382(6):554–561. https://doi.org/10.1056/NEJMra1907805

3. Rothman KJ, Michels KB. The continuing unethical use of placebo controls. *N Engl J Med.* 1994;331(6):394–398. https://doi.org/10.1056/NEJM199408113310611

4. Lariviere M, Vingtain P, Aziz M, et al. Double-blind study of ivermectin and diethylcarbamazine in African onchocerciasis patients with ocular involvement. *Lancet.* 1985;2(8448):174–177. https://doi.org/10.1016/s0140-6736(85)91496-5

5. Rickels K, Amsterdam J, Clary C, Fox I, Schweizer E, Weise C. The efficacy and safety of paroxetine compared with placebo in outpatients with major depression. *J Clin Psychiatry.* 1992;53(Suppl):30–32. https://pubmed.ncbi.nlm.nih.gov/1531820

6. World Medical Association. Declaration of Helsinki 1996. October 1996. https://www.wma.net/what-we-do/medical-ethics/declaration-of-helsinki/doh-oct1996

7. Skierka A-S, Michels KB. Ethical principles and placebo-controlled trials—interpretation and implementation of the Declaration of Helsinki's placebo paragraph in medical research. *BMC Med Ethics.* 2018;19(1):24. https://doi.org/10.1186/s12910-018-0262-9

8. Hill AB. Medical ethics and controlled trials. *Br Med J.* 1963;1(5337):1043–1049. https://doi.org/10.1136/bmj.1.5337.1043

9. Kroenke K, Spitzer RL, Williams JB. The PHQ-9: validity of a brief depression severity measure. *J Gen Intern Med.* 2001;16(9):606–613. https://doi.org/10.1046/j.1525-1497.2001.016009606.x

10. Wang B, Wang H, Tu XM, Feng C. Comparisons of superiority, non-inferiority, and equivalence trials. *Shanghai Arch Psychiatry.* 2017;29(6):385–388. https://doi.org/10.11919/j.issn.1002-0829.217163

11. Polack FP, Thomas SJ, Kitchin N, et al. Safety and efficacy of the BNT162b2 mRNA COVID-19 vaccine. *N Engl J Med.* 2020;383:2603–2615. https://doi.org/10.1056/NEJMoa2034577

12. U.S. Food and Drug Administration. Pfizer-BioNTech COVID-19 vaccine. 2020. https://www.fda.gov/news-events/press-announcements/fda-takes-key-action-fight-against-covid-19-issuing-emergency-use-authorization-first-covid-19

13. Majerus PW, Broze GJ, Miletich JP, et al. Anticoagulant thrombolytic, and antiplatelet drugs. In: Hardman JG, Limbird LE, eds. *Goodman and Gilman's the Pharmacological Basis of Therapeutics.* McGraw-Hill; 1996:1347–1351.

14. Landrigan CP, Rahman, SA, Sullivan, JP, et al. Effect on patient safety of a resident physician schedule without 24-hour shifts. *N Engl J Med.* 2020;382(26):2514–2523. https://doi.org/10.1056/NEJMoa1900669

15. Anton RF, O'Malley SS, Ciraulo DA, et al. Combined pharmacotherapies and behavioral interventions for alcohol dependence the COMBINE study: a randomized controlled trial. *JAMA.* 2006;295(17):2003–2017. https://doi.org/10.1001/jama.295.17.2003

16. Ciccozzi M, Menga R, Ricci G, et al. Critical review of sham surgery clinical trials: confounding factors analysis. *Ann Med Surg.* 2016;12:21–26. https://doi.org/10.1016/j.amsu.2016.10.007

17. Evidence for Contraceptive Options and HIV Outcomes Trial Consortium. HIV incidence among women using intramuscular depot medroxyprogesterone acetate, a copper intrauterine device, or a levonorgestrel implant for contraception: a randomised, multicentre, open-label trial. *Lancet.* 2019;394(10195):303–313. https://doi.org/10.1016/S0140-6736(19)31288-7

18. Tartof SY, Slezak JM, Fischer H, et al. Effectiveness of mRNA BNT162b2 COVID-19 vaccine up to 6 months in a large integrated health system in the USA: a retrospective cohort study. *Lancet.* 2021;398(10309):1407–1416. https://doi.org/10.1016/S0140-6736(21)02183-8

19. U.S. Food and Drug Administration. What does FDA regulate? 2021. https://www.fda.gov/about-fda/fda-basics/what-does-fda-regulate

20. Bhutta Z. Standards of care in research. *BMJ.* 2004;329(7475):1114–1115. https://doi.org/10.1136/bmj.329.7475.1114

21. van der Graaf R, van Delden JJ. What is the best standard for the standard of care in clinical research? *Am J Bioeth.* 2009;9(3):35–43. https://doi.org/10.1080/15265160802654129

22. Iunes R, Uribe MV, Torres JB, et al. Who should pay for the continuity of post-trial health care treatments? *Int J Equity Health.* 2019;18(1):26. https://doi.org/10.1186/s12939-019-0919-0

23. Zong Z. Should post-trial provision of beneficial experimental interventions be mandatory in developing countries? *J Med Ethics.* 2008;34(3):188–192. https://doi.org/10.1136/jme.2006.018754

24. CONSORT Group. The CONSORT statement. 2010. https://www.equator-network.org/reporting-guidelines/consort/

25. Beigel JH, Tomashek KM, Dodd LE, et al. Remdesivir for the treatment of COVID-19—final report. *N Engl J Med.* 2020;383:1813–1826. https://doi.org/10.1056/NEJMoa2007764

# CHAPTER 5

# COHORT DESIGNS

## KEY TERMS

closed cohort

cohort design

induction period

latency period

observational studies

open cohort

## LEARNING OBJECTIVES

5.1 Describe the basic design features of a cohort study.

5.2 Discuss the ways in which epidemiologic cohorts can be defined.

5.3 Understand the difference between open and closed cohorts.

5.4 Describe the different types of reference groups that may be defined in a cohort study.

5.5 Describe why induction and latency periods should be considered when designing a cohort study.

5.6 Describe the strengths and limitations of cohort designs.

## THE EVOLUTION OF NUTRITION SCIENCE

It may seem obvious today that what we eat has an important influence on our health; however, this wasn't always the case. The study of nutrition in the early 1900s was novel and focused on the so-called deficiency diseases, such as rickets, pellagra, beriberi, and scurvy, which were major contributors to mortality. Researchers noticed that individuals of lower socioeconomic status who had less varied diets experienced higher rates of these illnesses compared to individuals of higher socioeconomic status. These investigations laid the foundation for modern nutrition science, which has greatly improved public health. These investigations also importantly contributed to dispelling the racist and classist ideas of eugenics, which posited that certain people had ill health because of their weak or defective genes, which was a common belief in some countries in the early 1900s.

In the second half of the 20th century, nutrition science began to focus on the emerging leading killers: chronic diseases, such as heart disease, cancer, diabetes, and obesity. The Framingham Heart Study was one of the early cohort studies to begin to explore the role of saturated fat and cholesterol in the development of heart disease. As you will see in the case study explored in this chapter, elevated red meat consumption has been associated with coronary heart disease (CHD) in men in the United States.

As noted in **Chapter 4, "Randomized Controlled Trial Designs,"** controlled trials are useful as they allow researchers to isolate the health effect(s) of one or more exposures. However, controlled trials can only be used when it is both ethical and feasible for investigators to assign study participants to different exposure conditions. When a controlled trial is not feasible, investigators conduct observational research in which they measure exposure conditions that occur anyway (i.e., without assigning them to study participants). The **cohort design**—the focus of this chapter—has the same overarching design elements as a controlled trial: an at-risk group of individuals with different exposures are followed to see who develops the outcome of interest. The important difference between controlled trials and the cohort design is that in cohort designs, the exposure status is merely observed, not assigned, by the study investigators. This is what distinguishes the cohort design as an **observational study**.

## COHORT STUDY DESIGN BASICS (LEARNING OBJECTIVE 5.1)

Take some time to review **Figure 5.1**, which depicts the basic cohort study that you were briefly introduced to in **Chapter 3, "Introduction to Analytic Epidemiologic Study Designs and Measures of Association."** Recall that in this design, investigators first sample participants from a source population that is **at-risk** of developing the outcome(s) of interest. As with all study designs, it is imperative that investigators carefully define their **source population** (the group of people from which study participants will be selected) and then thoughtfully select participants to be included in the **sample population** (the people who are actually selected from the source population to participate in the study). You will learn more about defining the source population and sampling strategies in later chapters.

Participants are then classified by whether they are exposed or unexposed. Finally, study participants are followed longitudinally, meaning forward through time, to measure new (i.e., incident) cases of the outcome(s) of interest. Since investigators follow a group of at-risk participants to measure new cases of the outcome, we describe outcome frequency using a risk or rate. Consequently, the associations between exposures and health outcomes in a cohort study are often quantified using risk- and rate-based measures of association.

## FIGURE 5.1 SCHEMATIC OF A COHORT DESIGN

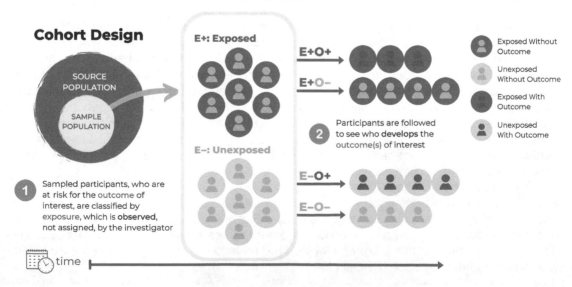

Now consider **Table 5.1**, which provides a more detailed view of the basic steps involved in conducting a cohort study, including formulating a research question, designing and conducting the cohort study, and analyzing and reporting the data. Each of the bolded terms in **Table 5.1** are discussed in detail throughout this chapter.

**TABLE 5.1 BASIC STEPS IN DESIGNING AND CONDUCTING A COHORT STUDY**

| **State the Research Question** |
| --- |
| State the study hypothesis(es) based on the research question. |
| **Design the Cohort Study** |
| Define outcome(s) with case definitions. |
| Define the cohort.<br>• Define who is eligible (who comprises the population at-risk for the outcome[s])<br>• General population or special exposure cohorts<br>• Open or closed cohort |
| Design a cohort study conducted in real time or using historical records. |
| Define the exposure and reference (comparison) group. |
| Decide whether you want to conduct matching. |
| Consider induction and latency periods. |
| **Conduct the Cohort Study** |
| Select subjects from an at-risk source population, obtain informed consent, and classify by exposure status. |
| Follow subjects and collect data on incident outcomes as well as key covariates. |
| **Analyze and Report Data** |
| Calculate measures of frequency and association. |
| Report findings using the STROBE reporting guidance. |
| Consider the strengths and limitations of the study. |

# DEVELOPING A HYPOTHESIS

Similar to a randomized trial, a cohort study may be designed to address a specific hypothesis about an association between an exposure and outcome(s) of interest. However, it is often the case that investigators designing and conducting cohort studies strive to learn many things about a particular broad research area such as cancer, cardiovascular disease, or HIV. In this case, investigators are not focused on a single study hypothesis; rather, a cohort study will be designed to explore the associations between many exposures on various health outcomes. Regardless of whether a cohort study is designed to evaluate one or many study hypotheses, all exposures and outcomes should be defined using rigorous case definitions, as described in **Chapter 2, "Descriptive Epidemiology, Surveillance, and Measures of Frequency."**

Examples of large cohort studies conducted in the United States include the Framingham Heart Study, the Black Women's Health Study, the Nurses' Health Study, and the Health Professionals Follow-Up Study. These studies include thousands of participants, and have been very productive, meaning that they have been used to answer many different research questions. In each of these studies, investigators were able to evaluate several hypotheses, even including the role of some exposures that were not of interest when the cohorts were originally designed:

- The Framingham Heart Study began in 1948 and, at the time of this writing, is enrolling its third generation of participants. This study was designed to identify many different risk factors for cardiovascular disease.[1]

- Similarly, the Black Women's Health Study, which began in 1995, was designed to identify many different risk factors for several chronic diseases which disproportionately affect Black women relative to their non-Black counterparts such as breast cancer and diabetes. Although the Black Women's Health Study was designed long before the emergence of SARS-CoV-2, it has recently been used to address the impact of COVID-19 in Black communities.[2]

- Two long-standing cohort studies of health professionals, the Nurses' Health Study,[3] which began in 1976, and the Health Professionals Follow-Up Study, which began in 1986,[4] were designed to identify many different risk factors for several major chronic diseases in women and men, respectively, including cardiovascular disease, diabetes, and various cancers.

As described in **Chapter 3** all study hypotheses should address the following key areas:

- What is the population of interest?
- What is the heath outcome of interest and how is it defined?
- What is the exposure of interest and how is it defined?
- What measures of frequency are being compared?
- What is the direction of the hypothesized association?

Once the research goals and hypotheses have been identified, investigators must define the cohort of subjects who are at-risk for the outcomes of interest.

## DEFINING THE COHORT (LEARNING OBJECTIVE 5.2)

In a very broad sense, the word **cohort** means a group of individuals who are followed or traced over a period of time, and for which membership is defined by some common criteria. For example, a **birth cohort** is a cohort of people defined by being born during a particular period of time. For example, all Australians born in 1990 and followed until death would comprise a birth cohort, with the common admissibility criteria being birth in 1990 and Australian nationality.

In epidemiology, cohorts are a **well-defined** group of individuals who are **at-risk for the outcome(s) of interest** at the start of the follow-up period. In epidemiologic cohorts, membership can be defined based on either (a) general population characteristics or (b) specific exposures.

If the goal of a cohort study is to evaluate the effect of exposures which commonly occur in large populations (such as smoking, alcohol, exercise, diet, and obesity), then a **general population cohort** may be defined. General population cohorts use very broad admissibility criteria to define membership, and thus findings from such cohorts are thought to be **generalizable** (i.e., applicable) to large groups of people. For example, in the Framingham Heart Study, one criterion for cohort membership was being a resident of Framingham, Massachusetts, with the rationale that men and women from this area would be broadly representative of middle-class adults in the United States. As the racial and ethnic profile of Framingham became more diverse, additional waves of cohort members were recruited to reflect that diversity for improved generalizability.[1] In the Nurses' Health Study and the Health Professionals

Follow-Up Study, one criterion for cohort membership was being a health professional. It was thought that health professionals would provide more accurate data on their exposures and health outcomes, that they would be relatively easier to follow than the general population, and that they would be more motivated to participate in a study lasting several years. A benefit of a general population cohort is that once participants have been selected, investigators can assess a wide range of exposures and outcomes occurring in the cohort.

Alternatively, investigators may be interested in studying the health effects of a particular exposure that only affects a certain group of individuals. In these cases, investigators may define a **special exposure cohort** where study participants are intentionally selected on the basis of their exposure status. This approach is useful when the exposure of interest is uncommon in the general population because a general population cohort may not contain any exposed people to study. For example, to study the effects of chrysotile, a type of asbestos, on mortality, a cohort study in Russia enrolled workers with varying levels of occupational exposure to chrysotile during mining activities.[5] These individuals comprised the exposed group in the cohort study, and a comparison group of individuals without chrysotile exposure were then selected to comprise the unexposed group.

Regardless of the cohort type, investigators must ensure that all participants included in a given analysis were at-risk for the outcomes(s) of interest at the beginning of the follow-up period. This can happen in one of two ways. First, investigators can only enroll individuals who are known to be at-risk for the outcomes of interest. For example, since investigators in the Framingham Heart Study were interested in learning about the causes of cardiovascular diseases, individuals with a history of heart attack, stroke, or other cardiovascular conditions were excluded from enrollment. Another approach is to identify a cohort where there is a mix of people with and without the outcomes of interest, and to make appropriate exclusions during the analysis phase of the study. This was the approach for the cohort studies of health professionals which considered many chronic disease outcomes. For a given research question, investigators would exclude any participants who reported a history of the outcome of interest at enrollment.

## OPEN AND CLOSED COHORTS (LEARNING OBJECTIVE 5.3)

Epidemiologic cohorts are further categorized as either open or closed (**Figures 5.2A** and **5.2B**). **Closed cohorts** are defined by a common start time, and no one is added to the cohort during the follow-up period. Individuals only exit the cohort when they get the outcome of interest, the study ends, or they die. A cohort is not closed if any participants are **lost to follow-up**, meaning that they leave the study population and investigators do not know whether they developed the outcome of interest. Competing risks, as defined in **Chapter 2, "Descriptive Epidemiology, Surveillance, and Measures of Frequency,"** can also prevent a cohort from being considered closed since individuals may experience some other event, like death from another cause, that prevents them from getting the outcome of interest. As you might imagine, it can be difficult to maintain a closed cohort, particularly when the follow-up period is very long, the study population is highly mobile, or the study population experiences high rates of morbidity or mortality.

**Figure 5.2A** illustrates an example of a closed cohort that includes a total of five study participants, all of whom entered the study on January 1, 2020. Investigators have complete outcome information on all five individuals for the entire 5-year study period: Participants 1, 2, and 4 all got the outcome of interest, Participant 3 completed the entire follow-up period, and Participant 5 died.

With certain conditions, the group of students enrolled in an epidemiology class could be considered a closed cohort. The start date of the follow-up period would be defined as the day after students can no longer change their schedules for the term. Additionally, it would have to be the case that no new students could enroll during the semester, and none of the students drop the course before the end of the term.

## FIGURE 5.2A CLOSED COHORT

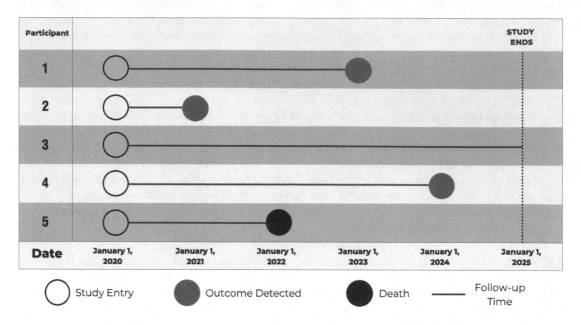

## FIGURE 5.2B OPEN COHORT

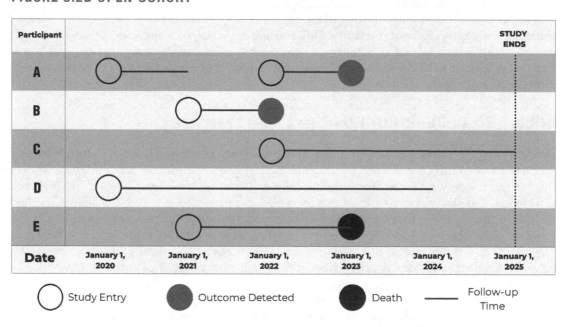

In contrast, **open cohorts,** also called dynamic cohorts, allow members to enroll and leave at different times. Since people can enter and exit the open cohort, it is possible that a person could enter, leave, and later re-enter the cohort. In an open cohort, study participants can contribute vastly different amounts of person-time during the follow-up period. Figure 5.2B illustrates an example of an open cohort that also includes a total of five study participants. Here, we see that participants entered the study at different time points, some were lost to follow-up (Participant D), and one even left and re-entered the study (Participant A). Returning to our epidemiology class example, we might have an open cohort if students were allowed to join the class in the middle of the term, or if some students dropped the class mid-way through.

## Open Versus Closed Cohorts: Why Does It Matter?

Whether a cohort is open or closed informs which measures of frequency (and therefore measures of association) can be validly calculated. Assuming the amount of time each individual contributed to the study has been recorded, rates can always be calculated in a cohort study. Whether a cohort is open or closed has an impact on whether it is appropriate to calculate risks.

- Data from *closed cohorts* may be analyzed using risks.
- Rates, not risks, should be calculated in *open cohorts*.

This concept ties back to the problems with calculating risk, discussed in **Chapter 2, "Descriptive Epidemiology, Surveillance, and Measures of Frequency."** If not everyone in a cohort is followed until they either get the outcome or complete the same study follow-up time, it can be difficult, if not impossible, to accurately estimate risk without advanced statistical techniques that are beyond the scope of this text.[6]

In short, you can always use rates to describe data in both open and closed cohorts. However, you can only calculate risk if everyone in a cohort is followed until they either get the outcome or complete the same study follow-up time (meaning that there is no [or very little] loss to follow-up and few competing risks). You will have the opportunity to practice calculating measures of frequency and association from open and closed cohorts later in this chapter.

## Highlights

### Cohort Design Basics: Defining the Cohort, Open Versus Closed Cohorts

- In the cohort design, the exposure status is observed, not assigned, which distinguishes the cohort design as an **observational study**.
- The basic components of a cohort study:
  - Participants are sampled from a source population that is at-risk for developing the outcome(s) of interest.
  - Participants are classified by whether they are exposed or unexposed.
  - Participants are followed longitudinally, meaning forward through time, to measure new cases of the outcome(s) of interest.
- In epidemiologic cohorts, membership can be defined based on either **general population** characteristics or **specific exposures**.
- Closed cohorts are defined by a common start time, and no one is added to the cohort during the follow-up period. Open cohorts allow members to enroll and leave at different times.
  - Data from closed cohorts may be analyzed using risks.
  - Rates, not risks, should be calculated using open cohort data.

## REAL-TIME AND HISTORICAL COHORT STUDIES

Some investigators distinguish between two different types of cohort studies: real-time and historical. In this context, these terms are differentiated by the investigator's perspective relative to the timing of the data collection. Under this definition, a **real-time cohort study** occurs when investigators identify and enroll a cohort of at-risk individuals and follow them forward in real-time to see who develops the outcome(s) of interest (**Figure 5.3A**). In contrast, a **historical cohort study** can be categorized as the use of historical records to understand what has happened to a cohort of individuals in the past (**Figure 5.3B**). Notably, real-time cohort

## FIGURE 5.3A COHORT STUDY CONDUCTED IN REAL-TIME

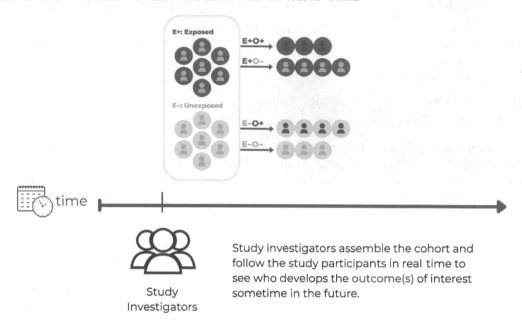

Study Investigators

Study investigators assemble the cohort and follow the study participants in real time to see who develops the outcome(s) of interest sometime in the future.

## FIGURE 5.3B COHORT STUDY CONDUCTED USING HISTORICAL DATA

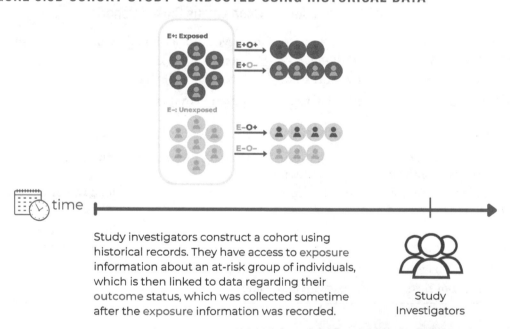

Study investigators construct a cohort using historical records. They have access to exposure information about an at-risk group of individuals, which is then linked to data regarding their outcome status, which was collected sometime after the exposure information was recorded.

Study Investigators

and historical cohort designs differ in terms of whether the data have been collected prior to the investigators' involvement; however, both designs study a cohort of at-risk individuals for whom outcome data are available after some time has elapsed. There is often a misconception that real-time cohort studies are inherently of greater quality than cohorts that use historical data. While investigators conducting a real-time cohort study do have the advantage of having control over how and which data are collected, the strengths of the cohort design remain relevant for a study that is conducted using historical records.

## Note on Terminology

It is important to note that investigators often use the term *prospective* to describe real-time cohort studies and the term *retrospective* to describe cohort studies that use historical data. However, we caution against the use of these terms since they have been used in various contexts with vastly different definitions.[7,8] A detailed discussion of the different definitions and uses of these terms is beyond the scope of this text; however, we caution new learners of epidemiology to be aware that these terms are used differently in different contexts, and we recommend that epidemiologists refrain from using these terms, and instead provide a description that clarifies what they mean.

The Framingham Heart Study, the Black Women's Health Study, and the Nurses' Health Study are all examples of cohort studies conducted in real-time.

In cohort studies using historical records, both the exposure and outcome have already occurred before the investigators begin the study (Figure 5.3B). To conduct this type of cohort study, investigators must be able to identify three important elements:

- A cohort of individuals who were initially at-risk for the outcome(s) of interest at some time point in the past
- A data source from which to abstract exposure status at the beginning of the observation period
- A data source from which to abstract subsequent outcome data

For example, historical cohort studies are useful for the study of occupational exposures where an employment register can be used to construct an at-risk cohort of employees. In the context of an accidental chemical exposure, a cohort could be defined as all individuals who were working at the facility at the time that the chemical spill occurred. Those with direct contact with the spilled chemical could comprise the exposed group, while the remaining employees could comprise the unexposed group. If the outcome of interest was mortality within 25 years, investigators could link the data from this cohort of employees to the U.S. National Death Index to determine who died during the 25 years following the chemical spill.

Historical cohort studies may also be designed using data from surveillance systems or health registries. For example, one recent historical cohort study evaluated the risk of breast cancer among transgender people in the Netherlands (a country with robust surveillance and registry data) who were receiving hormone treatment. The cohort was all individuals in the Netherlands without a previous breast cancer diagnosis. Using comprehensive medical records, investigators were able to identify transgender individuals receiving hormone treatment, who comprised the exposed group. The unexposed group was made up of cisgender individuals in the Dutch population. Breast cancer diagnoses were obtained using the Nationwide Network and Registry of Histopathology and Cytopathology in the Netherlands.[9]

## Comparing the Strengths and Limitations of Real-Time and Historical Cohort Studies

There are situations where a real-time cohort design is more appealing or appropriate than a historical design, and vice versa. In a real-time cohort study, study participant recruitment and data collection (including which data are collected, how often, and using what definitions) are entirely under the control of the study investigators. In contrast, in a historical cohort study, investigators must rely on the existing data, and thus cannot change how or which data were previously collected. The inability to influence the data collection process in a historical cohort study has the potential to yield poorer quality data relative to a real-time cohort study; however, this is not guaranteed. We will discuss this further in **Chapter 11, "Information Bias and Screening and Diagnostic Tests,"** when we describe how studies can be influenced by poor quality data; however, it is important to keep in mind that there is no inherent difference in data quality between real-time and historical cohort studies. If well-designed, valid conclusions may be drawn from either cohort type.

Given the resources that are required to identify, recruit, and actively follow a cohort of individuals, real-time cohort studies are generally much more costly than historical cohort studies. Additionally, investigators must wait for outcomes to occur in a real-time cohort study; thus, it can take a much longer time to obtain study results relative to a historical cohort study.

## Pause to Practice 5.1

### Design Considerations in the Health Professionals Follow-Up Study

The Health Professionals Follow-Up Study was a cohort study conducted among men in the United States which began in 1986.[4] This all-male cohort study was created to complement the research questions investigated in the Nurses' Health Study, which was conducted among women. Both cohort studies sought to investigate several exposures that are common in the general population (e.g., diet, smoking, obesity) and several chronic disease outcomes (e.g., cancer, heart disease). In 1986, the Health Professionals Follow-Up Study enrolled 51,529 men aged 40 to 75 years and had no ongoing enrollment of additional participants.

As described in **Pause to Practice 3.3**, one hypothesis explored by the Health Professionals Follow-Up Study was whether high (vs. lower) red meat consumption was associated with CHD among men in the United States. To explore this hypothesis, analyses were conducted using a subset of men enrolled in the study who did not have CHD at enrollment to explore the relationship between red meat consumption and new cases of CHD.[10]

1. Is the Health Professionals Follow-Up Study a general population or special exposure cohort? How do you know?

2. Is this an open or a closed cohort? How do you know, and what additional information would you like to have to confirm? What measures of outcome frequency do you think you can calculate?

3. Does this study use historical data, or were the data collected in real-time? How do you know? What might be some strengths of this approach?

## DEFINING THE EXPOSURE AND REFERENCE GROUPS
### (LEARNING OBJECTIVE 5.4)

In all analytic epidemiologic studies, we must define our exposure of interest, which for a dichotomous (i.e., two-level) exposure includes defining both an exposed group and an unexposed reference (or comparison) group. Thinking back to our discussions in **Chapter 3, "Introduction to Analytic Epidemiologic Study Designs and Measures of Association,"** about the counterfactual, the ideal unexposed reference group would be the exact same participants as those in the exposed group, except they would be unexposed. Since this ideal scenario is not possible, we define an unexposed reference group that is very similar to the exposed group in terms of any extraneous factors that may be associated with the outcome of interest. These factors are potential **confounders**, which we will discuss in **Chapter 9, "Error in Epidemiologic Research and Fundamentals of Confounding."**

For now, let's consider an example where our exposure of interest is smoking, and our outcome of interest is death. We learned in **Chapter 3, "Introduction to Analytic Epidemiologic Study Designs and Measures of Association,"** that exposed and unexposed groups are often defined not just by whether an exposure occurred, but also considering the dose and duration of the exposure. Suppose that we defined our exposure groups as follows:

- **Exposed group**: people who have smoked at least one pack of cigarettes a day for at least 10 years.

- **Unexposed reference group**: people who have never smoked.

Recall the benefits of randomization discussed in **Chapter 4, "Randomized Controlled Trial Designs,"** where the distribution of factors that might be associated with the outcome are balanced across the intervention and control groups. Although we cannot ethically randomize exposure to smoking, our goal is for unexposed "never smokers" to be similar to the exposed group of smokers for any factor that might be associated with death. Since smoking isn't assigned randomly, we can expect that our smokers may be different from our never smokers in important ways.

Consider an extreme example where all of the smokers were very young (younger than 20 years old) and all of the nonsmokers were very old (older than 99 years old). We know logically that age is associated with death, which means that our nonsmokers are much more likely to die during our study period simply due to their age. Similarly, given that they are young, we would expect lower mortality among the smokers. If we compare the group of young smokers to this older reference group, we could incorrectly conclude that smoking actually *prevents* death.

This extreme example helps illustrate the importance of selecting reference groups that are comparable to the exposed group in terms of any factors that may be associated with the outcome of interest (i.e., attempting to approximate the counterfactual). In randomized trials, we attempt to achieve this through randomization; in observational designs like cohort studies, more thought needs to go into defining and identifying the reference group. It is not always possible to enroll reference groups that are similar to the exposed groups on factors associated with the outcome. Fortunately, as you will learn in **Chapter 9, "Error in Epidemiologic Research and Fundamentals of Confounding,"** and **Chapter 13, "Introduction to Epidemiologic Data Analysis,"** imbalances that lead to bias may be adjusted for during data analysis.

## Sources of Reference (Comparison) Groups

In addition to thinking about the characteristics of the people who should comprise the reference group, there are different sources of comparison groups used in cohort studies: **internal** and **external reference groups**.

In a general population cohort, an **internal reference group** is comprised of the unexposed members of the cohort. This is a preferred reference group as members are generally similar to the exposed groups for factors that may influence the outcome. The Framingham Heart Study used internal reference groups; one example is in the evaluation of the association between smoking and cardiovascular diseases. Both the smoking and nonsmoking groups came from the same cohort and were likely to have shared characteristics for many extraneous factors that might introduce error in the study results, such as environmental exposures, lifestyle factors, and socioeconomic status.

An **external reference group** may be used in special exposure cohorts. In a special exposure cohort, selection into the cohort is based on an individual's exposure status, and thus everyone initially sampled is exposed. A group of unexposed people external to the exposed group is then identified and enrolled. For example, a study in New Zealand was interested in the quality of life experiences of medical students. Medical students were enrolled into a special exposure cohort, and an appropriate external reference group of nonmedical students were used as the comparison group.[11]

Whether using an internal or external reference group, careful consideration is needed regarding how any potential reference group may differ from the exposed group, which could be substantially different in ways that could introduce error.

## INDUCTION AND LATENCY PERIODS (LEARNING OBJECTIVE 5.5)

In a cohort study, measures of outcome frequency and measures of association should be calculated within a specified **risk period**, which is the time during which an exposure of interest could possibly cause an outcome and is conceptualized in relation to both **induction** and **latency periods** (Figure 5.4). As we discussed in **Chapter 3, "Introduction to Analytic Epidemiologic Study Designs and Measures of Association,"** for an exposure to have caused an outcome, the exposure must have occurred before that outcome. The concepts of induction and latency period take temporality one step further since there could still be a period of time after the exposure occurred during which it could not have plausibly caused the outcome. As an example, if a person smokes for the very first time on August 15 and receives a lung cancer diagnosis on August 20, it is nearly impossible for smoking to have caused their lung cancer since only 5 days passed between their first exposure and the occurrence of an outcome which typically takes a long time to develop.

## FIGURE 5.4 INDUCTION AND LATENCY PERIODS

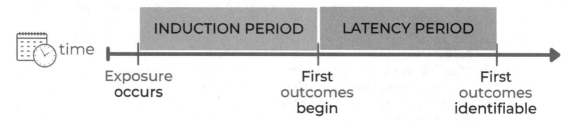

The **induction period** is the time it takes for an outcome to occur due to an exposure of interest. For example, the induction period between exposure to asbestos and pleural mesothelioma is thought to be around 25 years.[12] If a person developed pleural mesothelioma 6 months after first being exposed to asbestos, we would be suspicious about whether the asbestos exposure could have caused pleural mesothelioma since the outcome occurred well within the induction period. It is important to note that *outcomes* themselves do not have induction periods; induction periods are a function of the causal relationship between an exposure–outcome pair, reflecting the time between when a causal exposure occurs and the related outcome develops. Estimates of the induction periods for some exposure–outcome relationships may not be known, but can be reasonably estimated using what is known about disease etiology or explored using more advanced analytic techniques.

The **latency period** is the time during which an outcome exists but is not clinically or otherwise diagnostically detectable. The latency period for an outcome is a function of the state of existing diagnostic methods for the outcome of interest. For example, the latency period for diagnosis of HIV depends on the diagnostic test used: HIV genetic material can be detected via a nucleic acid amplification test (NAAT) within approximately 10 to 33 days of infection, HIV antigen can be detected via an antigen test within approximately 18 to 45 days of infection, and HIV antibodies can be detected via an antibody test within approximately 1 to 3 months of infection.[13]

Both induction and latency periods are important to consider when calculating measures of incidence (i.e., risk or rate) because they help define who is at-risk of developing the outcome *due to the exposure of interest*. If a study participant is not at-risk of developing the outcome due to the exposure measured in your study, then they should be excluded from the study's analysis.

## Pause to Practice 5.2

### Using Induction and Latency Periods to Define Who Is at Risk in Your Study

Use the information in **Figure 5.5** to answer the following questions.

1.  In *Panel A*, an outcome was *observed* among a member of the cohort during the induction period. Should that person be included in the calculations of risk or rate?

2.  In *Panel B*, an outcome was *detected* within the latency period. Should that person be included in the calculations of risk or rate?

**FIGURE 5.5 INDUCTION AND LATENCY PERIODS FOR OUTCOMES OCCURRING AT DIFFERENT TIMES DURING FOLLOW-UP**

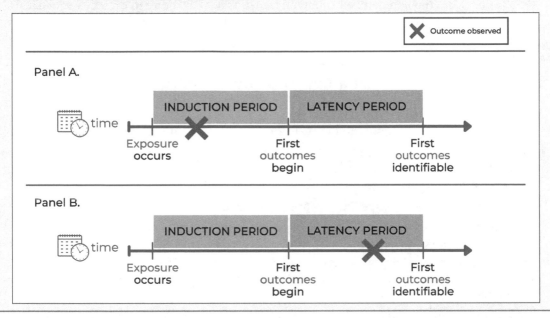

Induction and latency periods are important considerations for longitudinal studies such as cohort studies and controlled trials, because not all outcomes observed during the follow-up period should contribute to measures of incidence. It may be that outcomes that occur early in follow-up are not causally related to the exposure of interest that you measured. Alternatively, outcomes observed early in the follow-up period may have actually occurred prior to the start of your study, and simply weren't detectable until later. If the induction and latency periods for your outcome of interest are known, investigators may decide to exclude such cases. A related alternative is to exclude all outcomes that occurred within a particular time frame after follow-up starts.

### What Is the Incubation Period?

You may have heard the term ***incubation period***, which is reserved for infectious diseases and is defined as the time between when exposure to an infectious agent occurs and symptoms begin. For example, wildtype COVID-19 (i.e., the original strain that first emerged in 2019) has an incubation period up to 14 days (median 4 to 5 days)[13] and influenza has an incubation period ranging from 1 to 4 days.[14] Knowing the incubation period of infectious diseases can help investigators to estimate when people may become symptomatic (and possibly most infectious) during an outbreak, and it may also help to pinpoint the timing and/or source of an exposure. Importantly, people may pass on infectious diseases during the incubation period, before they even know they are sick.

## Pause to Practice 5.3

### Reference Groups and Induction and Latency Periods in the Health Professionals Follow-Up Study

1. Based on what you have learned, do you think this Health Professionals Follow-Up Study used internal, external, or general population reference groups?

2. As we have learned, it is important to consider induction and latency periods when calculating both risks and rates. The development of CHD occurs several years after exposure to nutritional risk factors. Think about the Health Professionals Follow-Up Study that we have been discussing. How should the induction and/or latency period be considered when determining who is at-risk for CHD due to dietary exposures?

## Highlights

### Use of Real-Time Versus Historical Cohort Data, Defining Reference Groups, Induction and Latency Periods

- Cohorts may be either conducted in real-time or by making use of historical data.
- In addition to thinking about the characteristics of the people who should comprise the **reference group**, there are different sources of comparison groups used in cohort studies: internal and external reference groups.
  - **Internal reference groups** are comprised of the unexposed members of the cohort.
  - **External reference groups** are comprised of unexposed individuals from some external group.
- Both **induction** and **latency periods** are important to consider when calculating risk or rate because they help define who is at-risk of developing the outcome *due to the exposure of interest*.
  - The **induction period** is the time it takes for an outcome to occur due to an exposure of interest.
  - The **latency period** is the time during which an outcome exists but is not clinically or otherwise diagnostically detectable.

## DATA LAYOUTS AND MEASURES OF FREQUENCY AND ASSOCIATION CALCULATED IN COHORT STUDIES

**Table 5.2** details the two different data layouts along with the measures of frequency and association commonly used in cohort studies, which are also summarized in **Table M.4**.

**TABLE 5.2 DATA LAYOUTS AND MEASURES OF OUTCOME FREQUENCY AND ASSOCIATION CALCULATED IN COHORT STUDIES**

| | Participants are followed until they either get the outcome or complete the same study follow-up time | Participants contribute different person-time during the study and outcome status is NOT known for everyone |
|---|---|---|
| **Data Layout (2×2 tables)** | <table><tr><td></td><td>Exposed (E+)</td><td>Unexposed (E−)</td><td>TOTAL</td></tr><tr><td>Outcome (O+)</td><td>A</td><td>B</td><td>$M_1$ (A+B)</td></tr><tr><td>No Outcome (O−)</td><td>C</td><td>D</td><td>$M_0$ (C+D)</td></tr><tr><td>TOTAL</td><td>$N_1$ (A+C)</td><td>$N_0$ (B+D)</td><td>N</td></tr></table> | <table><tr><td></td><td>Exposed (E+)</td><td>Unexposed (E−)</td><td>TOTAL</td></tr><tr><td>Outcome (O+)</td><td>A</td><td>B</td><td>$M_1$ (A+B)</td></tr><tr><td>Person-Time</td><td>$PT_1$</td><td>$PT_0$</td><td>$PT_{Total}$ ($PT_1$+$PT_0$)</td></tr></table> |
| **Measures of Outcome Frequency** | **Risk-Based Measures** <br><br> $Risk_{Cohort} = \dfrac{M_1}{N}$ <br><br> $Risk_{Exposed} = \dfrac{A}{N_1}$  $Risk_{Unexposed} = \dfrac{B}{N_0}$ | **Rate-Based Measures** <br><br> $Rate_{Cohort} = \dfrac{M_1}{PT_{Total}}$ <br><br> $Rate_{Exposed} = \dfrac{A}{PT_1}$  $Rate_{Unexposed} = \dfrac{B}{PT_0}$ |
| **Measures of Association and Interpretations** | **Risk Ratio (RR)**  $\left(\dfrac{A}{N_1}\right) / \left(\dfrac{B}{N_0}\right)$ <br><br> The [length of follow-up] risk of the outcome in the exposed is RR times the risk of the outcome in the unexposed. <br><br> **Risk Difference (RD)**  $\left(\dfrac{A}{N_1}\right) - \left(\dfrac{B}{N_0}\right)$ <br><br> The difference in the [length of follow-up] risk of the outcome in the exposed versus the unexposed is RD. | **Rate Ratio (IDR)**  $\left(\dfrac{A}{PT_1}\right) / \left(\dfrac{B}{PT_0}\right)$ <br><br> The rate of the outcome in the exposed is IDR times the rate of the outcome in the unexposed. <br><br> **Rate Difference (IDD)**  $\left(\dfrac{A}{PT_1}\right) - \left(\dfrac{B}{PT_0}\right)$ <br><br> The difference in the rate of the outcome in the exposed versus the unexposed is IDD. |

## Pause to Practice 5.4

### Data Analysis in the Health Professionals Follow-Up Study

Thus far, we have considered **dichotomous** (or **binary**) exposures, or those that are defined using only two levels: an exposed group and an unexposed reference group. Exposures can also be defined ordinally. An **ordinal** exposure is one with multiple levels which have a natural order, such as low, medium, and high. Data from the Health Professionals Follow-Up Study were used to evaluate whether higher red meat consumption was associated with a higher rate of CHD among men in the United States compared to those with lower red meat consumption.[10] Red meat consumption was categorized ordinally using quintiles (i.e., five evenly distributed, mutually exclusive categories). **Table 5.3** presents data on CHD diagnoses stratified by the ordinal categorization of the exposure.

1.  Rates of CHD in each quintile can be compared to rates within a specified reference group. What exposure level would you select as a reference group and why?

2.  Calculate the rate ratio that compares the incidence of CHD among men in the fifth quintile of red meat consumption to those in the first quintile.

3.  Write a one-sentence interpretation of the rate ratio. *Don't forget to provide details about your exposure and outcomes of interest.*

4. Calculate the rate ratio that compares the incidence of CHD among men in the fourth quintile of red meat consumption to those in the first quintile.

5. A summary of the findings for each quintile using the first quintile as the reference group is shown in **Table 5.4**. Compare the rate ratios. Is this trend what you would have expected? Why or why not?

6. The measures of association comparing the fourth, third, and second quintiles each to the first quintile are very similar. This may lead the investigators to consider dichotomizing the previous data, thereby "collapsing" or combining the data from quintiles 2–4 in order to create a dichotomous exposure as shown in **Table 5.5**. The rate ratio calculated from **Table 5.5** is 1.30. Use the data in the table to find this value.

**TABLE 5.3 DATA ON CORONARY HEART DISEASE DIAGNOSES STRATIFIED BY ORDINAL CATEGORIZATION OF RED MEAT CONSUMPTION**

| | Fifth Quintile* | Fourth Quintile | Third Quintile | Second Quintile | First Quintile** | TOTAL |
|---|---|---|---|---|---|---|
| CHD Diagnosis (O+) | 1,087 | 865 | 859 | 833 | 811 | 4,455 |
| Person–Years (PY) | 204,079 | 206,087 | 203,718 | 206,108 | 203,879 | 1,023,871 |

*Highest Quintile of Red Meat Consumption
**Lowest Quintile of Red Meat Consumption
CHD, coronary heart disease.
*Source*: Data from Al-Shaar L, Satija A, Wang DD, et al. Red meat intake and risk of coronary heart disease among US men: prospective cohort study. *BMJ*. 2020;371:m4141. Published 2020 Dec 2. https://doi.org/10.1136/bmj.m4141

**TABLE 5.4 ASSOCIATIONS BETWEEN QUINTILES OF RED MEAT CONSUMPTION AND CORONARY HEART DISEASE**

| Quintiles Compared | Rate Ratio |
|---|---|
| 5 vs. 1 | 1.34 |
| 4 vs. 1 | 1.06 |
| 3 vs. 1 | 1.06 |
| 2 vs. 1 | 1.02 |

**TABLE 5.5 DATA ON CORONARY HEART DISEASE DIAGNOSES STRATIFIED BY DICHOTOMOUS CATEGORIZATION OF RED MEAT CONSUMPTION**

| | High Red Meat Consumption *Highest Quintile* (E+) | Low Red Meat Consumption *Lowest Four Quintiles Combined* (E−) | TOTAL |
|---|---|---|---|
| CHD Diagnosis (O+) | 1,087 | 3,368 | 4,455 |
| Person–Years (PY) | 204,079 | 819,792 | 1,023,871 |

CHD, coronary heart disease.
*Source*: Data from Al-Shaar L, Satija A, Wang DD, et al. Red meat intake and risk of coronary heart disease among US men: prospective cohort study. *BMJ*. 2020;371:m4141. Published 2020 Dec 2. https://doi.org/10.1136/bmj.m4141

## Digging Deeper

### Analysis of Time-Varying Exposures

It may be the case that individuals' exposure statuses change during the course of a longitudinal study. For example, over a long follow-up period, a person's weight may change appreciably and meaningfully for a given research question. Thus, it may be important to not only measure study participants' weight at enrollment, but also at regular intervals throughout the study period. The effects of such **time-varying exposures** can be analyzed using person-time denominators with advanced statistical methods which are beyond the scope of this textbook.[15]

### Reporting Study Findings From Cohort Studies: The STROBE Statement

All study designs, whether experimental or observational, have standard reporting guidance. Many journals require investigators to use the **STROBE Statement** (STrengthening the Reporting of OBservational studies in Epidemiology) when presenting results from an observational study, including cohort studies.[16] The STROBE Statement is an evidence-based, minimum set of recommendations for reporting of observational studies. The statement consists of a checklist with items related to study design, analysis, and interpretation. Select items that are specific to the reporting of cohort studies. Include:

- "[E]ligibility criteria, and the sources and methods of selection of participants. Describe methods of follow up…
- …If applicable, explain how loss to follow-up was addressed…
- …Summarize follow-up time (e.g., average and total amount)…
- …Report numbers of outcome events or summary measures over time."

## STRENGTHS AND LIMITATIONS OF COHORT STUDIES
### (LEARNING OBJECTIVE 5.6)

### Strengths of Cohort Studies

**Temporality.** Given that the exposure status is observed and/or recorded prior to the occurrence of the outcome, the **temporality** between the exposure and outcome is established by the cohort design. As we discussed in **Chapter 3, "Introduction to Analytic Epidemiologic Study Designs and Measures of Association,"** temporality is a core tenet of causality (e.g., for the exposure to have caused the outcome, The exposure must have occurred before the outcome). As you will later see, this contrasts with other study designs which do not establish temporality between the exposure and outcome by design.

**Study of rare exposures.** Since investigators have the option to conduct a special exposure cohort study whereby individuals are selected on the basis of a shared exposure status, cohort studies are relatively well-suited for studying rare exposures, or exposures that would occur infrequently in the general population. As you will later see, there are some study designs that are not suitable for the study of rare exposures.

**Study of several outcomes.** Cohort studies allow study of associations between multiple exposures on several outcomes, allowing researchers to test multiple hypotheses.

**Calculation of measures of outcome frequency.** Cohort studies allow investigators to calculate the risk or rate of the health outcome(s) under study (in addition to the related measures of association). As you will soon learn in **Chapter 6, "Case-Control Designs,"** this is in contrast to case-control studies, which do not allow the direct calculation of measures of outcome frequency. Thus, cohort studies provide information on the risk or rate of outcomes to allow researchers to better understand changes in outcome frequency over time, including disease progression and the natural history of diseases.

### Limitations of Cohort Studies

**Loss to follow-up.** As with all longitudinal studies, or those that involve tracking participants over time, there is the potential for loss to follow-up. This can be a problem if those who are lost are different from those who stay in the study in important ways. This can lead to a phenomenon called **selection bias**, which will be discussed in detail in **Chapter 10, "Selection Bias."**

**Study of rare outcomes.** If the outcome of interest is rare, investigators may not observe enough individuals with the outcome(s) of interest to be able to detect differences in their occurrence across the exposure groups.

**Study of exposure–outcomes relationships with long induction periods or outcomes with long latency periods.** Similarly, longitudinal studies like cohorts may not be well-suited to study exposure–outcome relationships that have long induction periods or outcomes with long latency periods. If the induction and/or latency periods are long, investigators would have to wait a long time to accrue enough outcomes to be able to draw conclusions. Further, the longer the follow-up period, the more likely it is that participants will be lost to follow-up.

**Logistics.** Cohort studies, particularly those conducted in real-time, can be expensive, time-consuming, and resource intensive.

## Pause to Practice 5.5

### Strengths and Limitations of the Health Professionals Follow-Up Study

1.  What are some strengths of collecting data in real-time in the Health Professionals Follow-Up Study (relative to using historical data)?

2.  What are some limitations of collecting data in real-time in the Health Professionals Follow-Up Study (relative to using historical data)?

## Highlights

### Measures of Frequency and Association in Cohorts, Strengths, and Limitations

- Measures of frequency that may be calculated in cohort studies include risks and rates.
- Measures of association that may be calculated in cohort studies include risk- and rate-based measures of association.
- Main strengths and limitations of controlled trials include:
  - **Strengths**: clear temporality between exposure and outcome, ability to study rare exposures, ability to study several outcomes, and calculation of measures of outcome frequency
  - **Limitations**: potential for loss to follow-up, difficult to study rare outcomes or outcomes with long latency periods, and complicated logistics

## WHERE WE'VE BEEN AND WHAT'S UP NEXT

Cohort studies are often viewed as a very robust observational study design. However, as we note, it is not well-suited for all research questions. Up next, in **Chapter 6, "Case-Control Designs,"** you will learn about case-control studies, another observational design with strengths that complement the limitations of the cohort design. After that, we conclude our discussion of epidemiologic study designs with cross-sectional studies (**Chapter 7, "Cross-Sectional Designs"**). You will see that each study design has its own strengths and limitations, and you will be able to view those relative to the other designs.

# END OF CHAPTER PROBLEM SET

Assume you conducted a cohort study to explore multiple exposures (e.g., participant demographics, behaviors, and clinical factors) associated with incident HIV infections. Participants were enrolled over a 2-year period and were allowed to leave and re-enter the cohort. Exposures of interest are measured at study enrollment and participants are followed over several years to observe new cases of the outcome. In your study population, HIV is relatively rare (12.6/100,000 people).

1. Does this study design make use of historical data, or are the investigators collecting new data?

2. Is this an open or closed cohort study?

3. Which of the following are true for a cohort study that has a relatively long follow-up period? *Select all that apply.*
   a. Participants are more likely to experience competing risks over longer follow-up periods.
   b. Participants are more likely to be lost to follow-up over longer follow-up periods.
   c. A valid measure of association cannot be calculated.

4. Given your answers to Questions 2 and 3, what measure(s) of association do you think should be calculated in this study? Provide at least two reasons why you chose the measure(s) that you did.

## Questions 5 and 6 refer to the following description and Figure 5.6.

Recall that the *latency period* is the time during which an outcome exists but is not clinically or diagnostically detectable. Thus, the latency period for a given outcome will depend on the diagnostic methods used. For HIV, there is a 1- to 3-month latency period between infection with the virus and development of enough antibodies to be detectable (see Figure 5.6).

## FIGURE 5.6 LATENCY PERIOD FOR DETECTION OF HIV ANTIBODIES

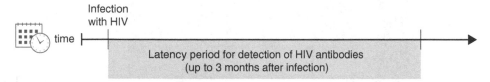

5. Recall that all individuals included in a cohort study should be at-risk for the outcome of interest at the time that they are enrolled. Would you have concerns about how the latency period could affect the eligibility of a study participant who...
   • tested negative for HIV antibodies at study enrollment, and after three months of follow-up, *and*
   • tested positive for HIV antibodies after 6 months of follow-up?

6. Would you have concerns about how the latency period could affect the eligibility of a study participant who...
   • tested negative for HIV antibodies at study enrollment, and
   • tested positive for HIV antibodies after 2 months of follow-up?

7. Refer to Figure 5.7. Recall that the induction period is the time it takes for an outcome to occur after and due to an exposure. Suppose we conduct a cohort study in real-time to explore whether exposure to extremely high levels of radiation is associated with leukemia. Assume that it is estimated that the induction period for this relationship is 10 years. If someone develops leukemia on the day after the high-level radiation exposure occurs, should they be included in the study?

## FIGURE 5.7 INDUCTION PERIOD FOR DEVELOPMENT OF LEUKEMIA DUE TO EXPOSURE TO HIGH LEVELS OF RADIATION

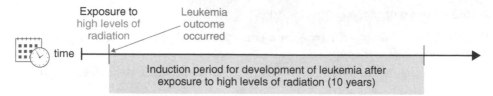

### Questions 8 to 10 refer to the following description and Figure 5.8.

Questions 8 to 10 will help you explore what happens analytically when induction (or latency) periods are not considered. Assume that it takes 10 years for leukemia to develop after high-level radiation exposure which occurred at enrollment and assume that leukemia is immediately detectable upon development of disease (no latency period).

8. Use the data presented in Figure 5.8 to calculate the rate ratio with NO consideration of the induction period (i.e., without excluding the outcome occurring during the induction period).

## FIGURE 5.8 STUDY DATA TO EVALUATE THE ASSOCIATION BETWEEN HIGH-LEVEL RADIATION AND LEUKEMIA

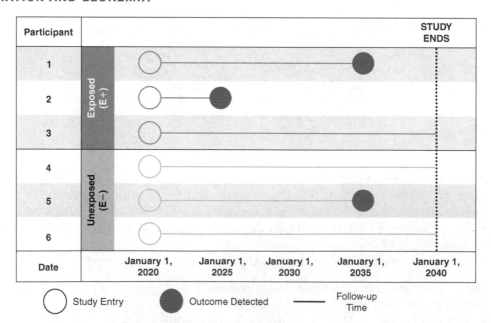

9. Use the data presented in **Figure** 5.8 to calculate the rate ratio WITH consideration of the induction period (i.e., excluding the outcome occurring during the induction period).

10. Compare your answers to Questions 8 and 9. How did the (inappropriate) inclusion of an outcome occurring in the induction period influence your results?

# REFERENCES

1. Tsao CW, Vasan RS. Cohort profile: the Framingham Heart Study (FHS): overview of milestones in cardiovascular epidemiology. *Int J Epidemiol*. 2015;44(6):1800–1813. https://doi.org/10.1093/ije/dyv337

2. Black Women's Health Study. About the Black Women's Health Study. 2022. https://www.bu.edu/bwhs

3. Colditz GA, Hankinson SE. The Nurses' Health Study: lifestyle and health among women. *Nat Rev Cancer*. 2005;5(5):388–396. https://doi.org/10.1038/nrc1608

4. Health H.T.C.S.o.P. Health Professionals Follow-Up Study. 2023. https://www.hsph.harvard.edu/hpfsni

5. Schüz J, Bukhtiyarov I, Olsson A, et al. Occupational cohort study of current and former workers exposed to chrysotile in mine and processing facilities in Asbest, the Russian Federation: cohort profile of the Asbest Chrysotile Cohort Study. *PLoS ONE*. 2020;15(7):e0236475. https://doi.org/10.1371/journal.pone.0236475

6. Lash T, VanderWeele TJ, Haneuse S, Rothman KJ. Measures of occurrence. In: Lash T, VanderWeele TJ, Haneuse S, Rothman KJ, eds. *Modern Epidemiology*. 4th ed. Wolters Kluwer; 2021:69.

7. Vandenbroucke JP. Prospective or retrospective: what's in a name? *BMJ*. 1991;302(6771):249–250. https://doi.org/10.1136/bmj.302.6771.249

8. Rothman KJ, Greenland S, Lash TL. *Modern Epidemiology*. 3rd ed. Wolters Kluwer Health/Lippincott Williams & Wilkins; 2008.

9. de Blok CJM, Wiepjes CM, Nota NM, et al. Breast cancer risk in transgender people receiving hormone treatment: nationwide cohort study in the Netherlands. *BMJ*. 2019;365:l1652. https://doi.org/10.1136/bmj.l1652

10. Al-Shaar L, Satija A, Wang DD, et al. Red meat intake and risk of coronary heart disease among US men: prospective cohort study. *BMJ*. 2020;371:m4141. https://doi.org/10.1136/bmj.m4141

11. Henning MA, Krägeloh CU, Hawken SJ, Zhao Y, Doherty I. The quality of life of medical students studying in New Zealand: a comparison with nonmedical students and a general population reference group. *Teach Learn Med*. 2012;24(4):334–340. https://doi.org/10.1080/10401334.2012.715261

12. Nurminen M, Karjalainen A, Takahashi K. Estimating the induction period of pleural mesothelioma from aggregate data on asbestos consumption. *J Occup Environ Med*. 2003;45(10):1107–1115. https://doi.org/10.1097/01.jom.0000091682.95314.01

13. Centers for Disease Control and Prevention. Clinical care considerations: clinical considerations for care of children and adults with confirmed COVID-19. January 27, 2023. https://www.cdc.gov/hiv/basics/hiv-testing/hiv-window-period.html#:~:text=A%20rapid%20antigen%2Fantibody%20test,to%2045%20days%20after%20exposure

14. Centers for Disease Control and Prevention. How flu spreads. 2018. https://www.cdc.gov/flu/about/disease/spread.htm

15. Robins JM, Hernan MA. Estimation of the causal effects of time-varying exposures. In: Fitzmaurice G, Davidian M, Laird NM, Ware JH, eds. *Longitudinal Data Analysis*. Taylor & Francis; 2009:553–599.

16. STROBE. What is STROBE. 2021. https://www.strobe-statement.org/checklists/

# CHAPTER 6

# CASE-CONTROL DESIGNS

## KEY TERMS

case-control design          matching                    source population
exposure odds ratio          observational studies

## LEARNING OBJECTIVES

6.1   Describe the basic design features of a case-control study.
6.2   Identify the source population in a case-control study.
6.3   Derive the formula for and correctly calculate and interpret the exposure odds ratio.
6.4   Explain why investigators cannot calculate the frequency of the outcome using 2×2 data from a case-control study.
6.5   Define and distinguish between primary- and secondary-base case-control studies.
6.6   Describe strategies for identifying cases.
6.7   Define and differentiate between incident and prevalent cases.
6.8   Describe strategies for identifying controls.
6.9   Describe how and why matching is used in a case-control study and how to calculate a pair-matched odds ratio.
6.10  Describe the strengths and limitations of case-control designs.

## EVERY DATA POINT TELLS A STORY

A couple arrives for their 38-week prenatal care visit. Despite some morning sickness early on, the pregnancy has been uncomplicated, and they eagerly await the arrival of their first child. The routine is familiar. The nurse requests a urine specimen, takes weight and blood pressure measurements, and they are walked to the exam room where they will wait for the obstetrician. It is at this point that things take an unexpected turn—when the doctor checks for the baby's heartbeat, the steady rhythm they've come to expect is replaced with static. Certain that the baby is simply awkwardly positioned, the obstetrician sends them for an ultrasound. In this room, the parents hear eight words that will shatter their world: *I am so sorry, there is no heartbeat*. The baby they longed for has died.

The news comes suddenly and brutally. How is this possible? No one had ever hinted that their pregnancy journey could end this way.

Stillbirth, defined in the United States as a pregnancy loss occurring at 20 weeks' gestation or later, is far more common in the United States than it should be, with over 21,000 families experiencing a loss each year.[1] However, from an epidemiologic standpoint, stillbirths are too rare of an outcome to reasonably study using a cohort design. With approximately 3.6 million annual births in the United States, this averages to approximately one stillbirth in every 170 deliveries. To study stillbirth using a cohort design, we would need to enroll a group of at least 17,000 pregnant people in order to end up with just 100 stillbirths. You'll learn more about the importance of having an adequate sample size in **Chapter 12, "Random Error in Epidemiologic Research,"** but suffice to say, this is not a practical design approach for studying the causes of stillbirth. Luckily, the case-control design provides the alternative that we need.

*It can be easy to get caught up in the details of each study design or their related analyses. However, we must remember that every number in our datasets represents an individual, each with their own story. The work that we do as epidemiologists has the potential to impact lives in immeasurable ways that we cannot imagine and will never know.*

---

When an exposure cannot be randomized, we now know that we can use a cohort design to study the association between that exposure and a health outcome. However, as we learned in **Chapter 5, "Cohort Designs,"** cohort designs have an important limitation in that they are not efficient for the study of rare outcomes or outcomes with long induction or latency periods. Fortunately, the **case-control design** provides an alternative observational design for the study of such outcomes. As you will learn, the case-control design is also useful for outbreak investigations since the outcomes have already occurred.

While case-control studies are a very useful tool to have in our epidemiologic toolbox, conceptually, they are less straightforward than any of the other observational designs. As you'll see throughout this chapter, it can be complicated to conceptualize the context in which a case-control study is occurring. Once you can grasp the premise underlying the case-control design, you will see their great utility, particularly since they can typically yield results quicker and at a lower cost relative to the cohort design.

## CASE-CONTROL STUDY DESIGN BASICS (LEARNING OBJECTIVES 6.1 & 6.2)

Review Figure 6.1, which provides a schematic of the case-control design that you were introduced to in **Chapter 3, "Introduction to Analytic Epidemiologic Study Designs and Measures of Association."** Recall that in a case-control design, investigators identify **cases**, or individuals with the health outcome of interest, and compare them to a suitable group of individuals *without* the outcome, called the **controls**. The purpose of the control group is to provide an estimate of the **frequency of the exposure(s) of interest** in the **source population**, or the population from which the cases came (sometimes referred to as the *population that gave rise to the cases*). As we will discuss later, the conceptualization of the source population is crucial for the success of a case-control study. At this stage, it is important to recognize that a case-control study must be envisioned as occurring within some defined source population. As an example, if investigators were studying stillbirth in the United States, the source population would be all U.S. pregnancies that made it to at least 20 weeks' gestation. If studying nosocomial infections (i.e., infections which occur within health facilities) in China, the source population would be all patients in health facilities in China.

## FIGURE 6.1 SCHEMATIC OF A CASE-CONTROL DESIGN

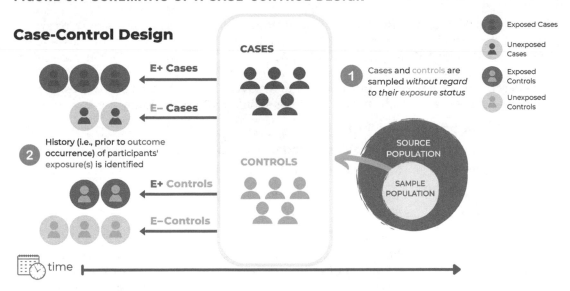

In a case-control study, the cases and controls comprise the **sample** population (also called the **study population)**. Once the sample has been identified, investigators ascertain the *history* of any exposures of interest among the cases and controls to determine whether there is a difference in the frequency of these exposures across these two groups. As we will describe in more detail in the text that follows, while the case-control design allows investigators to calculate a measure of association describing the relationship between an exposure and an outcome, this design cannot be used to calculate a measure of the *frequency* of the outcome.

Now consider **Table 6.1**, which provides a more detailed view of the basic steps involved in conducting a case-control study, including formulating a research question, designing and conducting the study, and analyzing and reporting the data. Each of the blue terms in **Table 6.1** will be discussed throughout this chapter.

### TABLE 6.1 BASIC STEPS IN DESIGNING AND CONDUCTING A CASE-CONTROL STUDY

| **State the Research Question** |
| --- |
| State the study hypothesis(es) based on the research question. <br> • Define outcome(s) with case definitions. <br> • Define the exposure and reference group. |
| **Design the Case-Control Study** |
| Determine whether you will conduct a primary or secondary-base case-control study. <br><br> Identify the sample population from the source population. <br> • Decide on a strategy to identify cases. <br> • Decide on a strategy to identify controls. <br><br> Decide whether you want to conduct matching. |
| **Conduct the Case-Control Study** |
| Select cases and controls, obtain informed consent, and measure the past exposure status of the participants. <br> Collect data on key covariates. |
| **Analyze and Report Data** |
| Calculate measures of association (and conduct a matched analysis, if appropriate). <br> Report findings using the STROBE reporting guidance. <br> Consider the strengths and limitations of the study. |

# DEVELOPING A HYPOTHESIS

The case-control design is used when investigators are interested in studying a particular health outcome and wish to identify the cause(s) of that outcome. Often, the case-control design is used to investigate the source of an outbreak or to identify risk factors for a health outcome that is rare or has a long latency or induction period.

As described in **Chapter 3, "Introduction to Analytic Epidemiologic Study Designs and Measures of Association,"** all study hypotheses should address the following key areas:

- What is the population of interest?
- What is the heath outcome of interest and how is it defined?
- What is the exposure of interest and how is it defined?
- What measures of frequency are being compared?
- What is the direction of the hypothesized association?

When developing a hypothesis for a case-control study, investigators begin with a case definition which details who is eligible for enrollment as a case in the study. As discussed in **Chapter 2, "Descriptive Epidemiology, Surveillance, and Measures of Frequency,"** the case definition should be as rigorous as possible and should align with a generally accepted definition of the outcome.

Once the health outcome has been identified and a case definition has been established, investigators must identify and define their exposure(s) of interest. A case-control design is a bit like detective work: investigators are trying to solve the mystery of *why* an outcome has occurred, and thus will often consider several different exposures in order to identify which may be the culprit(s). Exposures that are considered in a case-control design should be factors that could plausibly be linked to the outcome of interest. As with defining the outcome, investigators should be as rigorous as possible when defining their exposure(s) of interest and should use definitions that are consistent with previous literature.

For example, after receiving notifications of 31 cases of *Salmonella* Havana, a bacterial disease that infects the intestinal tract, investigators undertook a case-control study in South Australia to identify the source of the outbreak.[2] Cases were defined using a **gold standard** case definition as individuals with a laboratory-confirmed case of *S.* Havana reported to the Communicable Disease Control Branch in South Australia between June 1 and June 20, 2018. Salmonella infection, also called salmonellosis, is mostly attributable to consumption of contaminated water or food, including raw meat, poultry, seafood, eggs, and select fruits and vegetables. To narrow down the list of potential foods that may have caused the outbreak, investigators conducted hypothesis-generating interviews with the cases to learn about where they had been and what they had eaten 7 days prior to their illness. Foods that were identified during these interviews, such as eggs, almonds, lettuce, alfalfa sprouts, and broccoli, were then considered as potential exposures in the case-control study.

## Gold Standard

The term *gold standard* is often used in epidemiology to describe a measurement method that is widely accepted as being the best or most reliable way to measure an exposure or health outcome.

In the *S.* Havana outbreak, investigators could have considered identifying cases by asking residents of South Australia if they recently reported having symptoms consistent with the infection (e.g., diarrhea, fever, and stomach cramps). This could be problematic because they might accidentally miss some asymptomatic people who really did have *S.* Havana, or they might accidentally include some people as having *S.* Havana when they really didn't. By incorporating gold standard laboratory confirmation in their case definition, the investigators could feel confident that those who were included as cases truly had *S.* Havana.

The term *gold standard* will return when we discuss the importance of accurate measurement of both exposures and health outcomes in detail in **Chapter 11, "Information Bias and Screening and Diagnostic Tests."**

## Pause to Practice 6.1

### Identifying Study Exposure, Outcome, and Source Population in a Case-Control Study

Let's return to the example introduced in **Chapter 3, "Introduction to Analytic Epidemiologic Study Designs and Measures of Association,"** which described a case-control study of stillbirth.[3] The case-control design is ideal for studying stillbirth since it only occurs in approximately one in every 170 deliveries in the United States.[4]

This particular study was conducted by the Stillbirth Collaborative Research Network, with the goal of identifying risk factors for stillbirth using information known at the time of pregnancy confirmation. Before enrolling participants in the study, investigators identified five distinct geographic areas, called catchment areas, from which study participants would be selected. They then selected all stillbirths (pregnancy losses occurring at 20 weeks' gestation or later) and a sample of livebirths born to residents of those geographic areas. Investigators then reviewed their medical records and administered questionnaires to see whether there were any factors (e.g., age at conception, obesity/overweight, smoking prior to pregnancy) that were associated with stillbirth.[3,5]

1. What is the outcome and how is it defined?
2. What is (are) the exposure(s) of interest?
3. What is the source population?

## DATA LAYOUT AND MEASURE OF ASSOCIATION CALCULATED IN CASE-CONTROL STUDIES

Before jumping into the details about the identification of study participants, we will revisit the case-control data layout and analysis that you learned in **Chapter 3, "Introduction to Analytic Epidemiologic Study Designs and Measures of Association."** This will help motivate why careful selection of cases and controls is so important, and also provide a more detailed explanation for why we cannot estimate the frequency of the *outcome* using case-control data.

As summarized in **Table 6.2** and **Table M.4**, data for a case-control design can be organized using a traditional 2×2 table, where a number of study participants are organized by their exposure and outcome statuses. Recall that the measure of association calculated using data from a case-control design is the **exposure odds ratio** (EOR), a measure that compares the frequency of the exposure in cases to the frequency of that exposure in controls.

### How Do You Derive the Exposure Odds Ratio? (LEARNING OBJECTIVE 6.3)

In **Chapter 3, "Introduction to Analytic Epidemiologic Study Designs and Measures of Association,"** we introduced the following formula for calculating the exposure odds ratio:

$$\text{Exposure odds ratio (EOR)} = \frac{A/B}{C/D} \qquad (6.1)$$

**TABLE 6.2 DATA LAYOUT AND MEASURES OF FREQUENCY AND ASSOCIATION FOR CASE-CONTROL STUDIES**

| Data Layout | | Exposed (E+) | Unexposed (E−) | TOTAL |
|---|---|---|---|---|
| | Cases | A | B | $M_1$ (A+B) |
| | Controls | C | D | $M_0$ (C+D) |

| Measure of Outcome Frequency | None |
|---|---|
| Measure of Exposure Frequency[a] | Odds of **exposure** among cases $= \dfrac{A/M_1}{B/M_1} = \dfrac{A}{B}$ <br><br> Odds of exposure among controls $= \dfrac{C/M_0}{D/M_0} = \dfrac{C}{D}$ |
| Measure of Association and Interpretation | Exposure odds ratio $= \dfrac{\text{Odds of exposure among cases}}{\text{Odds of exposure among controls}} = \dfrac{A/B}{C/D} = \dfrac{A \times D}{B \times C}$ <br><br> The odds of exposure among cases are [insert value for **EOR**] times the odds of exposure among controls. |

EOR, exposure odds ratio.

[a]Note that measures of exposure frequency are not typically reported in a case-control study. Rather, they are a required step to calculate the measure of association.

This formula simplifies to what epidemiologists sometimes refer to as the **cross-product**, calculated as:

$$\text{Exposure odds ratio (EOR)} = \frac{A \times D}{B \times C} \tag{6.2}$$

Let's spend some time to understand where the exposure odds ratio comes from.

Thinking back to the detective analogy that we used earlier, the case-control design allows investigators to learn which exposure(s) may be causing a particular health outcome. They begin looking for clues among a group of people who *have* that outcome of interest and collect information about their past exposures. In the case of the S. Havana outbreak investigation, investigators learned that of the 18 cases, six (33%) had eaten alfalfa sprouts and eight (44%) had eaten almonds in the 7 days prior to their illness.[2] At this stage, we don't have enough information to know whether either of these foods led to the outbreak. To make this determination, we need to know how common eating alfalfa sprouts and almonds were among the general population in South Australia (for this study, that was the source population from which the cases arose). If people who were sick were *more likely* to have eaten almonds compared to the general population, this is a clue that almonds may have caused the outbreak.

In the case-control design, the purpose of the *cases* is to provide an estimate of how common the exposure was *among those with the outcome of interest in the source population*. The purpose of the *control group* is to provide a comparison: specifically, an estimate of the frequency of the exposure *in the source population*, or the population from which the cases came.

To motivate the derivation of the exposure odds ratio, we begin by examining the probability (here, the frequency) of the exposure among the cases and the probability of the exposure among the controls. These probabilities are calculated by dividing the number of exposed individuals in each group by their corresponding total, as shown in **Equations 6.3** and **6.4**. These measures correspond to the proportion of the cases and controls who were exposed, respectively.

$$\text{Probability of exposure among } cases = p_{\text{cases}} = \frac{A}{M_1} \tag{6.3}$$

$$\text{Probability of exposure among } controls = p_{\textbf{controls}} = \frac{C}{M_0} \qquad (6.4)$$

For the S. Havana outbreak investigation, we already know these values for our cases:

$$\text{Probability of eating alfalfa sprouts among } cases = \frac{6}{18} = 33\%$$

$$\text{Probability of eating almonds among } cases = \frac{8}{18} = 44\%$$

Of course, we need comparison information from a control group. In the S. Havana outbreak, investigators identified 54 controls, and found that only one of them had recently eaten alfalfa sprouts, while 24 had recently eaten almonds.[2] The probability of each exposure among the controls is thus calculated as follows:

$$\text{Probability of eating alfalfa sprouts among } controls = \frac{1}{54} = 2\%$$

$$\text{Probability of eating almonds among } controls = \frac{24}{54} = 44\%$$

The probabilities of exposure are then transformed into the **odds** of exposure. The odds is a measure of frequency that describes the probability of an event occurring (denoted as $p$) divided by the probability of that event *not* occurring (denoted as $1-p$). The general formula for the odds is shown in **Equation 6.5**.

$$\text{Odds} = \frac{\text{Probability of an event occurring}}{\text{Probability of an event NOT occurring}} = \frac{p}{1-p} \qquad (6.5)$$

We can use the probabilities of exposure shown in **Equations 6.3** and **6.4** to calculate the odds of exposure among cases and controls as shown in **Equations 6.6** and **6.7**, respectively.

$$\text{Odds of } exposure \text{ among } cases = \frac{\text{Probability of being } exposed \text{ among } cases}{\text{Probability of being } unexposed \text{ among } cases} \qquad (6.6)$$

$$= \frac{p_{\textbf{cases}}}{1-p_{\textbf{cases}}} = \frac{A/M_1}{B/M_1} = \frac{A}{B}$$

$$\text{Odds of } exposure \text{ among } controls = \frac{\text{Probability of being } exposed \text{ among } controls}{\text{Probability of being } unexposed \text{ among } controls} \qquad (6.7)$$

$$= \frac{p_{\textbf{controls}}}{1-p_{\textbf{controls}}} = \frac{C/M_0}{D/M_0} = \frac{C}{D}$$

Data for the investigation of the associations between eating alfalfa sprouts and almonds and salmonellosis are summarized in **Table 6.3**. We can use this information to calculate the odds of each exposure (eating alfalfa sprouts and almonds) for cases and controls as follows:

$$\text{Odds of } eating\ alfalfa\ sprouts \text{ among } cases = \frac{6/18}{1-6/18} = \frac{6/18}{12/18} = \frac{6}{12}$$

$$\text{Odds of } eating\ alfalfa\ sprouts \text{ among } controls = \frac{1/54}{1-1/54} = \frac{1/54}{53/54} = \frac{1}{53}$$

$$\text{Odds of } eating\ almonds \text{ among } cases = \frac{8/18}{1-8/18} = \frac{8/18}{10/18} = \frac{8}{10}$$

$$\text{Odds of } eating\ almonds \text{ among } controls = \frac{24/54}{1-24/54} = \frac{24/54}{30/54} = \frac{24}{30}$$

**TABLE 6.3 DATA LAYOUT AND MEASURES OF FREQUENCY AND ASSOCIATION FOR THE *SALMONELLA* HAVANA OUTBREAK INVESTIGATION OF ALFALFA SPROUTS AND ALMONDS**

| | Association Between Alfalfa Sprout Consumption and Salmonellosis | | | | Association Between Almond Consumption and Salmonellosis | | | |
|---|---|---|---|---|---|---|---|---|
| **Data Layout** | | Exposed (Ate alfalfa sprouts) (E+) | Unexposed (Did not eat alfalfa sprouts) (E−) | TOTAL | | Exposed (Ate almonds) (E+) | Unexposed (Did not eat almonds) (E−) | TOTAL |
| | Cases | 6 | 12 | 18 | Cases | 8 | 10 | 18 |
| | Controls | 1 | 53 | 54 | Controls | 24 | 30 | 54 |
| **Measures of Exposure Frequency** | Odds of eating alfalfa sprouts among cases $= \dfrac{6/18}{12/18} = \dfrac{6}{12}$  Odds of eating alfalfa sprouts among controls $= \dfrac{1/54}{53/54} = \dfrac{1}{53}$ | | | | Odds of eating almonds among cases $= \dfrac{8/18}{10/18} = \dfrac{8}{10}$  Odds of eating almonds among controls $= \dfrac{24/54}{30/54} = \dfrac{24}{30}$ | | | |
| **Measure of Association and Interpretation** | $\text{EOR}_{\text{alfalfa sprouts}} = \dfrac{6/12}{1/53} = \dfrac{6\times53}{12\times1} = 26.5$  The odds of eating alfalfa sprouts among those with salmonellosis were 26.5 times the odds of eating alfalfa sprouts among controls. | | | | $\text{EOR}_{\text{almonds}} = \dfrac{8/10}{24/30} = \dfrac{8\times30}{10\times24} = 1.0$  The odds of eating almonds among those with salmonellosis were 1.0 times the odds of eating almonds among controls. | | | |

## The Odds Are Odd

Odds are an unusual measure that can take some time to wrap your mind around. Odds are defined as the probability of an event *happening* divided by the probability of that event *not happening*.

A common application of odds is in the context of sports betting, where the "event" is, perhaps counterintuitively, *losing* the game. Thus, the *greater* the odds, the *more* likely it is that a particular team will lose. The odds in sports are often described as "X to 1"; this means that a person can expect to win $X for every $1 that they wager. Thus, the higher the odds are, the less likely a team is to win, *but* the greater the payout will be.

When calculating odds, here are some tips to help you check your work:

• Since probabilities are bound between 0 and 1, the odds can never be negative.

• The numerator and the denominator of an odds expressed as a fraction should always sum to 1.

As its name suggests, the exposure odds ratio is calculated by taking the ratio of the (odds of exposure among cases) and the (odds of exposure among controls), as shown in **Equation 6.1**, which is equivalent to the cross-product formula shown in **Equation 6.2**.

$$\text{Exposure odds ratio (EOR)} = \frac{A/B}{C/D} = \frac{A\times D}{B\times C}$$

The exposure odds ratios that quantify the association between eating alfalfa sprouts and salmonellosis, as well as between eating almonds and salmonellosis, are thus calculated as follows:

$$\text{EOR}_{\text{alfalfa sprouts}} = \frac{\text{Odds of eating alfalfa sprouts among cases}}{\text{Odds of eating alfalfa sprouts among controls}} = \frac{6/12}{1/53} = \frac{6 \times 53}{12 \times 1} = 26.5$$

$$\text{EOR}_{\text{almonds}} = \frac{\text{Odds of eating almonds among cases}}{\text{Odds of eating almonds among controls}} = \frac{8/10}{24/30} = \frac{8 \times 30}{10 \times 24} = 1.0$$

Recall from **Chapter 3, "Introduction to Analytic Epidemiologic Study Designs and Measures of Association,"** that the null value for a ratio measure of association is 1, which signals that there is no association between the exposure and outcome. With an exposure odds ratio of 1, the data suggest that almonds were unlikely to be the source of the outbreak. However, with an exposure odds ratio of 26.5, there is strong evidence that alfalfa sprouts contributed to the *S.* Havana outbreak.

## Compared to What?

At first glance, you may have thought that almonds were likely to be the source of the *S.* Havana outbreak since more cases reported eating almonds (44%) than alfalfa sprouts (33%). However, we didn't have enough information at that stage to know how the consumption of almonds and alfalfa sprouts among those with salmonellosis compared to consumption among the source population (which in this study was the general population of South Australia).

Once we compared the frequency of the consumption of these foods in those with salmonellosis to the controls, we saw that both groups had the same frequency of consumption of almonds (44%); however, the consumption of alfalfa sprouts was much more common among cases than controls (33% vs. 2%, respectively).

Remember that when evaluating the potential link between an exposure and an outcome, you must always ask yourself: *compared to what?* In this case, we wanted to know how the consumption of certain foods among those with salmonellosis compared to the consumption among a sample of people from the source population. Without this comparison, we cannot determine whether there is an association between an exposure and an outcome.

Once we have calculated an exposure odds ratio, we must interpret it. The general structure for interpreting an exposure odds ratio is as follows **(Learning Objective 6.3)**:

The odds of *exposure* among *cases* is [insert value of **EOR**] times the odds of *exposure* among *controls*.

When reporting the results from a given analysis, it is important to specify the exposure and outcome categories associated with the research question. Returning to the *S.* Havana outbreak investigation, we would interpret our exposure odds ratios as follows:

$\text{EOR}_{\text{alfalfa sprouts}}$:

The odds of having eaten alfalfa sprouts among those with *S.* Havana infection were 26.5 times the odds of having eaten alfalfa sprouts among the controls.

$\text{EOR}_{\text{almonds}}$:

The odds of having eaten almonds among those with *S.* Havana infection were 1.0 times the odds of having eaten almonds among the controls. *Alternatively...*

The odds of having eaten almonds among those with *S.* Havana infection were the same as the odds of having eaten almonds among the controls.

These interpretations put words to what we saw before—consumption of alfalfa sprouts was much more common among the cases than the controls, whereas the frequency of almond consumption was the same for both groups.

## Common Mistakes in Interpreting the Exposure Odds Ratio

When first learning about the case-control design, it can be tempting to interpret the exposure odds ratio using the structure of a risk or rate ratio calculated from a clinical trial or cohort design. Since the case-control design is fundamentally different from those longitudinal studies, we must remember that the interpretation of the measure of association is different as well.

Recall that the purpose of a case-control study is to ascertain whether a particular exposure is more (or less) common in those with the outcome compared to the source population. For this reason, our interpretation should only reference the exposed condition, the cases, and the controls. We do *not* include the non-exposure condition in the interpretation.

As an example, the following interpretation would *not* be correct because it compares exposure in cases to non-exposure in controls:

✗ The odds of having eaten alfalfa sprouts among those with *S.* Havana infection were 26.5 times the odds of not having eaten alfalfa sprouts among the controls.

As previously noted, the correct interpretation is:

✓ The odds of having eaten alfalfa sprouts among those with *S.* Havana infection were 26.5 times the odds of having eaten alfalfa sprouts among the controls.

## Digging Deeper

### Why Does the Exposure Odds Ratio Work?

The case-control design is useful because it allows investigators to evaluate the association between one or more exposures and a single health outcome without (a) having exposure information about everyone in the source population and (b) requiring a follow-up period.

When selecting a comparison group, it would be inefficient, and frankly unnecessary, to collect information about the exposure status of *everyone* in the source population. Instead, investigators can obtain all the information that they need from a group of controls who are sampled from the source population.

The controls selected for the *S.* Havana outbreak case-control study should have been just as likely to have eaten alfalfa sprouts and almonds as those living in South Australia (the source population for the outbreak investigation). Among the controls that the investigators selected, 1/54 or 1.85% reported eating alfalfa sprouts during the relevant time frame. In 2018, the population of South Australia was 1,736,422[6]; if one out of every 54 South Australians had eaten alfalfa sprouts during the study period, we would expect that 32,123 of them would have recently eaten alfalfa sprouts. If we assume that the cases identified for the outbreak investigation comprised all individuals with a *S.* Havana infection during the study period, we can use this information to populate a 2×2 table that would reflect the data that would have been captured had investigators conducted a (massive!) cohort study on all individuals living in South Australia (**Table 6.4**).

The risk ratio for the association between eating alfalfa sprouts and salmonellosis in our hypothetical cohort study is 26.5 (you can use the data in **Table 6.4** to practice calculating this yourself). To illustrate why the exposure odds ratio works, we will use our hypothetical cohort as the source for our case-control study. We will select everyone who had salmonellosis ($n =$ 18) as cases and will select a random fraction (0.01%) of the population of South Australia as controls. It may seem strange that this approach yields a total of 173.6 controls since we know that we can't observe a fraction of an individual. However, we retain the decimal places here just to illustrate how the math works. In this case, 3.2 of our controls would have recently eaten alfalfa sprouts while 170.4 would not have eaten alfalfa sprouts. The exposure odds ratio for the association between alfalfa sprouts and salmonellosis calculated in this case-control study is 26.5 (again, we encourage you to use the data in **Table 6.4** to practice calculating this yourself).

**TABLE 6.4 WHY THE EXPOSURE ODDS RATIO WORKS**

| | Data From a Hypothetical Cohort Study of the Association Between Alfalfa Sprout Consumption and Salmonellosis | | | Data From a Hypothetical Case-Control Study of the Association Between Alfalfa Sprout Consumption and Salmonellosis | | |
|---|---|---|---|---|---|---|
| **Data Layout** | | Exposed (E+) | Unexposed (E−) | TOTAL | | Exposed (E+) | Unexposed (E−) | TOTAL |
| | Outcome (O+) | 6 | 12 | 18 | Cases | 6 | 12 | 18 |
| | No Outcome (O−) | 32,117 = 32,123 − 6 | 1,704,287 = 1,704,299 − 12 | 1,736,404 = 1,736,422 − 18 | | | | |
| | Total Source Population | 32,123 = 0.0185 × 1,736,422 | 1,704,299 = 1,736,422 − 32,123 | 1,736,422 | Controls | 3.2 | 170.4 | 173.6 |

Select 0.01% of the **source population** to be controls

| | | |
|---|---|---|
| **Measure of Association** | Risk Ratio = $\dfrac{\text{Risk of salmonellosis among those who ate alfalffa sprouts}}{\text{Risk of salmonellosis among those who did not eaat alfalfa sprouts}}$ <br><br> $= \dfrac{A/N_1}{B/N_0} = \dfrac{6/32,123}{12/1,704,299} = 26.5$ | Exposure Odds Ratio = $\dfrac{\text{Odds of eating alfalfa sprouts among thhose with salmonellosis}}{\text{Odds of eating alfalfa sprouts amonng the controls}}$ <br><br> $= \dfrac{A/B}{C/D} = \dfrac{A \times D}{B \times C} = \dfrac{6 \times 170.4}{12 \times 3.2} = 26.5$ |

In comparing the measures of association across these two studies, we see that the risk ratio and the exposure odds ratio are identical.

The take-home message is that when a case-control study contains all of the cases from the source population, and a sample of controls whose exposure frequency matches the source population, the exposure odds ratio will be the same as the risk ratio. This is great news because it allows investigators to estimate a risk ratio without having to enroll and follow a large cohort of individuals!

## Odds Ratios Are Not Unique to Case-Control Studies

When reading excerpts from published studies, many new learners of epidemiology will mistakenly think that any study that reports an odds ratio is a case-control study. While the odds ratio is the *only* measure of association that can be calculated in a case-control study, other study designs may also calculate an odds ratio.

The cross-product can be calculated in any study with 2×2 data. In a cohort study, the value of the cross-product is called a **risk odds ratio**, and in a cross-sectional study it is called a **prevalence odds ratio**. It is common to see odds ratios reported in epidemiologic literature because there is an analysis technique popular among epidemiologists, called logistic regression, which generates odds ratios. Some logistic regression basics will be introduced in **Chapter 13, "Introduction to Epidemiologic Data Analysis"**; however, at this stage, it's important to know that odds ratios are not unique to case-control studies.

To determine whether investigators have conducted a case-control study, look for clues that study participants have been selected based on their outcome status!

## Why Can't We Calculate the Risk, Rate, or Prevalence of the Outcome in a Case-Control Study? (LEARNING OBJECTIVE 6.4)

Unlike other analytic study designs, we cannot calculate a measure of outcome frequency using case-control study data. Investigators choose the relative number of cases to controls for inclusion in a case-control study, and therefore they cannot obtain measures of the risk, rate, or prevalence of the outcome when analyzing case-control study data. **Table 6.5** shows two different scenarios where cases and controls are sampled from a population where the prevalence of the exposure in those with the outcome is 75% and the prevalence of the exposure in the controls is 50%. What is different about these studies is that Study A includes one control for every case (called a 1:1 case-control study), while Study B includes two controls for every case (called a 2:1 case-control study).

We obtain the same exposure odds ratio, regardless of which study we use:

$$\text{EOR}_{\text{Study A}} = \frac{75 \times 50}{25 \times 50} = \text{EOR}_{\text{Study B}} = \frac{75 \times 100}{25 \times 100} = 3$$

**TABLE 6.5 AN ILLUSTRATION OF WHY MEASURES OF OUTCOME FREQUENCY CANNOT BE CALCULATED USING 2×2 DATA FROM A CASE-CONTROL STUDY**

| | STUDY A — 1 Control for Every Case | | | | | STUDY B — 2 Controls for Every Case | | | | |
|---|---|---|---|---|---|---|---|---|---|---|
| | | Exposed (E+) | Unexposed (E−) | TOTAL | | | Exposed (E+) | Unexposed (E−) | TOTAL | |
| **Data Layout** | Cases | 75 | 25 | 100 | | Cases | 75 | 25 | 100 | |
| | Controls | 50 | 50 | 100 | | Controls | 100 | 100 | 200 | |
| **Prevalence of Exposure Among Cases** | $= \frac{75}{100} = 75\%$ | | | ✓ | | $= \frac{75}{100} = 75\%$ | | | | |
| **Prevalence of Exposure Among Controls** | $= \frac{50}{100} = 50\%$ | | | ✓ | | $= \frac{100}{200} = 50\%$ | | | | |
| **Exposure Odds Ratio (EOR)** | $= \frac{75 \times 50}{25 \times 50} = 3$ | | | ✓ | | $= \frac{75 \times 100}{25 \times 100} = 3$ | | | | |
| **INCORRECT Frequency of Outcome** | $= \frac{100}{200} = 50\%$ | | | ✗ | | $= \frac{100}{300} = 33\%$ | | | | |

However, if we were to *incorrectly* attempt to calculate the frequency of the outcome in each of these studies, we would end up with different results for each:

$$\text{Frequency of outcome}_{\text{Study A}} = \frac{100 \text{ cases}}{200 \text{ participants}} = 50\%$$

$$\text{Frequency of outcome}_{\text{Study B}} = \frac{100 \text{ cases}}{300 \text{ participants}} = 33\%$$

These outcome frequencies only tell us about the *ratio* of cases to controls that the study investigators decided to include in the study; they do not provide meaningful information about the actual frequency of the outcome in the source population. The decision about how many controls to enroll for each case relates to the concept of study power, which will be discussed in **Chapter 12, "Random Error in Epidemiologic Research."**

## Pause to Practice 6.2

### Calculating Exposure Odds Ratios in a Case-Control Study of Stillbirth

Two of the many risk factors that the Stillbirth Collaborative Research Network considered were older age of the birthing parent at delivery and smoking in the 3 months prior to the pregnancy. Among the 614 stillbirth cases, 28 of the birthing parents were aged 40 years or older, and 119 reported smoking in the 3 months prior to the pregnancy. Among the 1,354 livebirth controls, 28 of the birthing parents were aged 40 years or older, and 181 reported smoking in the 3 months prior to the pregnancy.

1.  Use this information to populate **Tables 6.6** and **6.7**.

2.  Calculate the probability of each exposure among the cases.

3.  Calculate the probability of each exposure among the controls.

4.  Calculate the odds of each exposure among the cases.

5.  Calculate the odds of each exposure among the controls.

6.  Use your answers to Questions 4 and 5 to calculate the exposure odds ratio. Compare your answers to those obtained using the cross-product method. *Note that your answers should be close to one another, but they may not be identical due to rounding.*

7.  Provide a one-sentence interpretation of each of the exposure odds ratio you calculated using the cross-product method. Which exposure is more strongly associated with stillbirth?

**TABLE 6.6 DATA LAYOUT FOR THE ASSOCIATION BETWEEN OLDER AGE AT DELIVERY AND STILLBIRTH**

|  | E+ Aged 40 Years or More | E− Aged Less Than 40 Years | TOTAL |
|---|---|---|---|
| Cases |  |  |  |
| Controls |  |  |  |

**TABLE 6.7 DATA LAYOUT FOR THE ASSOCIATION BETWEEN SMOKING IN THE 3 MONTHS PRIOR TO PREGNANCY AND STILLBIRTH**

|  | E+ Smoked | E− Did Not Smoke | TOTAL |
|---|---|---|---|
| Cases |  |  |  |
| Controls |  |  |  |

## Case-Control Study Design Basics, Data Layout, and Measure of Association

- In the case-control design, the exposure status is observed, not assigned, which distinguishes the case-control design as an **observational study**.

- The **source population** is defined as the population from which the cases came.

- The basic components of a case-control study:
  - Participants are classified by whether they have the outcome of interest (cases vs. controls) and their *history* of one or more exposures is assessed.
  - The exposure frequency in individuals with the outcome of interest (cases) is compared to the exposure frequency among a group of people sampled from the source population (controls).

- Since investigators determine how many cases and controls to enroll in their study, the frequency of the outcome cannot be calculated.

- The measure of association in a case-control study is the **exposure odds ratio (EOR)**, which is calculated as:

$$\frac{\text{Odds of exposure among cases}}{\text{Odds of exposure among controls}}$$

# PRIMARY VERSUS SECONDARY BASE CASE-CONTROL STUDIES
## (LEARNING OBJECTIVE 6.5)

We can distinguish between two different types of case-control studies: **primary-** and **secondary base** case-control studies. Though the approach for identification and selection of cases and controls differs between these two, the underlying goal remains the same: the conceptualization of the source population.

To motivate the utility of identifying the source population, recall that the ultimate goal of a case-control study is to determine whether the frequency of the exposure among those who have the outcome of interest is more (or less) common compared to the frequency of the exposure in the source population. Investigators answer this question by comparing the exposure frequency in the cases to the exposure frequency in the controls. This leads us to consider the primary purposes of the cases and controls:

- **Purpose of the cases**: Provide an estimate of the frequency of the exposure among those who have the outcome of interest in the source population.

- **Purpose of the controls**: Provide an estimate of the frequency of the exposure in the source population.

Primary and secondary base case-control studies will be discussed in detail in the text that follows. Briefly, in a **primary base** case-control study, the source population is first well-defined, and cases and controls are then selected from that population. This makes it more likely that those who are selected into the sample population as cases and controls will fulfill their respective purposes as previously outlined. When the source population is harder to clearly define and sample from, a **secondary base** case-control study may be conducted in which we begin by identifying the cases. From there, investigators attempt to identify an appropriate source for the controls. This approach may yield a control group that doesn't quite fulfill its purpose to provide an estimate of the frequency of the exposure in the source population.

## Primary Base Case-Control Studies

As previously described, the **primary base case-control design** begins with the identification of the source population before cases and controls are sampled from that population (**Learning Objective 6.5**). This strategy ensures that cases and controls are sampled from the same source population, making the primary base case-control design the most robust approach.

The *S.* Havana outbreak investigation is an example of a primary base case-control study, where the source population was defined as all residents of South Australia. Both cases and controls were sampled from this population, with cases coming from reports made to the Communicable Disease Control Branch of South Australia, and controls selected from an existing database that is representative of South Australian residents.[2] By using a primary base case-control design, investigators can be more confident that the cases are providing an estimate of the frequency of the exposures in those with *S.* Havana in South Australia, while the controls are providing an estimate of the exposures among all South Australians.

## Secondary Base Case-Control Studies

Although it is preferable to conduct a primary base case-control study, there are times when it may not be feasible to clearly define and sample from the source population that gave rise to the cases. When this is the case, investigators begin with identifying a feasible mechanism for selecting cases from the source population, such as selecting all individuals being treated for a particular condition at a specific healthcare facility. Without a well-defined source population, investigators must attempt to identify an appropriate comparison group of individuals who *would have been identified as cases had they developed the outcome of interest*. This type of case-control design is called a **secondary base case-control design** (**Learning Objective 6.5**).

For example, consider a secondary base case-control study of the association between use of personal care products containing aluminum and breast cancer conducted in Austria.[7] In this study, investigators were unable to clearly define and sample from the entire source population of Austria. Therefore, they began by identifying all breast cancer patients aged 20 to 85 years who were treated by the Department of Obstetrics and Gynecology at the Medical University of Innsbruck. The investigators then went to a different department at the same hospital (Department of Plastic, Reconstructive and Aesthetic Surgery), where they selected a sample of controls. The investigators made a key assumption that these controls would have been treated at the Medical University of Innsbruck if they had breast cancer. By using a secondary base case-control design, we are less confident that the cases are providing an estimate of the frequency of exposure to aluminum-containing personal products in everyone with breast cancer in Austria or that the controls are providing an estimate of exposure to aluminum-containing personal products among all Austrians. Another way to think about this, we are less confident that the cases and controls come from the same source population.

## Pause to Practice 6.3

### Identifying the Study Base in a Case-Control Study

Let's revisit the description of how the Stillbirth Collaborative Research Network identified study participants as described in **Pause to Practice 6.1**.

> … investigators identified five distinct geographic areas, called catchment areas, from which study participants would be selected. They then selected all stillbirths (pregnancy losses occurring at 20 weeks' gestation or later) and a sample of livebirths born to residents of those geographic areas.…[3]

1. This is an example of a primary base case-control study. What are the defining features that make it a primary base case-control study?

2. If all stillbirths delivered at one particular hospital were selected as cases, how could controls have been selected to make this a secondary base case-control study?

### The Role of the Source Population in Case-Control Studies

- It is preferable to identify the source population for a case-control study to ensure that all study participants (both cases and controls) are selected from the same population.
- Case-control studies are classified on the basis of whether the source population can be identified and sampled from:
  - **Primary base.** The source population is identified prior to the selection of cases or controls. Subsequently, cases and controls are sampled from this source population.
  - **Secondary base.** Investigators begin with selecting the mechanism for identifying cases and then attempt to identify a suitable control group. It is more difficult to determine whether these cases and controls come from the same source population. Often, investigators conceptualize this group to be individuals who would have been identified as cases in the study *had they developed the outcome of interest*.

## IDENTIFICATION AND SELECTION OF PARTICIPANTS INTO THE SAMPLE POPULATION

Thoughtful consideration about how cases and controls will be identified and selected for a case-control study cannot be overstated. As we begin to think about this process, we will once again keep the purposes of the case and control groups at the forefront:

- **Purpose of the cases**: Provide an estimate of the frequency of the exposure among those who have the outcome of interest in the source population.
- **Purpose of the controls**: Provide an estimate of the frequency of the exposure in the source population.

The sections that follow provide information that investigators must keep in mind when identifying and selecting individuals for inclusion in a case-control study.

### Strategies to Identify Cases (LEARNING OBJECTIVE 6.6)

Once investigators have identified and defined the outcome for their case-control study, they must then determine how they will select cases for inclusion. This process differs depending on whether investigators have access to, or can create, a listing of all of the cases in a source population. However, either of the approaches noted in the text that follows can be used for a primary or secondary base case-control study. We will begin our discussion of case identification by considering the situation where a listing of all individuals with the outcome in the source population is available.

#### SAMPLING CASES AFTER ENUMERATION OF ALL CASES IN THE SOURCE POPULATION

This approach begins by identifying a list of all cases occurring in the source population and including all of these individuals as cases in the study. This strategy is common when conducting a case-control study of health outcomes that are systematically collected and/or reportable (e.g., using registry data, vital records, or a previously conducted cohort study), and can be employed in either a primary or secondary-base case-control study. Many countries or research centers maintain registries that include detailed clinical information about individuals with a particular health outcome, such as cancer or cerebral palsy. For example, to investigate whether statins prevent endometrial cancer, investigators in Denmark used the Danish Cancer Registry, "which contains virtually complete and accurate data on all incident cancer cases in Denmark"(p. 145)[8] to identify cases of endometrial cancer for inclusion in a case-control study.[8] Recall that the purpose of the cases in a case-control study is to provide an estimate of the frequency of the exposure(s) among those with the outcome in the source population. Thus, if *all* of the cases from the source population are included, as in the Danish Cancer Registry study, then this goal is achieved.

After enumeration of all cases in the source population, there may be instances where it is not possible to enroll all the cases that were identified. This is common when resources are limited and it would be too costly to enroll all of the cases in the source population. For example, this could occur if the study protocol required additional follow-up with the cases or collection of expensive biological specimens from the cases. In these situations, investigators can instead enroll a **random sample** (meaning each case has the same probability of being selected) of the cases. In fact, investigators don't always *need* to enroll all of the cases in their study to address the study hypothesis. If the cases are sampled randomly from the source population, the frequency of the exposure(s) in this group should be very similar to all of those with the outcome. This is illustrated in **Figure 6.2**, where a source population includes a total of 100 cases, 60 of whom have the exposure of interest. **Figure 6.2** illustrates what we would expect to see if we randomly sampled 30 cases from this source population, which is that 18 (60%) of the cases in the sample population would be exposed.

## FIGURE 6.2 SCHEMATIC ILLUSTRATING RANDOM SELECTION OF CASES FOR A CASE-CONTROL STUDY

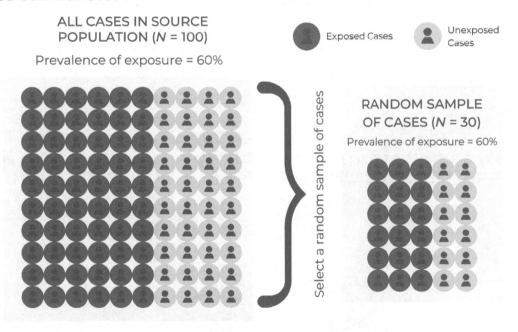

### SAMPLING CASES WITHOUT ENUMERATION OF ALL CASES IN THE SOURCE POPULATION

If there is no registry or some other way to identify all individuals with the health outcome of interest in the source population, investigators will need to consider other approaches to identify cases. Often, this will involve identifying patients receiving care at a particular healthcare facility. This was the approach that the investigators in Austria took when identifying cases for their secondary base case-control study of the association between personal care products containing aluminum and breast cancer.[7] Cases included in this study were all breast cancer patients aged 20 to 85 years who were treated by the Department of Obstetrics and Gynecology at the Medical University of Innsbruck between January 2013 and October 2016. Although this study identified all cases of breast cancer treated by this department during the study period, it is likely that some breast cancer patients living in Innsbruck, Austria, during the study period would have been missed due to being treated somewhere else.

While this strategy allows investigators to enroll cases when they cannot identify all individuals with the health outcome in the source population, sampled cases may be different in meaningful ways from those that would have been selected if investigators had a complete listing of everyone in the source population with the health outcome of interest. Thus, it is possible that the cases in the study may not provide an accurate estimate of the frequency of the exposure(s) among everyone with the outcome in the source population.

Consider **Figure 6.3**, which contains the same source population of cases as shown in **Figure 6.2**, except these cases receive treatment at two different hospitals. The frequency of exposure among all cases in this source population is still 60%; however, the frequency of the exposure among those receiving treatment at Hospital A (86%) is very different from the frequency of the exposure among those receiving treatment at Hospital B (41%). If investigators had only sampled cases for their case-control study from one of these facilities, they would end up with an estimate of the frequency of exposure among people with the outcome in the source population that was either too high (recruiting only from Hospital A) or too low (recruiting only from Hospital B).

Returning to the study of breast cancer in Austria, if some breast cancer patients receive treatment somewhere other than the Department of Obstetrics and Gynecology at the Medical University of Innsbruck, or do not receive care at all, they would not be eligible for inclusion in this case-control study. This situation becomes problematic if those receiving treatment for breast cancer by the Department of Obstetrics and Gynecology at the Medical University of Innsbruck are different in important ways (i.e., have a different prevalence of exposure) from those receiving care elsewhere or not receiving care at all. This touches on an important epidemiologic concept called **selection bias**, where those in the *sample* population are different in meaningful ways from those in the *source* population. We will discuss selection bias in detail in **Chapter 10, "Selection Bias."**

## FIGURE 6.3 SCHEMATIC ILLUSTRATING POTENTIAL FOR ERROR WHEN CASES ARE SELECTED FROM AN INCOMPLETE LISTING OF CASES IN THE SOURCE POPULATION

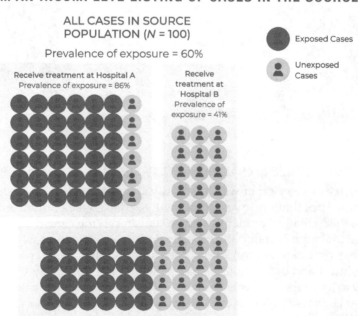

## Sampling Incident Versus Prevalent Cases (LEARNING OBJECTIVE 6.7)

When identifying cases for a case-control study, investigators must be mindful of whether they are selecting **incident** (i.e., new) or **prevalent** (i.e., existing) **cases** of the health outcome. **Figure 6.4** illustrates why it is preferable to enroll incident cases. In this population, there are a total of 10 incident cases of the outcome. If investigators identified and selected these individuals at the time that the health outcome occurred, they would obtain an accurate estimate of the frequency of exposure for those with this outcome (i.e., 5/10 = 50%). However, if they did not enroll incident cases, but rather identified and selected prevalent cases sometime after the outcomes occurred, they would obtain an inaccurate estimate of the frequency of the exposure for those with this outcome (i.e., 1/5 = 20%). We will discuss this further in **Chapter 10, "Selection Bias;"** however, the problem is that the exposure is associated with survival among those with the outcome. In other words, unexposed cases live longer than exposed cases, and thus will be overrepresented in a sample of prevalent cases measured at a later time point. Thus, if exposure is associated with survival, prevalent cases may not provide an accurate estimate of the frequency of the exposure(s) among those with the outcome in the source population.

## FIGURE 6.4 SELECTING INCIDENT VERSUS PREVALENT CASES FOR A CASE-CONTROL STUDY

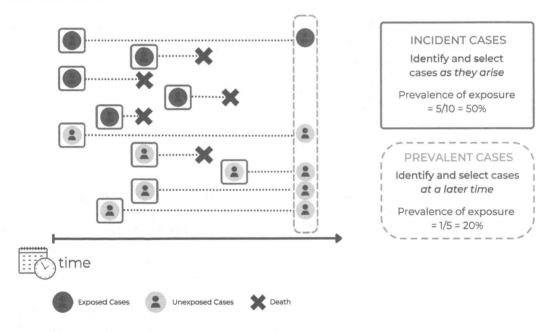

## Strategies to Identify Controls (LEARNING OBJECTIVE 6.8)

Thoughtful consideration is also required for the identification and selection of controls for inclusion in a case-control study, which can be very difficult to do without introducing error. Controls are a group of individuals who should be selected from the same source population as the cases. As previously described, the purpose of the control group is to provide investigators with an estimate of the frequency of the exposure(s) in the source population.

Consider, for example, that a team of investigators was designing a case-control study of the association between smoking and pancreatic cancer where the source population was all U.S. adults. For this study, it would be important for the control group to have the same frequency of smoking as all U.S. adults. In 2021, this prevalence was 11.5%,[9] thus, 11.5% of the controls should have a history of smoking.

In the text that follows, we discuss three different sources from which investigators might select controls for a case-control study, alongside their relative strengths and limitations.

## POPULATION-BASED CONTROLS

Primary base case-control studies employ the most robust approach for identifying controls, which is the use of **population-based controls**. In these studies, investigators have access to a complete roster of individuals in the source population, which is typically defined by a geographic area. Such a roster would exist for a source population of births occurring to residents of a particular state, where the roster is generated by a state health department using birth certificates. Another example where a complete roster could be identified is in a source population defined by students enrolled in schools within the same district, where the roster includes all enrolled students. In the case of the S. Havana outbreak, the controls were randomly selected from a list of residents of South Australia generated from an existing surveillance system. Although this surveillance system did not include *all* residents of South Australia, these controls are still considered population-based because the surveillance system included a random sample of South Australian residents. The main benefit of this method of control identification is that when controls are randomly selected from a population-based roster (or a random subset of a roster, as in the S. Havana outbreak investigation), the frequency of exposure in the controls should closely mirror that of the source population.

While population-based control selection is the most robust method, there are potential drawbacks. Since controls are selected outside of a healthcare setting, they may be less likely to agree to participate. This can become problematic if a substantial number (e.g., more than 20%) of sampled controls decline to participate. In these instances, there is a chance that those who decline to participate have a different frequency of the exposure(s) than those who agree to participate. When this happens, the controls may not provide an accurate estimate of the frequency of the exposure(s) in the source population, and error will be introduced in the study results. Additionally, although this may be the most desirable method of control selection, it may not always be feasible if investigators are unable to identify a roster (or a random subset of a roster) for the source population.

## HOSPITAL- AND CLINIC-BASED CONTROLS

When cases are identified at hospitals or clinics, investigators may enroll **hospital- or clinic-based controls**. The source population is thus conceptualized as a group of individuals who would be treated at the facility where the cases were identified if they were to develop the outcome of interest.

The study of use of personal care products containing aluminum and breast cancer conducted in Austria enrolled clinic-based controls.[7] Recall that cases were those being treated for breast cancer by the Department of Obstetrics and Gynecology at the Medical University of Innsbruck. The controls were a sample of female patients from a different department in the same hospital. The assumption underlying the selection of this control group is that patients receiving care for something other than breast cancer at the Medical University of Innsbruck would receive treatment there *if they were to develop breast cancer*.

Not only are hospital- or clinic-based controls easier to find than population-based controls, but they may also be more motivated to participate since they are contacted in a healthcare setting. Additionally, given that cases and controls are seeking care at similar facilities, it is likely that they could be similar on other important factors, called confounders, that could explain the relationship between the exposure(s) and outcome of interest (more on confounding in **Chapter 9, "Error in Epidemiologic Research and Fundamentals of Confounding"**).

Although this approach can be a convenient way to identify controls, it is not without limitations. As with the selection of cases when there is no enumeration of all cases in a source population, the use of hospital- or clinic-based controls carries a risk of selecting a group of controls whose frequency of exposure(s) is different from the source population. Since the role of the control group is to provide an accurate estimate of the frequency of exposure(s) in the source population, investigators must be careful about which hospitals or clinics they select when identifying controls.

## RELATIVES, NEIGHBORS, OR FRIENDS OF CASES

In instances where controls cannot be identified using population-, hospital-, or clinic-based approaches, investigators may select relatives, neighbors, or friends of the cases as controls. A study of the association between malnutrition and disability in children living in Turkana, Kenya, employed this approach, whereby siblings (the closest in age to the cases) and neighbors (within 1 year of age of the cases) of children with disabilities were selected for inclusion in the study as controls.[10]

This approach avoids having to enumerate the entire source population. Additionally, given the controls' social connection to the cases, these controls may have increased motivation to agree to participate. As with hospital- and clinic-based controls, controls who have some known relationship to the cases may be similar with respect to other confounding factors that could explain the relationship between the exposure(s) and the outcome of interest.

There are two important limitations to consider when selecting controls who are relatives, neighbors, or friends of cases. First, investigators may have to rely on cases to provide contact information for potential controls. Depending on the nature of the health outcome or the relationship between the case and potential controls, cases may have reservations about sharing this information. For example, disability is unfortunately stigmatized in many communities. Depending on how a family perceives their position in the community, they may not be interested in involving their neighbors in a study. Another limitation is that, given their proximity to the cases, the frequency of the exposure(s) among these controls may be more similar to that of the cases than to the source population. This, of course, is problematic since the purpose of the control group is to provide an estimate of the frequency of the exposure(s) in the source population. If the controls are too similar to the cases with respect to their frequency of the exposure, the measure of association will be weaker than it should be.

A summary of where to identify controls in a case-control study, and the advantages and challenges to these strategies, is shown in **Table 6.8**.

## TABLE 6.8 SOURCES OF CONTROLS IN A CASE-CONTROL STUDY

|  | **Population-Based Controls** | **Hospital- or Clinic-Based Controls** | **Relatives, Neighbors, and Friends of Cases** |
|---|---|---|---|
| **Description** | Controls are sampled from a roster that includes all individuals in the source population. | Used when the source population is conceptualized as a group of people who would be treated in a given clinic or hospital if they developed the outcome of interest. | If the source population isn't easily enumerated, individuals who are known to the cases may be sampled. |
| **Advantages** | The exposure **distribution** of the controls should be the same as the **source population** (given random sampling and high participation). | No need to enumerate the entire source population.<br>Many confounding factors may be similar between cases and controls (e.g., SES/education/neighborhood).<br>Relative to population-based controls:<br>• Easier and lower cost to identify<br>• May be more willing to participate | |
| **Challenges** | Population-based controls may be less motivated to participate in a study.<br><br>Must be able to enumerate entire source population. | The exposure **distribution** of the controls may not be the same as the **source population**. | The exposure **distribution** of the controls may not be the same as the **source population**.<br><br>Cases may not be willing to share contact information with investigators. |

SES, socioeconomic status.

### Identification of Cases and Controls

Given that the vast majority of U.S. births occur in hospitals, the Stillbirth Collaborative Research Network targeted hospitals for the identification of stillbirth cases and livebirth controls.[3] Investigators selected hospitals for participation such that they would capture at least 90% of all stillbirths and livebirths occurring to residents of each predefined catchment area (recall these were five distinct geographic areas from which study participants were selected). While many residents delivered their babies in hospitals that were located in the same catchment area where they lived, some residents traveled outside of this area to deliver their babies. For this reason, the investigators needed to include hospitals both inside and outside of the catchment areas to obtain a representative sample of births occurring to residents of those catchment areas.

Study team members reviewed the delivery logs at each of the participating hospitals to identify stillbirths and livebirths occurring to residents of the catchment areas. All stillbirths were reviewed for potential inclusion in the study, and a sample of the live births were selected. Both cases and controls were identified and approached before being discharged from the hospital to allow for collection of biological specimens and administration of questionnaires.

1. What strategy did the investigators use to identify cases?
2. How and where were the controls selected?

## Case-Control Studies Versus Cohort Studies

A common misconception among new students of epidemiology is that case-control studies are interchangeable with cohort studies that make use of historical data. While case-control and cohort studies have shared goals of estimating the associations between exposures and outcomes, they take two very different approaches to get there!

Recall that a defining feature of the cohort design is that a group (i.e., cohort) of individuals who are at-risk for the outcome of interest are followed over some period of time to see who *develops* the outcome(s) of interest. Even if investigators use historical data to conduct a cohort study, the underlying structure remains the same: an at-risk group is followed for some period of time and outcome frequency can be measured.

Although the case-control design often makes use of historical data, it does not involve following a cohort of at-risk individuals over time. Thus, calculation of measures of outcome frequency is not possible in a case-control study.

## Identifying and Selecting Study Participants for a Case-Control Study

Selecting cases

- Regardless of the method of selection, the goal is to obtain a group of cases who have the same frequency of the exposure(s) as those *with* the outcome in the source population.
- There are two strategies for selecting cases:
  - Enumeration of all individuals with the health outcome in the source population. When investigators have a listing of everyone in the source population who has the outcome of interest, they have two options:
    - Select all of these individuals as cases.
    - Take a random sample.

- Sampling cases without complete enumeration. If a complete listing of all individuals with the outcome of interest in the source population is not available, investigators must select cases from a source that only captures some of those with the outcome in the source population, such as patients being treated at a particular hospital.

- Investigators must also decide whether to enroll **incident** (i.e., newly occurring) or **prevalent** (i.e., existing) **cases**. It is preferable to enroll incident cases, particularly if the exposure(s) of interest are likely to be associated with survival.

<u>Selecting controls</u>

- Regardless of the method of selection, the goal is to obtain a group of controls who have the same frequency of the exposure(s) as everyone in the source population.

- The most robust method is to choose **population-based controls**, which are used in a **primary base case-control study**. Population-based controls are randomly selected from a roster of all individuals in the source population, which is typically defined by a particular geographic area.

- When investigators do not have access to a roster of all individuals in the source population, they may select **hospital- or clinic-based controls**, or controls who are **relatives, neighbors, or friends of the cases**. There is a risk that individuals belonging to these groups may have a higher or lower frequency of the exposure(s) than the entire source population.

## MATCHING IN CASE-CONTROL STUDIES (LEARNING OBJECTIVE 6.9)

Investigators may select controls with specific attributes that correspond to those of the cases. This process is called **matching** and is only done for factors that are likely to be confounders of the relationship between the exposure and the outcome. We will discuss confounding in detail in **Chapter 9, "Error in Epidemiologic Research and Fundamentals of Confounding"**; however, at this stage, it is important to know that confounders are factors that are associated with both the exposure and the outcome of interest and may partially explain the association between the exposure and outcome. If these factors are ignored in the analysis, the exposure odds ratio will be biased, meaning incorrect.

It is common for investigators to match controls to cases on factors such as the participants' age, sex, and/or race. Cases and controls may be **pair-matched**, meaning that one control is matched to each case; however, investigators may choose to match more than one control to each case, which is called *n*-to-one matching, where *n* is the number of controls that are matched to each case.

Once a case is identified in a case-control study employing matching, investigators will seek a control or a set of controls that has the same matching factors as the case. For example, if a 36-year-old female case were enrolled in a study matching on age and sex, investigators would need to find a 36-year-old female control to enroll in the study. In this instance, it could be challenging to find an exact match, since seeking a person who is exactly 36 years old drastically limits the pool of controls eligible for selection. Instead of using exact matching for a variable like age, investigators may employ one of two different matching strategies: **category matching** or **caliper matching**.

In **category matching**, investigators begin by defining mutually exclusive categories for the matching factor of interest (e.g., for age, they might define groups as 18–24, 25–29, 30–39, 40–49, 50+). Once a case is identified, investigators will select a control whose age falls within the same category as the case. Given these categories, the investigators in the previous example would select a female control between the ages of 30 and 39.

In contrast, **caliper matching** allows for the identification of controls with a value within a specified range of that of the case. For example, investigators might decide to select controls whose ages are within 3 years of the corresponding case. Investigators in the study seeking a control for a 36-year-old female would look for a female control between the ages of 33 and 39 (36 ± 3).

## Advantages of Matching in a Case-Control Study

Matching in a case-control study can help prevent confounding by the matched factors. Additionally, matching in case-control studies can reduce the influence of random error, which will be discussed further in **Chapter 12, "Random Error in Epidemiologic Research"** While this is a primary reason investigators employ matching in a case-control design, these specifics are beyond the scope of this text and are described elsewhere.[11]

## Limitations of Matching in a Case-Control Study

While there are certainly benefits to the use of matching in case-control studies, matching makes it more difficult to identify controls for inclusion in the study and can be both time-consuming and costly. Investigators must spend time identifying and recruiting controls who have the specific characteristics required to be matched to a given case. Additionally, once investigators have matched on a particular factor (e.g., sex), they can no longer consider that factor as a potential exposure in their analysis. By matching, they have forced the cases and controls to have the same frequency of the matched factors, and thus any exposure odds ratio estimating the association between a matched factor and the outcome will always be 1. We will explore this phenomenon further in **Chapter 9, "Error in Epidemiologic Research and Fundamentals of Confounding."**

## Calculating the Exposure Odds Ratio in a Pair-Matched Analysis

The data layout for a pair-matched case-control study differs from that of an unmatched case-control study, as does the calculation of the exposure odds ratio. Once cases and controls have been matched on the factor(s) of interest, investigators evaluate the **exposure pattern** of each pair, meaning they determine whether the exposure status of the case and control are **concordant** (the same) or **discordant** (different). The data layout for a pair-matched case-control study is shown in **Table 6.9**. The information in the columns corresponds to the exposure status of the control, while the information in the rows corresponds to the exposure status of

**TABLE 6.9 DATA LAYOUT AND MEASURES OF FREQUENCY AND ASSOCIATION FOR PAIR-MATCHED CASE-CONTROL STUDIES**

| | | | CONTROL | |
| --- | --- | --- | --- | --- |
| | | | Exposed (E+) | Unexposed (E−) |
| Data Layout[a] | CASE | Exposed (E+) | W | X |
| | | Unexposed (E−) | Y | Z |
| Measure(s) of Association and Interpretation | Pair-matched odds ratio [insert value of mOR] $= \dfrac{X}{Y}$ | | | |
| | After controlling for the matched factors, the odds of exposure among cases are [insert value of **mOR**] times the odds of exposure among controls. | | | |

[a]The numbers in a pair-matched 2×2 table correspond to the number of *matched pairs* with each exposure pattern. Thus, the total number of study participants = 2×(W+X+Y+Z).

the case. This table differs from a traditional 2×2 table in that the numbers in each cell represent the number of *pairs* with a given exposure pattern, rather than the number of *individuals* with a given exposure/outcome pattern.

When the exposure status of the case and control pair are *concordant*, that is, both the case and control are exposed (cell W) or they are both unexposed (cell Z), we don't gain any additional information to help us evaluate the relationship between the exposure and the outcome.

However, when the exposure status of the case and control are *discordant*—either the case is exposed and the control isn't (cell X) or the control is exposed and the case isn't (cell Y)—we are able to evaluate whether there is an association between the exposure and the outcome.

The measure of association for a pair-matched case-control study is the **pair-matched odds ratio** and is calculated as shown in **Equation 6.8**.

$$\text{Pair-matched odds ratio (moR)} = \frac{X}{Y} \tag{6.8}$$

The pair-matched odds ratio is often described as the **ratio of discordant pairs**. The pair-matched odds ratio will only be greater than its null value of one (thus suggesting a positive association between the exposure and outcome) if we have many more pairs where the case is exposed and the control is not. Conversely, the pair-matched odds ratio can only be less than one (suggesting a negative association between the exposure and outcome) if there are many more pairs where the control is exposed while the case is not.

The interpretation of a pair-matched odds ratio is very similar to that of an exposure odds ratio; however, investigators must be sure to include that they have employed matching in the design of their study. Consider the example of a pair-matched case-control study conducted in South India where investigators matched controls to patients with chronic kidney disease on age and sex.[12] They considered many potential exposures that might cause chronic kidney disease, including hypertension. There were 33 pairings where the case had hypertension but the control did not ($X = 33$), and there were only three pairings where the control had hypertension but the case did not ($Y = 3$). The pair-matched exposure odds ratio calculated in this study is 11 (= 33/3). An appropriate interpretation of this odds ratio would be:

*After matching on (or controlling for) age and sex, the odds of hypertension among patients with chronic kidney disease were 11 times the odds of hypertension among the controls.*

## Digging Deeper

### What Happens if We Ignore the Matching in a Pair-Matched Case-Control Study?

When analyzing a pair-matched case-control study, it is important to account for the matching using a pair-matched odds ratio as previously described. To illustrate the importance of retaining the matching in the analysis of a pair-matched case-control study, we will revisit the study of chronic kidney disease from South India.[12] **Table 6.10** shows complete data for the distribution of hypertension for the case and control pairs.

Recall that the numbers in this table correspond to the number of *pairs* enrolled in the study; thus, these data include a total of 80 individuals. We can (incorrectly!) break the matching by using the pair-matched data to populate a traditional 2×2 table (**Table 6.11**) as shown in the text that follows.

To obtain the number of exposed and unexposed cases, we ignore the exposure status of their matched controls and sum the values in the rows of the pair-matched table. Similarly, to obtain the number of exposed and unexposed controls, we ignore the exposure status of their matched cases, and sum the values in the columns of the pair-matched table.

We can compare the results of the odds ratios obtained from each method:

$$\text{Pair-matched odds ratio} = \frac{X}{Y} = \frac{33}{3} = 11.0$$

$$\text{Exposure odds ratio} = \frac{A \times D}{B \times C} = \frac{38 \times 72}{42 \times 8} = 8.1$$

We see that these methods do not yield the same measure of association. The unmatched exposure odds ratio provides a **biased** (i.e., incorrect) estimate of the association between hypertension and chronic kidney disease because it does not account for the fact that cases and controls were matched on age and sex.

For this reason, it is important to retain the matching when analyzing pair-matched case-control data!

**TABLE 6.10 PAIR-MATCHED 2X2 TABLE FOR THE ASSOCIATION BETWEEN HYPERTENSION AND CHRONIC KIDNEY DISEASE**

| | | Exposure (Hypertension) Status of the Control | |
| --- | --- | --- | --- |
| | | Exposed | Unexposed |
| Exposure (Hypertension) Status of the Case | Exposed | 5 | 33 |
| | Unexposed | 3 | 39 |

**TABLE 6.11 TRADITIONAL 2X2 TABLE DATA AFTER INCORRECTLY IGNORING THE PAIR-MATCHING**

| | Exposed | Unexposed |
| --- | --- | --- |
| Case | 38 (= 5+33) | 42 (= 3+39) |
| Control | 8 (= 5+3) | 72 (= 33+39) |

# STRENGTHS AND LIMITATIONS OF CASE-CONTROL STUDIES (LEARNING OBJECTIVE 6.10)

## Strengths of Case-Control Studies

**Study of multiple exposures.** The case-control design allows for the study of multiple exposures. This is particularly useful when the cause of a particular outcome is unknown, such as in an outbreak investigation, and thus there is a need to consider several exposures at once.

**Study of rare outcomes.** The case-control design is well-suited for the study of rare outcomes, as well as outcomes with long induction or latency periods and outcomes that have already occurred. In the case of a rare outcome, investigators would have to enroll a very large cohort to have enough individuals who develop the outcome of interest to be able to make meaningful comparisons. Similarly, for outcomes that take a very long time to develop or be detectable, a case-control design is preferable because investigators conducting a cohort study would need to follow the cohort for a very long time and could risk substantial loss-to-follow-up during the study period.

**Logistics.** With appropriate selection of the control group, investigators can obtain an estimate of the frequency of the exposure in the source population without actually having to measure the exposure status of everyone in the source population. Thus, the case-control design requires a smaller sample size than the cohort design. Therefore, these studies are generally less resource intensive. Additionally, case-control studies can often be conducted more quickly than a randomized controlled trial or a cohort study.

## Limitations of Case-Control Studies

**Study of rare exposures.** The case-control design is not well-suited for the study of rare exposures. If an exposure is rare, investigators would need to enroll a very large number of cases and controls to have an adequate number of exposed individuals to be able to make meaningful comparisons.

**Limited to a single outcome.** Since the sample population for a case-control study is selected based on the individual's outcome status, investigators are restricted to only studying that particular outcome. Thus, the case-control design is not suitable for the study of multiple outcomes.

**Examining outcome frequency**. Given that investigators decide how many cases and how many controls to enroll in a case-control study, it is not possible to estimate the frequency of the outcome. Despite this limitation, investigators can still calculate a measure of *association* to describe the relationship between exposures of interest and the outcome.

**Temporality.** Recall that a necessary criterion when establishing whether an exposure causes an outcome is that the exposure must have occurred *prior to* the outcome. There are numerous ways to establish temporality between the exposure and the outcome in a case-control study, such as using medical records to identify information about potential exposures *before* the outcome occurred. However, there are times when investigators must rely on self-report of exposures after the outcome has occurred, which make it more difficult to establish temporality between the exposure and outcome relative to a controlled trial or a cohort study.

**Biased participant selection**. The case-control design provides an excellent opportunity to consider outcomes that are challenging to study using a cohort design. This comes at a cost, however, which is that the case-control design is particularly susceptible to selection bias if studies are not carefully designed. We will discuss selection bias in detail in **Chapter 10, "Selection Bias"**; however, in short, it is a phenomenon that leads to errors in our studies due to the way participants either enter or leave the sample population. The success of a case-control study relies on the appropriate selection of cases and controls from the source population. If the source population has not been properly identified, or if there is bias in the selection of either cases or controls, the results may be incorrect.

The case-control design may also be susceptible to selection bias if investigators select prevalent (vs. incident) cases. Prevalent cases may have a different frequency of the exposure than incident cases, which can influence our results. This topic will be discussed further in **Chapter 10, "Selection Bias."**

**Biased exposure measurement**. Since the case-control design often relies on historical records or self-report for the collection of exposure information, it may be particularly susceptible to errors in the reporting of the exposure, which will be discussed further in **Chapter 11, "Information Bias and Screening and Diagnostic Tests."**

## Reporting Study Findings From Case-Control Studies: The STROBE Statement

As discussed in **Chapter 5, "Cohort Designs,"** there is standardized reporting guidance for reporting the results from observational studies.[12] Items that are specific to the reporting of case-control studies include:

- "[E]ligibility criteria, and the sources and methods of case ascertainment and control selection..."
- "...[R]ationale for the choice of cases and controls..."
- "...[F]or matched studies...matching criteria and the number of controls per case, and how this was addressed in the analysis..."
- "...[R]eporting of the number of individuals in each exposure category, or summary measures of exposure."

## WHERE WE'VE BEEN AND WHAT'S UP NEXT

The case-control design is a great alternative to the cohort design when investigators are using an observational design to study a rare outcome, one with a long latency or induction period, or an outbreak. However, great care is needed to ensure that the sample population is selected appropriately to yield valid results! Up next, you will learn about the third and final observational study design discussed in this textbook: cross-sectional studies (**Chapter 7, "Cross-Sectional Designs"**).

---

## END OF CHAPTER PROBLEM SET

**Questions 1 to 4 refer to one of the earliest and most well-known case-control studies, which examines the association between smoking and lung cancer.**

During the 1940s, when smoking was very common and the link between smoking and lung cancer had not yet been established, Richard Doll and Bradford Hill undertook a case-control study to evaluate this association.[13] They enrolled both men and women patients with lung cancer as their cases along with control patients who had diseases other than lung cancer. They analyzed the data for males and females separately, and for the purpose of this exercise we will just consider the data for males. **Table 6.12** shows the distribution of five different levels of smoking for male cases and controls.[13]

**TABLE 6.12 DISTRIBUTION OF FIVE DIFFERENT LEVELS OF SMOKING FOR MALE CASES AND CONTROLS**

| | Average Number of Cigarettes Smoked Daily | | | | | TOTAL |
| --- | --- | --- | --- | --- | --- | --- |
| | 1–4 | 5–14 | 15–24 | 25–49 | ≥ 50 | |
| Lung Cancer Cases | 33 | 250 | 196 | 136 | 32 | 647 |
| Controls | 55 | 293 | 190 | 71 | 13 | 622 |

1. Using those who smoked one to four cigarettes per day as the reference group, calculate the exposure odds ratio that describes the association between smoking five or more cigarettes per day and lung cancer. Provide a one-sentence description of this finding. *Hint, you may want to create a 2×2 table to help you answer this question.*

2. Calculate the exposure odds ratio that evaluate the associations between smoking and lung cancer for each of the four higher smoking categories compared to those who smoked one to four cigarettes per day. *Hint, you may want to create four new 2×2 tables to help you answer this question.*

3. What do you notice about the association between smoking and lung cancer as the number of cigarettes smoked per day increases? Why is your answer for Question 1 insufficient to understand this trend?

4. Your friend who is not studying epidemiology takes a look at your assignment and remarks that the occurrence of lung cancer was really high in this study with 647/1,269 (51%) of the study participants having lung cancer. They remember a conversation from a recent study session where you described the concept of the risk of a health outcome and ask you why you think the risk of lung cancer is so high in this study. Provide a brief explanation for why your friend is mistaken in thinking about the risk of lung cancer in the context of this particular study design.

## Questions 5 to 9 refer to a Danish study of endometrial cancer, described in the text that follows.

Denmark is an ideal place to conduct some epidemiologic research because the Danish Health Data Authority maintains a number of national health registers which provide nearly complete data on healthcare-related encounters that occur among all individuals living in Denmark.[14]

The questions that follow are adapted from a case-control study of the association between statin use (medications which can help lower LDL or "bad" cholesterol) and endometrial cancer among female residents of Denmark[8] and will evaluate the association between highest level of education attained and endometrial cancer.

In this study, cases were identified using the Danish Cancer Registry "which contains virtually complete and accurate data on all incident cancer cases in Denmark" (p. 145).[8] Cases were all individuals who were aged 30 to 84 years who had a verified endometrial cancer diagnosis between 2000 and 2009. Controls were sampled from Denmark's Civil Registration System, which contains information about all individuals living in Denmark.[15]

For all individuals in the sample population, investigators obtained information about their highest level of educational attainment by linking to the Population Education Register, which includes education information for 96% of the Danish population aged 15 to 69 years.[16] The sample population included 5,173 women who had confirmed endometrial cancer—among these, 4,217 had achieved a basic or vocational level of education at the time of the study. Additionally, the sample population included 68,348 women who had no history of endometrial cancer—among these, 56,045 had achieved a basic or vocational level of education at the time of the study. The remaining cases and controls had achieved a higher level of education at the time of the study.

5. What is the source population for this study?

6. Use this information to construct a 2×2 table for this study that classifies individuals by their highest level of educational attainment and endometrial cancer status. Calculate the exposure odds ratio that describes the association between educational attainment and endometrial cancer, where those with higher educational attainment are compared to those with a basic or vocational level of attainment. What do you conclude about this association?

7. Using the data from this study, what is our best estimate of the proportion of the source population that has a higher level of educational attainment?

8. Compare your answers to Questions 6 and 7 and comment on why you observed different results.

9. Suppose that the investigators used the same strategy described previously to identify cases; however, instead of using Denmark's Civil Registration System to identify controls, suppose they recruited women employed at local businesses such as hotels, grocery stores, and garden shops. A total of 68,348 controls were still recruited; however, 11.2% of them had a higher level of educational attainment. Use this information to construct a 2×2 table for this scenario. Calculate and interpret the odds ratio from this new sample population.

**Questions 10 to 12 explore matching in a case-control study.**

Let's return to the example of a matched case-control study described earlier in this chapter, which investigated the relationship between hypertension and chronic kidney disease.[12] Men are *more* likely than women to have hypertension[17]; however, they are *less* likely than women to have chronic kidney disease.[18] It is possible that these imbalances could prevent investigators from teasing out the true association between hypertension and chronic kidney disease. For this reason, investigators matched their cases and controls on sex—such that each male case was matched with a male control and each female case was matched with a female control.

This study identified a total of 59 men with chronic kidney disease and 21 women with chronic kidney disease.[12]

10. Use the previously detailed information to construct a 2×2 table that classifies the study participants by sex and outcome status.

11. Using your table from Question 10, calculate the ratio that describes the association between sex and chronic kidney disease in this sample population. Provide a one-sentence interpretation of this finding.

12. You should have found in Question 11 that there is no association between sex and chronic kidney disease in this sample population. By matching on sex, we have forced its relationship with chronic kidney disease to equal one—the null value for a ratio measure of association. Does this mean that sex isn't really associated with chronic kidney disease in the source population?

# REFERENCES

1. Centers for Disease Control and Prevention. Fetal deaths 2005–2018, as compiled from data provided by the 57 vital statistics jurisdictions through the vital statistics cooperative program. 2022. https://wonder.cdc.gov/controller/datarequest/D150

2. Harfield S, Beazley R, Denehy E, et al. An outbreak and case-control study of *Salmonella* Havana linked to alfalfa sprouts in South Australia, 2018. *Commun Dis Intell*. 2019;43. https://doi.org/10.33321/cdi.2019.43.45

3. Parker CB, Hogue CJ, Koch MA, et al. Stillbirth Collaborative Research Network: design, methods and recruitment experience. *Paediatr Perinat Epidemiol*. 2011;25(5):425–435. https://doi.org/10.1111/j.1365-3016.2011.01218.x

4. Macdorman MF, Kirmeyer S. The challenge of fetal mortality. *NCHS Data Brief*. 2009(16):1–8. https://www.cdc.gov/nchs/products/databriefs/db16.htm

5. Stillbirth Collaborative Research Network Writing Group. Association between stillbirth and risk factors known at pregnancy confirmation. *JAMA*. 2011;306(22):2469–2479. https://doi.org/10.1001/jama.2011.1798

6. Australian Bureau of Statistics. Regional population growth, Australia, 2017–18. March 27, 2019. https://www.abs.gov.au/AUSSTATS/abs@.nsf/Lookup/3218.0Main+Features12017-18?OpenDocument=

7. Linhart C, Talasz H, Morandi EM, et al. Use of underarm cosmetic products in relation to risk of breast cancer: a case-control study. *EBioMedicine*. 2017;21:79–85. https://doi.org/10.1016/j.ebiom.2017.06.005

8. Sperling CD, Verdoodt F, Friis S, Dehlendorff C, Kjaer SK. Statin use and risk of endometrial cancer: a nationwide registry-based case-control study. *Acta Obstet Gynecol Scand*. 2017;96(2):144–149. https://doi.org/10.1111/aogs.13069

9. Centers for Disease Control and Prevention. Current cigarette smoking among adults in the United States. 2023. https://www.cdc.gov/tobacco/data_statistics/fact_sheets/adult_data/cig_smoking/index.htm

10. Kuper H, Nyapera V, Evans J, et al. Malnutrition and childhood disability in Turkana, Kenya: results from a case-control study. *PLoS One*. 2015;10(12):e0144926. https://doi.org/10.1371/journal.pone.0144926

11. Lash VT, Lash TL, Haneuse S, Rothman KJ. *Modern Epidemiology* (4th ed.). Wolters Kluwer, 2021;176–179

12. Akkilagunta S, Premarajan KC, Parameswaran S, Kar SS. Association of non-allopathic drugs and dietary factors with chronic kidney disease: A matched case-control study in South India. *J Family Med Prim Care*. 2018;7(6):1346–1352. https://doi.org/10.4103/jfmpc.jfmpc_166_18

13. Doll R, Hill AB. Smoking and carcinoma of the lung; preliminary report. *Br Med J*. 1950;2(4682): 739–748. https://doi.org/10.1136/bmj.2.4682.739

14. Danish Health Data Authority. List of national health registers. September 4, 2022. https://sundhedsdatastyrelsen.dk/da/english/health_data_and_registers/national_health_registers/list-of-national-health-registers

15. Pedersen CB. The Danish civil registration system. *Scand J Public Health*. 2011;39(suppl 7):22–25. https://doi.org/10.1177/1403494810387965

16. Jensen VM, Rasmussen AW. Danish education registers. *Scand J Public Health*. 2011;39(suppl 7):91–94. https://doi.org/10.1177/1403494810394715

17. Ostchega Y, Fryar CD, Nwankwo T, Nguyen DT. Hypertension prevalence among adults aged 18 and over: United States, 2017–2018. *NCHS Data Brief*. 2020(364):1–8. https://www.cdc.gov/nchs/data/databriefs/db364-h.pdf

18. Charles C, Ferris AH. Chronic kidney disease. *Prim Care*. 2020;47(4):585–595. https://doi.org/10.1016/j.pop.2020.08.001

# CHAPTER 7

# CROSS-SECTIONAL DESIGNS

## KEY TERMS

cross-sectional design          observational studies          prevalence

## LEARNING OBJECTIVES

7.1  Know the basic design features of a cross-sectional study.
7.2  Describe the use of a cross-sectional study for prevalence estimation and hypothesis testing.
7.3  Distinguish between the source and sample population for a cross-sectional study.
7.4  Calculate measures of frequency and association in a cross-sectional study.
7.5  Interpret measures of frequency and association in a cross-sectional study.
7.6  Know the public health utility of conducting serial cross-sectional studies.
7.7  Describe the strengths and limitations of cross-sectional designs.

## RURAL HEALTH IN AMERICA

According to the U.S. Census Bureau, one in every five Americans lives in a rural area, defined as places that are "sparsely populated, have low housing density, and are far from urban centers"(para. 3).[1] While approximately 20% of U.S. residents live in rural areas, these areas account for 97% of the country's land mass.[2] If you were tasked with figuring out where to place healthcare facilities in rural areas, you can imagine the challenges that would arise as you tried to ensure that each facility had enough patients to stay in business, while also being within a reasonable distance to anyone requiring care.

Unfortunately, these are challenges that rural hospitals have faced for a long time, and in recent decades have led to a wave of rural hospital closures.[3] Rural hospitals in the United States serve a high proportion of patients with Medicaid or Medicare insurance or no insurance at all. The reimbursement for services that these patients receive isn't enough to cover the cost of their care. Since rural hospitals serve a smaller patient population, they do not have the advantage that urban hospitals do, whereby they can make up the difference through revenue generated by reimbursement from private insurance.

This problem has been particularly dire in the state of Georgia, where 12 rural hospitals closed between 2013 and 2020.[4] Vital care, such as obstetric services, is no longer available in many of Georgia's rural counties.[5] Rural hospital closures are of course devastating for the affected communities, but the challenges don't stop there. The safety and sustainability of U.S. agriculture is impacted by rural hospital closures given the important role that rural communities play in this arena.[6]

One way to address the rural health crisis is through legislation. In 2022, Georgia senators Raphael Warnock and Jon Ossoff championed rural health and secured nearly $450 million for rural healthcare providers and community health centers through the American Rescue Plan.[7,8] These resources will allow rural healthcare providers to stay in business and provide the care that their patients deserve. Keeping Georgia farmers healthy will have downstream effects on both the economy and food security.[9]

Given these unique challenges for those living in rural settings in the United States, it is important to continually monitor health outcomes across urban and rural settings to determine whether programs like the American Rescue Plan are working, and also to identify any emerging barriers for rural residents. As you'll see throughout this chapter, the cross-sectional design is well suited to assess the health of a population and can be used to make comparisons over time by conducting multiple cross-sectional studies.

---

We are concluding our series of observational study designs with a close-up look at cross-sectional studies. On the surface, this study design is straightforward: simply administer a questionnaire to a group of people at a particular point in time to simultaneously collect exposure and outcome data. However, as you'll see, there are important considerations to bear in mind when conducting a cross-sectional study. Further, this design is an incredibly powerful tool for us to have in our epidemiologic toolkit as it can be used to assess the health status of a population *and* to track changes in a population over time. That's public health!

## CROSS-SECTIONAL STUDY DESIGN BASICS (LEARNING OBJECTIVE 7.1)

Review **Figure 7.1**, which provides a schematic of the **cross-sectional design** that you were introduced to in **Chapter 3, "Introduction to Analytic Epidemiologic Study Designs and Measures of Association."** In a cross-sectional design, the exposure(s) and outcome(s) are measured at the same time. Unlike the cohort design, study participants are not followed over time; and unlike the case-control design, participants are not selected on the basis of their outcome status and assessed for historical exposures. Rather, the cross-sectional design provides a "snapshot" of the health status of the study population at a *single point in time*.

You are likely already familiar with cross-sectional studies, even if you haven't realized it. Course evaluations, internet surveys, and customer service feedback ratings are all examples of sources of cross-sectional data used in everyday life.

Cross-sectional studies are designed to estimate the prevalence of an exposure or a health outcome in a particular population (descriptive epidemiology) as well as to compare the presence of an existing (i.e., prevalent) outcome among those with and without an exposure of interest (analytic epidemiology).

Now consider **Table 7.1**, which provides a more detailed view of the basic steps involved in conducting a cross-sectional study, including formulating a research question, designing and conducting the study, and analyzing and reporting the data. Each of the blue terms in **Table 7.1** are discussed in detail in the text that follows.

## FIGURE 7.1 SCHEMATIC OF A CROSS-SECTIONAL DESIGN

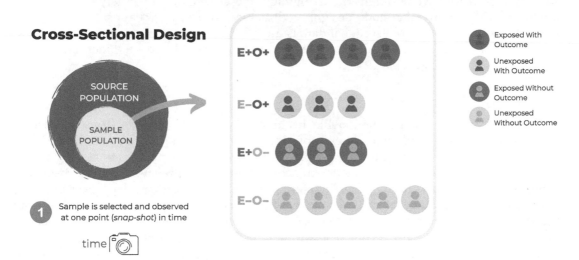

## TABLE 7.1 BASIC STEPS IN DESIGNING AND CONDUCTING A CROSS-SECTIONAL STUDY

| |
|---|
| **State the research question** |
| State the study hypothesis(es) based on the research question. |
| • Define **outcome(s)** with case definitions.<br>• Define the **exposure(s)** and their **reference group**. |
| **Design the cross-sectional study** |
| Identify the source and sample populations. |
| • Determine whether to select individuals based on their **group membership** or based on their **exposure** status. |
| **Conduct the cross-sectional study** |
| Select the sample population, obtain informed consent, and measure the **exposure** and outcome statuses of the participants. |
| Collect data on key covariates. |
| **Analyze and report data** |
| Calculate measures of frequency and association. |
| Report findings using the STROBE reporting guidance. |
| Consider the strengths and limitations of the study. |

# USING A CROSS-SECTIONAL STUDY FOR DESCRIPTIVE AND ANALYTIC ANALYSES (LEARNING OBJECTIVE 7.2)

There are two goals for undertaking a cross-sectional study. The first goal aligns with descriptive epidemiology, whereby investigators aim to estimate the prevalence of health-related exposures and/or outcomes in a particular population. The second goal aligns with analytic epidemiology, whereby investigators test one or more hypotheses to understand the relationship between exposures and health outcomes. Although these two goals aren't mutually exclusive (cross-sectional studies often estimate the prevalence of exposures and outcomes *and* test hypotheses), we find it helpful to highlight these scenarios separately to underscore the utility of this particular study design. As discussed in previous chapters, regardless of whether the analysis of cross-sectional data is intended to be descriptive or analytic, investigators must carefully define all exposures and outcomes, including the identification of appropriate reference groups.

## Prevalence Estimation

To improve health in a population, public health officials must first understand the current health status of that population. For example, they may want to know how common HIV is in the community, or how frequently people report having limited access to healthy foods. These questions can be answered by obtaining estimates of the **prevalence** of health-related exposures or outcomes. Recall from **Chapter 2, "Descriptive Epidemiology, Surveillance, and Measures of Frequency,"** that prevalence is the measure of frequency that describes how common a given characteristic is at one particular point in time. Estimating the prevalence of a health-related exposure or outcome will help us begin to understand the scope of the problem. We can then use this information to see whether certain groups of individuals are more likely to be affected, and then identify potential strategies to improve health outcomes.

An example of the use of a cross-sectional study to estimate the prevalence of a health-related exposure comes from a study that aimed to determine the proportion of babies born in Alberta, Canada, who were ever breastfed as well as the proportion who were exclusively breastfed at 6 months.[10] The World Health Organization recommends exclusive breastfeeding for the first 6 months, meaning waiting to introduce formula or other supplemental foods, if possible, until after 6 months of life.[11] This is important because breastfeeding has health benefits for both the lactating parent and the baby, including a reduced risk of breast cancer and an enhanced immune system, respectively.[12] Given these health benefits, it is helpful for health officials to understand how common this practice is at various points in an infant's life.

## Hypothesis Testing

Beyond their utility to obtain descriptive measures of the prevalence of health-related exposures and outcomes, cross-sectional designs are analytic designs that test one or more hypotheses about the association between exposures and health outcomes. To get the most out of a single cross-sectional study, investigators often explore multiple relationships between many exposures and outcomes.

As described in **Chapter 2, "Descriptive Epidemiology, Surveillance, and Measures of Frequency,"** all study hypotheses should address the following key areas:

- What is the population of interest?
- What is the heath outcome of interest and how is it defined?
- What is the exposure of interest and how is it defined?
- What measures of frequency are being compared?
- What is the direction of the hypothesized association?

In addition to obtaining estimates of the frequency of breastfeeding among infants in Alberta, Canada, public health officials may also be interested in using a cross-sectional study to identify ways to increase breastfeeding among new parents. Since it is important to initiate breastfeeding as soon as possible after delivery, the ideal time to provide expectant parents with information about breastfeeding is during the prenatal period, when most pregnant people in Canada have at least eight encounters with their healthcare providers.[13] These prenatal care visits not only provide an opportunity to evaluate the health of the birthing parent and the developing fetus, but also allow healthcare providers to provide education about important topics, including breastfeeding. While most patients in Canada have one-on-one visits with their healthcare providers during pregnancy, some patients in select healthcare facilities may also be offered group prenatal care visits, which offer additional time for patient education and discussion.[14] In one cross-sectional study, Canadian investigators tested the hypothesis that those who attended group prenatal care would be more likely to perceive having received sufficient information about breastfeeding during their prenatal care compared with those who only attended traditional individual prenatal care.[15]

## Can an Exposure Also Be Used as an Outcome in a Cross-Sectional Design?

Yes! Previously, we saw that breastfeeding can be treated as either an exposure or an outcome, depending on the study hypothesis.

When estimating the prevalence of breastfeeding, investigators may think about this factor as an exposure since it can prevent negative health outcomes in both the lactating parent and the baby.

At the same time, investigators may want to know what exposures are associated with an increased likelihood of breastfeeding. For example, investigators compared those who attended group prenatal care to those who only received traditional individual prenatal care on their perceptions about having received adequate information about breastfeeding. Receiving adequate information about breastfeeding is an important step toward increasing breastfeeding rates.

# IDENTIFY THE SOURCE AND SAMPLE POPULATIONS
## (LEARNING OBJECTIVE 7.3)

As with all study designs, it is imperative that investigators carefully define their **source population** (the group of people from which study participants will be selected) and then thoughtfully select participants to be included in the **sample population** (the people who are actually selected from the source population to participate in the study). As we discuss in detail in **Chapter 10, "Selection Bias,"** careful identification of the source and selection of the sample populations allow epidemiologists to use their study findings to learn something about a larger population.

Similar to the cohort design, the sample population may be identified in one of two ways. The first, and most common, approach is that individuals are selected based on their **group membership**, such as a study of patients receiving cancer treatment or students attending a particular university. This was the approach that investigators used to estimate the prevalence of ever breastfeeding and exclusive breastfeeding at 3 months, where the source population was "pregnant women from Edmonton and Calgary, Alberta."[10] The sample population was then chosen from this source population.

The second way that the sample population might be identified for a cross-sectional study is by their **exposure status**. This was the case in the study that compared the experiences of individuals who received group versus individual prenatal care.[15] Here, the source population was defined as low-risk pregnant individuals receiving prenatal care in a particular urban setting in Alberta, Canada. Since the focus of this study was on the impact of two different prenatal care models, the investigators needed to ensure that their sample included adequate numbers of individuals who received each type of prenatal care. To do this, they selected their exposed and unexposed groups separately. The exposed group was selected from a group of "women participating in [group prenatal care] at a community-based health centre in urban Alberta... [that serves] low-income and vulnerable populations" while their unexposed (i.e., comparison) group was selected from a group of "women who...received individual prenatal care at a low-risk maternity clinic run by the same physician group in the same geographic area of the city."[15]

We will return to the importance of appropriate selection of the source and sample populations when we discuss issues of selection bias and generalizability in **Chapter 10, "Selection Bias."**

## Pause to Practice 7.1

### Identifying Exposures, Outcomes, and Source and Sample Populations in a Cross-Sectional Study

Given differences in access to healthcare services across urban and rural areas, public health officials are often interested in comparing patterns of health-related outcomes by urbanicity, which considers factors such as population size and density.

An analysis of the 2019 National Health Interview Survey—a cross-sectional survey designed to understand health behaviors of U.S. adults—explored whether influenza vaccination prevalence differed across three categories of urbanicity: large metropolitan, small or medium metropolitan, and nonmetropolitan areas.[16]

Since influenza-related mortality rates are higher (on average) in rural counties compared with urban counties,[17] investigators hypothesized that the prevalence of influenza vaccination would be *lower* among those living in nonmetropolitan areas compared with those living in large metropolitan areas *and* that the prevalence of influenza vaccination would be *lower* among those living in nonmetropolitan areas compared with those living in small or medium metropolitan areas.

1. What are the study design features that indicate this is a cross-sectional study?
2. What is the exposure of interest in this study? What are the different levels of the exposure?
3. What is the outcome of interest in the study? What are the different levels of the outcome?
4. The investigators made two different comparisons, where the exposed group was compared with two different reference groups. Describe each of the comparisons that were made.
5. What is the source population for this study?
6. What is the sample population for this study?

## DATA LAYOUT AND MEASURES OF FREQUENCY AND ASSOCIATION CALCULATED IN CROSS-SECTIONAL DESIGNS (LEARNING OBJECTIVES 7.4 & 7.5)

As summarized in **Tables 7.2** and **M.4**, data for the cross-sectional design are organized using a traditional R×C table, where the number of study participants are organized by their exposure and outcome status. Recall that since a cross-sectional design only captures *prevalent* outcomes, the related measures of frequency and association must be prevalence-based.

In the cross-sectional design, the frequencies of the exposures and outcomes are described using measures of prevalence. Investigators may be interested in the prevalence of both the exposure and the outcome in the sample population. These measures may be referred to as the **prevalence of exposure** or **prevalence of outcome** and are shown in **Equations 7.1 and 7.2.**

$$\text{Prevalence of } \textit{exposure} \text{ in the sample population} = \frac{\text{Total } \textit{exposed}}{\text{Total in sample population}} = \frac{N_1}{N} \quad (7.1)$$

$$\text{Prevalence of } \textit{outcome} \text{ in the sample population} = \frac{\text{Total } \textit{with outcome}}{\text{Total in sample population}} = \frac{M_1}{N} \quad (7.2)$$

**TABLE 7.2 DATA LAYOUT AND MEASURES OF FREQUENCY AND ASSOCIATION FOR THE CROSS-SECTIONAL DESIGN**

| Data Layout | | Exposed (E+) | Unexposed (E−) | TOTAL |
|---|---|---|---|---|
| | Outcome + (O+) | A | B | $M_1$ (A+B) |
| | Outcome − (O−) | C | D | $M_0$ (C+D) |
| | TOTAL | $N_1$ (A+C) | $N_0$ (B+D) | N |

| Measures of Outcome Frequency | Prevalence of outcome $= \dfrac{M_1}{N}$ <br><br> Prevalence of outcome among exposed $= \dfrac{A}{N_1}$ <br><br> Prevalence of outcome among unexposed $= \dfrac{B}{N_0}$ |
|---|---|
| Measure of Exposure Frequency | Prevalence of exposure $= \dfrac{N_1}{N}$ |

| Measures of Association and Interpretations | Prevalence ratio (PR) $= \dfrac{A/N_1}{B/N_0}$ | The prevalence of the outcome among the exposed is [insert value of **PR**] times the prevalence of the outcome among the unexposed. |
|---|---|---|
| | Prevalence difference (PD) $= \dfrac{A}{N_1} - \dfrac{B}{N_0}$ | The difference in the prevalence of the outcome among the exposed versus the unexposed is [insert value of **PD**]. |
| | Prevalence odds ratio (POR)[*] <br><br> $= \dfrac{\text{Odds of a \textbf{prevalent outcome} among the exposed}}{\text{Odds of a \textbf{prevalent outcome} among the unexposed}}$ <br><br> $= \dfrac{A/C}{B/D} = \dfrac{A \times D}{B \times C}$ | The odds of a prevalent outcome among the exposed are [insert value of **POR**] times the odds of a prevalent outcome among the unexposed. |

\* The prevalence odds ratio is only suitable when the prevalence of the outcome in the exposed and unexposed groups is rare (i.e., ≤ 10%)

Consider the study designed to estimate the prevalence of ever having breastfed and exclusive breastfeeding at 6 months.[10] Adapting slightly from the study, let's assume investigators found that 396 of the 402 individuals in the sample population had ever breastfed their baby, while 62 of the 402 individuals reported that they were exclusively breastfeeding their babies at 6 months. We can use this information to calculate the prevalence of both ever having breastfed and exclusive breastfeeding at 6 months in the sample population:

Prevalence of *ever having breastfed* in the sample population

$$= \frac{396 \text{ people reported ever having breastfed their baby}}{402 \text{ people in the sample population}}$$

$$= \frac{396}{402} = 0.99 = 99\%$$

Prevalence of *exclusive breastfeeding at 6 months* in the sample population

$$= \frac{62 \text{ people reported exclusive breastfeeding at 6 months}}{402 \text{ people in the sample population}}$$

$$= \frac{62}{402} = 0.15 = 15\%$$

To put these numbers in context, we see that the vast majority (99%) of individuals in the sample population had ever breastfed their baby, while the prevalence of exclusive breast-feeding at 6 months dropped considerably to 15%. Information like this can be useful for public health officials to learn more about the needs of the community.

When evaluating the association between an exposure and an outcome, investigators typically compare the prevalence of the outcome in the exposed (**Equation 7.3**) to the prevalence of the outcome in the unexposed (**Equation 7.4**).

Prevalence of the *outcome* among the *exposed*

$$= \frac{\text{Total } \textit{with outcome} \text{ who are } \textit{exposed}}{\text{Total } \textit{exposed}} = \frac{A}{N_1} \tag{7.3}$$

Prevalence of the *outcome* among the *unexposed*

$$= \frac{\text{Total } \textit{with outcome} \text{ who are } \textit{unexposed}}{\text{Total } \textit{unexposed}} = \frac{B}{N_0} \tag{7.4}$$

**Table 7.3** shows data adapted from the study comparing the experiences of those who received group versus individual prenatal care with respect to their perceptions about having received sufficient information about breastfeeding during their pregnancies.[15] We can use this information to separately calculate the prevalence of having received sufficient information about breastfeeding for those who received group or individual prenatal care.

**TABLE 7.3 DATA ADAPTED FROM A STUDY OF THE ASSOCIATION BETWEEN RECEIVING GROUP VERSUS INDIVIDUAL PRENATAL CARE AND PERCEPTIONS ABOUT HAVING RECEIVED SUFFICIENT INFORMATION ABOUT BREASTFEEDING DURING PREGNANCY**

| | Group Prenatal Care | Individual Prenatal Care Only |
|---|---|---|
| Reported receiving **sufficient** information about breastfeeding during pregnancy | 43 | 64 |
| Reported receiving **insufficient** information about breastfeeding during pregnancy | 2 | 28 |
| TOTAL | 45 | 92 |

*Source:* https://doi.org/10.1007/s10995-018-2559-1

Prevalence of reporting receiving sufficient information about breastfeeding among those in...

$$\text{Group prenatal care} = \frac{43}{45} = 0.96 = 96\%$$

$$\text{Individual prenatal care only} = \frac{64}{92} = 0.70 = 70\%$$

The prevalence of the outcome across two exposure groups can be compared by division or subtraction, yielding the **prevalence ratio (PR; Equation 7.5)** and the **prevalence difference (PD; Equation 7.6)**, respectively. These measures of association compare the prevalence of the outcome in the exposed to the prevalence of the outcome in the unexposed.

Prevalence ratio (PR)

$$= \frac{\text{Prevalence of } \textit{outcome} \text{ among } \textit{exposed}}{\text{Prevalence of } \textit{outcome} \text{ among } \textit{unexposed}}$$

$$= \frac{A/N_1}{B/N_0} \tag{7.5}$$

Prevalence difference (PD)

= Prevalence of *outcome* among *exposed* − prevalence of *outcome* among *unexposed*

$$= \frac{A}{N_1} - \frac{B}{N_0}$$ (7.6)

Investigators compared the prevalence of reporting receiving sufficient information about breastfeeding among those in group prenatal care to the prevalence of reporting receiving sufficient information about breastfeeding among those who only received individual prenatal care.

$$\text{Prevalence ratio (PR)} = \frac{43/45}{63/92} = 1.40$$

$$\text{Prevalence difference (PD)} = \frac{43}{45} - \frac{63}{92} = 0.27 = 27\%$$

We can interpret these measures of association as follows:

**Prevalence Ratio:** Those who received group prenatal care had 1.4 times the prevalence of reporting having received sufficient information about breastfeeding during pregnancy compared with those who only received individual prenatal care.

**Prevalence Difference:** The difference in the prevalence of reporting having received sufficient information about breastfeeding during pregnancy among those who received group prenatal care versus those who received individual prenatal care was 27%.

Using the information that we have available at this stage, we can conclude that breastfeeding information was better communicated to those who received group prenatal care compared with those who only received individual prenatal care.

## Prevalence Odds Ratio

As described in **Chapter 6, "Case-Control Designs,"** there are times when investigators will report an odds ratio, even when they haven't conducted a case-control study. When an odds ratio is calculated using data from a cross-sectional study, it is called a **prevalence odds ratio (POR),** and is interpreted as follows:

The odds of a prevalent *outcome* among the *exposed* is [insert value of POR] times the odds of a prevalent *outcome* among the *unexposed*.

### Where There Are Odds Ratios, There May Not Always Be Case-Control Studies

In the following Digging Deeper, we share more detail about situations when the prevalence odds ratio is appropriate to calculate and when it is not. Depending on where you are in your epidemiologic journey, you may or may not be ready for these specifics. Regardless, as you are calculating measures of association for cross-sectional studies, we urge you to use the prevalence ratio and prevalence difference, as they are always appropriate for the analysis of cross-sectional data.

However, as we described in **Chapter 6, "Case-Control Designs,"** it is important for you to know that investigators sometimes report odds ratios, even when they have conducted a cross-sectional study. As you read peer-reviewed literature, be sure to read the study methods carefully to discern the study design, and do not rely on the reported measure(s) of association to make this determination!

## Caution Against Calculating an Odds Ratio When the Outcome of Interest Is Not Rare

While investigators *can* calculate an odds ratio whenever the outcome of interest is dichotomous, that doesn't mean that they always *should*. When the outcome of interest is rare (typically 10% or less) in both the exposed and unexposed groups, the prevalence odds ratio will be reasonably close to the prevalence ratio calculated using the same data. However, when the outcome is *not* rare, the prevalence odds ratio will provide an overestimate of the corresponding prevalence ratio, meaning that the effect of the exposure on the outcome will appear stronger than it really is.

**Table 7.4** shows an example where the prevalence odds ratio is a suitable substitute for the prevalence ratio.

TABLE 7.4 **AN EXAMPLE WHERE THE PREVALENCE ODDS RATIO IS A SUITABLE SUBSTITUTE FOR THE PREVALENCE RATIO**

|  | Exposed (E+) | Unexposed (E−) |
|---|---|---|
| Outcome + | 10 | 5 |
| Outcome − | 190 | 195 |
| TOTAL | 200 | 200 |

Prevalence of outcome among the...

$$\text{Exposed} = \frac{10}{200} = 0.05 = 5.0\%$$

$$\text{Unexposed} = \frac{5}{200} = 0.025 = 2.5\%$$

$$\text{Prevalence ratio (PR)} = \frac{A/N_1}{B/N_0} = \frac{10/200}{5/200} = 2.00 \qquad \text{Prevalence odds ratio (POR)} = \frac{A \times D}{B \times C} = \frac{10 \times 195}{5 \times 190} = 2.05$$

In this case, the prevalence of the outcome in the exposed (5%) and unexposed (2.5%) groups was less than 10%, and the prevalence odds ratio (POR = 2.05) was a close approximation to the prevalence ratio (PR = 2.00).

**Table 7.5** shows an example where the prevalence odds ratio is *not* a suitable substitute for the prevalence ratio and may not be appropriate to calculate in a cross-sectional study.

TABLE 7.5 **AN EXAMPLE WHERE THE PREVALENCE ODDS RATIO IS NOT A SUITABLE SUBSTITUTE FOR THE PREVALENCE RATIO**

|  | Exposed (E+) | Unexposed (E−) |
|---|---|---|
| Outcome + | 100 | 50 |
| Outcome | 100 | 150 |
| TOTAL | 200 | 200 |

Prevalence of outcome among the...

$$\text{Exposed} = \frac{100}{200} = 0.50 = 50\%$$

$$\text{Unexposed} = \frac{50}{200} = 0.25 = 25\%$$

$$\text{Prevalence ratio (PR)} = \frac{A/N_1}{B/N_0} = \frac{100/200}{50/200} = 2.00 \qquad \text{Prevalence odds ratio (POR)} = \frac{A \times D}{B \times C} = \frac{100 \times 150}{50 \times 100} = 3.00$$

In this case, the prevalence of the outcome in the exposed (50%) and unexposed (25%) groups was greater than 10%; thus, the prevalence odds ratio (POR = 3.00) was much larger than the prevalence ratio (PR = 2.00).

Investigators may choose to report odds ratios for data obtained from a cohort or cross-sectional study since the odds ratio is the measure of association produced by a standard, more advanced analytic technique that is popular among epidemiologists, called logistic regression. At this stage, it is best for you to continue calculating and reporting the appropriate risk- or prevalence-based measure of association to help reinforce the difference between the observational study designs. At the same time, it is important for you to understand why you might see PORs reported from a cross-sectional study (and in fact, they may just be labeled *odds ratios*!).

## Pause to Practice 7.2

### Calculating Measures of Frequency and Association in a Cross-Sectional Study

**Table 7.6** shows adapted data from the influenza vaccination study described previously, which classifies the study population by their household urban–rural classification and their influenza vaccine prevalence.[16] We can use this information to calculate measures of frequency to describe the distribution of influenza vaccination, and we can use it to understand the associations between urbanicity and influenza vaccination prevalence.

**TABLE 7.6 ADAPTED DATA FROM A STUDY OF THE ASSOCIATION BETWEEN HOUSEHOLD URBAN–RURAL CLASSIFICATION AND INFLUENZA VACCINATION**

| | | Household Urban–Rural Classification | | |
| --- | --- | --- | --- | --- |
| | | Large Metropolitan | Small and Medium Metropolitan | Nonmetropolitan |
| Received influenza vaccine in the 12 months preceding the survey | Yes | 7,920 | 4,642 | 2,192 |
| | No | 8,546 | 5,405 | 2,836 |
| TOTAL | | 16,466 | 10,047 | 5,028 |

*Source*: Data from Jain B, Paguio JA, Yao JS, et al. Rural-Urban Differences in Influenza Vaccination Among Adults in the United States, 2018-2019. *Am J Public Health*. 2022;112(2):304-307. https://doi.org/10.2105/AJPH.2021.306575

1. Name and calculate the epidemiologic measure that describes the frequency of the outcome in the sample population. Is this an example of a descriptive or an analytic epidemiologic measure? How can you tell?

2. Name and calculate the epidemiologic measures that describe the frequency of the outcome in each of the exposure groups.

3. Name and calculate the prevalence ratio that compares vaccination prevalence among those in nonmetropolitan (nonmetro) areas to those living in large metropolitan (large metro) areas. Is this an example of a descriptive or an analytic epidemiologic measure? How can you tell?

4. Name and calculate the prevalence ratio that compares vaccination prevalence among those in nonmetro areas to those living in medium and small metropolitan (medium/small metro) areas. Is this an example of a descriptive or an analytic epidemiologic measure? How can you tell?

5. Is the association between vaccination coverage and urbanicity stronger when comparing those living in nonmetro areas to those living in large metro areas or when comparing to those living in medium/small metro areas? How can you tell? How would you interpret this result?

# SERIAL CROSS-SECTIONAL STUDIES (LEARNING OBJECTIVE 7.6)

Cross-sectional surveys are often used to conduct public health surveillance, whereby a sample of individuals is taken periodically (e.g., every year or every 5 years) from a source population to obtain estimates of the prevalence of health behaviors and health outcomes. These surveys are particularly useful for tracking changes in trends over time. A prominent example of this in the United States is the Centers for Disease Control and Prevention's Behavioral Risk Factor Surveillance System (BRFSS). Each year, more than 400,000 U.S. adults are sampled for inclusion in BRFSS and are asked questions about their health-related behaviors and chronic health conditions.[18]

Although each sample contains different individuals, the sampling method employed by these studies ensures that those included in the sample population are *representative* of the source population. In the case of BRFSS, although only a fraction of the U.S population is included in the annual surveys, these results can be used to infer how health behaviors change across the source population of the United States.

Trends in the prevalence of smoking and smokeless tobacco use (chewing tobacco, snuff, or snus) using BRFSS data are shown in **Figure 7.2**. The prevalence of smoking declined from 21.2% in 2011 to 15.5% in 2020. Although the prevalence of smokeless tobacco use was consistently lower than the prevalence of smoking, its prevalence remained relatively stable during this same period (approximately 4%).[19]

## FIGURE 7.2 USING SERIAL CROSS-SECTIONAL STUDIES TO ASSESS THE PREVALENCE OF SMOKING AND SMOKELESS TOBACCO USE OVER TIME

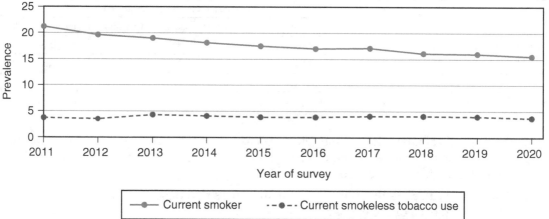

*Source*: Centers for Disease Control and Prevention. *BRFSS prevalence & trends data.* https://nccd.cdc.gov/BRFSSPrevalence/rdPage.aspx?rdReport=DPH_BRFSS.ExploreByTopic&irbLocationType=StatesAndMMSA&islClass=CLASS17&islTopic=TOPIC15&islYear=2020&rdRnd=6747

We are able to track the prevalence of both smoking and smokeless tobacco use during this time period because there were neither changes to the way that BRFSS identified and recruited participants nor to the wording of the questions about these factors. In contrast, while BRFSS has asked questions about fruit and vegetable consumption for several years, they made a change to the way that they asked these questions in 2017 to make them easier to understand.[20] In 2015, BRFSS participants were asked:

"During the past month, not counting juice, how many times per day, week, or month did you eat fruit? Count fresh, frozen, or canned fruit."

In 2017, this question was updated as follows:

"Not including juices, how often did you eat fruit? You can tell me times per day, per week, or per month."

While these questions both aim to understand how often individuals were eating fruit, results from before and after the wording change may not be comparable because of differences in how survey participants may have interpreted the question. Similar challenges arise when the survey methodology is updated, as was the case in 2011 when BRFSS employed new statistical techniques and expanded their recruitment strategy to include cellphone users.[21] These changes were necessary to improve how well BRFSS captured the current health status of U.S. adults; however, they did come at a cost to understanding trends over time since BRFSS results from 2011 onward are not comparable to previous years.

## STRENGTHS AND LIMITATIONS OF CROSS-SECTIONAL DESIGNS (LEARNING OBJECTIVE 7.7)

### Strengths of Cross-Sectional Studies

**Study of multiple exposures.** The cross-sectional design allows for the study of multiple exposures. This is particularly useful when there is interest in learning about many different factors that may influence health in a particular population.

**Study of multiple outcomes.** Similarly, the cross-sectional design also allows for the study of multiple health-related outcomes.

**Logistics.** In general, cross-sectional studies are less expensive and can be conducted more quickly compared with the other epidemiologic study designs.

**Avoids loss to follow-up**. Given that a cross-sectional study observes study participants at one point in time, there is no risk of losing individuals to follow-up.

**Utility for public health practice.** Cross-sectional studies are ideal for evaluating the burden of exposures or outcomes in a particular population. This information can be used to inform public health action, including the allocation of funding, targeted prevention strategies, and even public health policy.

**Aids with future study planning.** Cross-sectional studies may be used by investigators to obtain preliminary data to support proposals to fund more robust studies that are better suited to establish temporality between the exposure and outcome. Additionally, they may be used as exploratory studies that generate new hypotheses that are subsequently tested using other study designs.

### Limitations of Cross-Sectional Studies

**Temporality.** It can be very difficult to establish cause and effect using data from a cross-sectional study. The **temporality** between the exposure and the outcome may not always be evident, meaning that we may not know whether the exposure is known to have occurred before the outcome or vice versa. For example, in a cross-sectional study assessing current sleep quality and prevalent mental health, the temporality between the variables may be unclear: Does poor sleep lead to mental distress, or does mental distress lead to poor sleep? Let's think back to the randomized trial or cohort designs in which an at-risk group of exposed and unexposed individuals are followed over time to determine who develops new outcome(s) of interest. This structure of the measurement of the exposure *prior to* the outcome's occurrence establishes temporality between the exposure and the outcome, which is a required for a relationship to be causal. Even case-control studies are designed to establish temporality by looking back at previous exposures and/or enrolling cases with an incident outcome. In contrast, the exposure and outcome are measured at the same time in the cross-sectional design; thus, temporality is not established in the same way.

However, there are times when it is reasonable to assume that an exposure *did* precede the outcome. For example, the effects of hereditary traits such as blood type logically temporally precede health outcomes experienced over the life course. Additionally, survey questions used in cross-sectional studies may be designed to ask about distinct time periods to make clear that the exposure occurred before the health outcome. As an example, a cross-sectional study could explore the association between childhood sleep quality and current mental health in adults. Although it may not be possible to ascertain whether childhood sleep quality *caused* poor mental health in adulthood, we can feel confident that we have established temporality given that our exposure occurred during childhood and the outcome occurred during adulthood.

**Study of outcomes or exposures with short duration.** If an exposure or outcome has a short duration, such as temporary use of a sleep aid or strep throat, investigators may obtain an underestimate of exposure or outcome prevalence if studied using a cross-sectional design, which only captures measures at a particular point in time. For example, the challenges of measuring the prevalence of an exposure with a short duration are shown in **Figure 7.3**, using the example of temporary use of a sleep aid. The same issue applies to health-related outcomes with a short duration.

## FIGURE 7.3 ILLUSTRATING THE CHALLENGES OF STUDYING EXPOSURES* WITH A SHORT DURATION USING A CROSS-SECTIONAL DESIGN

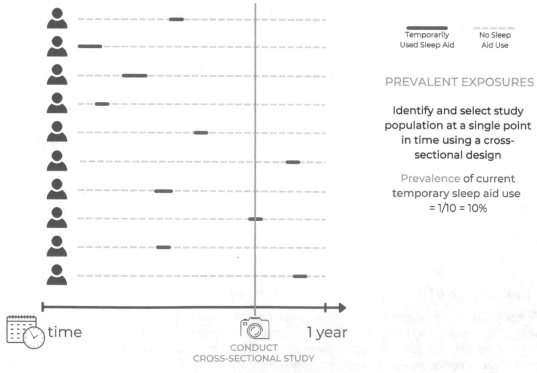

Temporarily Used Sleep Aid    No Sleep Aid Use

PREVALENT EXPOSURES

Identify and select study population at a single point in time using a cross-sectional design

Prevalence of current temporary sleep aid use = 1/10 = 10%

time    1 year

CONDUCT CROSS-SECTIONAL STUDY

*The same concerns arise for **outcomes** with short durations.

During the 1-year period, all 10 of the individuals in the sample population had temporarily used a sleep aid at some time or another. However, at the time that the cross-sectional study was conducted, there was only one person currently using a sleep aid. The prevalence of current temporary sleep aid use (1/10 = 10%) grossly underestimates the frequency of temporary sleep aid use during this year (10/10 = 100%).

In truth, this may not be a limitation if the goal of the study is to estimate how common temporary sleep aid use is at a particular moment in time. However, if the study goal was to understand the use of temporary sleep aids more broadly, a snapshot of *current* temporary sleep aid use wouldn't be very useful. To circumvent this problem, investigators might change how they ask the question. Instead of asking, "Are you currently using a sleep aid to temporarily help you sleep?" investigators may instead ask, "Have you temporarily used a sleep aid to help you sleep anytime in the last 12 months?" Since the data are collected at a single point in time, this would still be classified as a cross-sectional study. However, investigators are able to obtain a more accurate understanding of the frequency of temporary sleep aid use by expanding the time frame during which participants are asked to consider various health behaviors.

**Survival bias.** The cross-sectional design may be ill-equipped to study exposures that tend to either increase or decrease someone's likelihood of survival. We began to introduce this concept in **Chapter 6, "Case-Control Designs,"** when we discussed the importance of enrolling incident rather than prevalent cases of the outcome of interest in case-control studies. In the context of the cross-sectional design, where all outcomes are prevalent, we may be concerned about survival bias, which occurs when those who survive and are available to be included in the study are meaningfully different from those who die and thus are not available to be included. **Figure 7.4** is an adaptation of **Figure 6.4**, which, for simplicity, considers only those who have the outcome of interest. Among this group, those who are exposed are much more likely to die (4/5) compared with those who are unexposed (1/5). Although we started with an equal number of exposed and unexposed individuals (true prevalence of exposure among those with the outcome = 5/10 = 50%), differential mortality between these groups led to a **biased** (i.e., incorrect) assessment of the prevalence of the exposure among those with the outcome at the time that a cross-sectional study was conducted (prevalence of exposure after differential survival = 1/5 = 20%). As you will learn in **Chapter 10, "Selection Bias,"** differential survival can bias the measure of association calculated in a cross-sectional study only when this survival imbalance differs for those with and without the outcome.

## FIGURE 7.4 ILLUSTRATING THE IMPACT OF SURVIVAL BIAS WHEN ESTIMATING THE PREVALENCE OF THE EXPOSURE AMONG INDIVIDUALS WITH THE OUTCOME

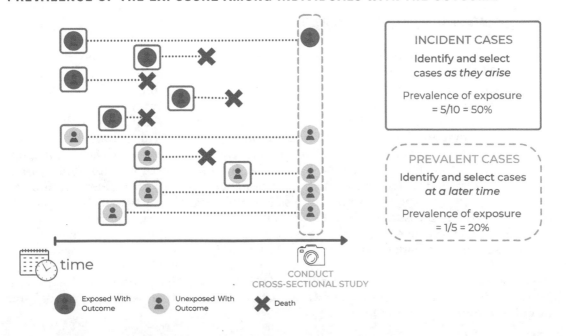

## Pause to Practice 7.3

### From a Cross-Sectional Study to Public Health Action

As we showed, the 2019 U.S. National Health Interview Survey found that influenza vaccination coverage is lower in nonmetropolitan areas. This is concerning since influenza-related mortality rates tend to be higher in rural counties than in urban counties.[17]

1. What are some possible reasons why the prevalence of influenza vaccination may be lower for those living in nonmetropolitan areas compared with those in metropolitan areas?

2. What types of public health actions might public health officials or policy makers undertake in response to these findings?

3. Do you have concerns about the temporality between the exposure and the outcome of interest in this particular study?

### Reporting Study Findings From Cross-Sectional Studies: The STROBE Statement

As discussed in **Chapter 5, "Cohort Designs,"** there is standardized reporting guidance for reporting the results from **observational studies**.[22] Items that are highlighted as being important for reporting data from cross-sectional studies include:

- "The eligibility criteria and the sources and methods of selection of participants"
- "Characteristics of study participants separately for exposed and unexposed groups"
- "If applicable, describe analytical methods taking account of sampling strategy"
- "Report numbers of outcome events or summary measures"

## WHERE WE'VE BEEN AND WHAT'S UP NEXT

This chapter concludes our discussion of the four main epidemiologic study designs. By now, you should have a good understanding of the different ways that epidemiologists collect information to study the patterns of health and disease in populations, and how to calculate and interpret appropriate measures of frequency and association.

Thus far, we have calculated measures of association that describe exposure–outcome relationships that apply to everyone in the sample population. This means that we have assumed that the exposure of interest has the same effect on everyone in the sample population, which may not always be the case. In **Chapter 8, "Effect Measure Modification and Statistical Interaction,"** we explore the phenomenon called **effect measure modification**, in which an exposure is more or less harmful for different subsets of the sample population. Effect measure modification is not an error to correct, but rather allows us to explore whether the effect of an exposure is different for different groups of people in your sample population. After this, we will take a deep dive into all the ways that epidemiologic studies can be influenced by error (**Chapter 9, "Error in Epidemiologic Research and Fundamentals of Confounding"**; **Chapter 10, "Selection Bias"**; **Chapter 11, "Information Bias and Screening and Diagnostic Tests"**; and **Chapter 12, "Random Error in Epidemiologic Research"**).

# END OF CHAPTER PROBLEM SET

**Questions 1 to 11 refer to the description of a study of COVID-19–related discrimination, described in the text that follows.**

Investigators conducted a study during the first year of the COVID-19 pandemic to learn about the experience of COVID-19–related discrimination among major racial and ethnic groups in the United States.[23] This was an important undertaking because the COVID-19 pandemic was unfortunately accompanied by surges in discrimination and xenophobia, as is often the case with infectious disease outbreaks. Since the experience of discrimination is known to have negative effects on both mental and physical health,[24] it is important to understand the pattern and scope of the experience of pandemic-related discrimination.

Eligible participants were individuals living in the United States who self-identify as belonging to "all major US racial/ethnic groups (as defined by the US Bureau of the Census)." The sample population included 5,500 U.S. residents, all of whom reported their race and ethnicity on the survey instrument. The stated objectives of this study were to[23]:

**Objective 1**: "Determine the prevalence of COVID-19–related discrimination among major US racial/ethnic groups"

**Objective 2**: "Estimate associations between discrimination, race/ethnicity, and other sociodemographic characteristics"

1. Does the study's first objective align with descriptive or analytic epidemiology? How do you know?

2. Does the study's second objective align with descriptive or analytic epidemiology? How do you know?

3. What are the source and sample populations for this study?

4. To assess respondents' experience of COVID-19–related discrimination, investigators asked whether, since the start of the pandemic, participants had experienced any of the following: people acting afraid of them; called them names or insulted them; threatened/harassed them; and/or made racist comments to them.[23]

   Explain why it is the case that this study still employs a cross-sectional design, even though this question is asking about an individual's experience of COVID-19–related discrimination over a span of several months.

Table 7.7 provides information adapted from the previously described study.

**TABLE 7.7 DATA ADAPATED FROM A STUDY OF THE ASSOCIATIONS BETWEEN RACE/ETHNICITY AND ENGLISH PROFICIENCY AND EXPERIENCE OF COVID-19-RELATED DISCRIMINATION**

| Characteristic | Number Who Reported Having Frequently[a] Experienced COVID-19–Related Discrimination |
|---|---|
| Race/Ethnicity | |
| Native American/Alaska Native ($n = 500$) | 84 |
| Asian ($n = 1,000$) | 126 |
| Black/African American ($n = 1,000$) | 91 |
| Latino ($n = 1,000$) | 106 |
| Hawaiian/Pacific Islander ($n = 500$) | 54 |
| White ($n = 1,000$) | 54 |
| Multiracial ($n = 500$) | 19 |

*(continued)*

**TABLE 7.7 DATA ADAPTED FROM A STUDY OF THE ASSOCIATIONS BETWEEN RACE/ETHNICITY AND ENGLISH PROFICIENCY AND EXPERIENCE OF COVID-19-RELATED DISCRIMINATION** (*continued*)

| Characteristic | Number Who Reported Having Frequently[a] Experienced COVID-19–Related Discrimination |
|---|---|
| English Proficiency | |
| Limited (*n* = 618) | 141 |
| Not limited (*n* = 4,852) | 393 |

[a]Survey participants were asked how frequently they experienced COVID-19–related discriminatory behaviors. Those who reported that they "sometimes" or "always" experienced COVID-19–related discrimination were considered as having frequently experienced COVID-19–related discrimination. Those who responded "rarely" or "never" were considered as not having frequently experienced COVID-19–related discrimination.

*Source*: Data from Strassle PD, Stewart AL, Quintero SM, et al. COVID-19-related discrimination among racial/ethnic minorities and other marginalized communities in the United States. *Am J Public Health*. 2022;112(3):453–466. https://doi.org/10.2105/AJPH.2021.306594

5. What is the prevalence of reporting having frequently experienced COVID-19–related discrimination for each of the seven race/ethnicity groups?

   The authors of this study compared the prevalence of frequently experiencing COVID-19–related discrimination in each of the race/ethnicity groups to the prevalence of COVID-19–related discrimination among White individuals.

6. What is the exposure of interest? What are the different levels?

7. What is the outcome of interest? What are the different levels?

8. Calculate the six relevant PRs and provide a written summary of the findings.

9. Your friend notices that 54 Hawaiian/Pacific Islander individuals and 54 White individuals reported having "sometimes" or "always" experienced COVID-19–related discrimination and remarks that the experience of COVID-19–related discrimination was the same for these two groups. Provide a response that you would give to your friend to help them understand their mistake.

10. The authors of this study also compared the prevalence of COVID-19–related discrimination among those with limited English proficiency to those who did not have limited English proficiency. Calculate this prevalence ratio and provide a written summary of the findings.

11. Compare the direction and magnitude of the prevalence ratios that you calculated in Questions 8 and 10. Which exposure was more strongly associated with COVID-19-related discrimination?

**Questions 12 to 14 refer to estimating the prevalence of autism spectrum disorder, described in the text that follows.**

Autism Spectrum Disorder (ASD), a developmental disability, impacts the way an individual communicates and experiences the world around them.[25] Although ASD has different manifestations, some common signs include avoiding eye contact, not knowing how to relate to others, difficulties adapting to changes in routines, and repetitive motions.[25]

The prevalence of autism has increased over time, potentially due to changes in risk factors, but also largely attributable to changes in autism detection and awareness over time.[26]

For each of the scenarios that follow, explain whether the prevalence estimates obtained from such a study are likely to be an overestimate, underestimate, or accurate estimate of the true prevalence of autism among children in the United States.

12. A study to estimate the prevalence of autism reviews a sample of records from U.S. pediatricians' offices to identify children whose medical records indicate that they meet the criteria consistent with an autism diagnosis.

13. A study to estimate the prevalence of autism selects a random sample of children living in the United States and conducts a multidisciplinary diagnostic assessment to determine whether the children meet the criteria consistent with an autism diagnosis.

14. Suppose that you are on a team that conducts autism surveillance in the United States and you have made no changes to your methods for estimating the prevalence of autism. However, during the 2 years between surveys, there happens to be increased media attention about autism and the importance of early detection. What is likely to happen when the results for your next surveillance cycle are available? What does this mean about the results for the previous cycle?

# REFERENCES

1. U.S. Census Bureau. What Is Rural America? 2017. https://www.census.gov/library/stories/2017/08/rural-america.html#:~:text=What%20is%20urban%20and%20what,are%20far%20from%20urban%20centers

2. America Counts Staff. One in five Americans live in rural areas. August 9, 2017. https://www.census.gov/library/stories/2017/08/rural-america.html

3. Scotti S. Tracking rural hospital closures. *NCSL Legisbrief*. 2017;25(21):1–2. https://pubmed.ncbi.nlm.nih.gov/28613458

4. Georgia Hospital Association. Georgia hospital closure list. 2022. https://www.gha.org/Advocacy

5. Zertuche AD. Georgia's obstetric care crisis. Presentation at: *South Carolina Birth Outcomes Initiative Symposium*. October 30, 2019. Columbia, SC. https://www.scdhhs.gov/sites/default/files/Georgia%27s%20Obstetric%20Care%20Crisis.pdf

6. National Agricultural Statistics Service. *Agricultural Statistics 2020*. United States Department of Agriculture; 2020.

7. Warnock RR. *Senators Reverend Warnock, Ossoff Secure $306 Million for Rural Georgia Health Care Providers*. Jon Ossoff; 2021.

8. Ossoff J. *Sens. Ossoff & Warnock Announce Over $143 Million for Georgia's 35 Community Health Centers*. Jon Ossoff; 2021.

9. U.S. Department of Agriculture Economic Research Service. Ag and food statistics: charting the essentials. March 22, 2022. https://www.ers.usda.gov/data-products/ag-and-food-statistics-charting-the-essentials

10. Jessri M, Farmer AP, Maximova K, Willows ND, Bell RC; APrON Study Team. Predictors of exclusive breastfeeding: observations from the Alberta pregnancy outcomes and nutrition (APrON) study. *BMC Pediatr*. 2013;13:77. https://doi.org/10.1186/1471-2431-13-77

11. World Health Organization. *Guideline: Counselling of Women to Improve Breastfeeding Practices 2018*. World Health Organization; 2018.

12. Department of Health and Human Services Office on Women's Health. Benefits of breastfeeding. *Nutr Clin Care*. 2003;6(3):125–131. https://pubmed.ncbi.nlm.nih.gov/14979457

13. Schuurmans AL. *Healthy Beginnings: Your Handbook for Pregnancy and Birth*. The Society of Obstetricians and Gynecologists of Canada; 2000.

14. Reid J. Centering pregnancy: a model for group prenatal care. *Nurs Womens Health*. 2007;11(4):382–388. https://doi.org/10.1111/j.1751-486X.2007.00194.x

15. Hetherington E, Tough S, McNeil D, Bayrampour H, Metcalfe A. Vulnerable women's perceptions of individual versus group prenatal care: results of a cross-sectional survey. *Matern Child Health J*. 2018;22(11):1632–1638. https://doi.org/10.1007/s10995-018-2559-1

16. Jain B, Paguio JA, Yao JS, et al. Rural-Urban differences in influenza vaccination among adults in the United States, 2018–2019. *Am J Public Health*. 2022;112(2):304–307. https://doi.org/10.2105/AJPH.2021.306575

17. Centers for Disease Control and Prevention. QuickStats: age-adjusted death rates for influenza and pneumonia, by urbanization level and sex—National Vital Statistics System, United States, 2019. *MMWR Morb Mortal Wkly Rep*. 2021;70(12):456. https://doi.org/10.15585/mmwr.mm7012a5

18. Centers for Disease Control and Prevention. About BRFSS. May 16, 2014. https://www.cdc.gov/brfss/about/index.htm

19. Centers for Disease Control and Prevention. *BRFSS prevalence & trends data*. https://nccd.cdc.gov/BRFSSPrevalence/rdPage.aspx?rdReport=DPH_BRFSS.ExploreByTopic&irbLocationType=StatesAndMMSA&islClass=CLASS17&islTopic=TOPIC15&islYear=2020&rdRnd=6747

20. Arrazola R. *Change request 2017 Behavioral Risk Factor Surveillane System (BRFSS)*. September 13, 2016. https://omb.report/icr/202011-0920-001/doc/105866901

21. Centers for Disease Control and Prevention. Methodologic changes in the Behavioral Risk Factor Surveillance System in 2011 and potential effects on prevalence estimates. *MMWR Morb Mortal Wkly Rep*. 2012;61(22):410–413. https://www.cdc.gov/mmwr/preview/mmwrhtml/mm6122a3.htm

22. Vandenbroucke JP, von Elm E, Altman DG, et al. Strengthening the Reporting of Observational Studies in Epidemiology (STROBE): explanation and elaboration. *Epidemiology*. 2007;18(6):805–835. https://doi.org/10.1097/EDE.0b013e3181577511

23. Strassle PD, Stewart AL, Quintero SM, et al. COVID-19-related discrimination among racial/ethnic minorities and other marginalized communities in the United States. *Am J Public Health*. 2022;112(3):453–466. https://doi.org/10.2105/AJPH.2021.306594

24. Pascoe EA, Smart Richman L. Perceived discrimination and health: a meta-analytic review. *Psychol Bull*. 2009;135(4):531–554. https://doi.org/10.1037/a0016059

25. Centers for Disease Control and Prevention. What is autism spectrum disorder? 2022. https://www.cdc.gov/ncbddd/autism/facts.html

26. Lai MC, Lombardo MV, Baron-Cohen S. Autism. *Lancet*. 2014;383(9920):896–910. https://doi.org/10.1016/S0140-6736(13)61539-1

# CHAPTER 8

# EFFECT MEASURE MODIFICATION AND STATISTICAL INTERACTION

## KEY TERMS

biologic interaction

effect measure modification

effect modifier

interaction

scale dependence

statistical interaction

## LEARNING OBJECTIVES

8.1 Understand the concept of effect measure modification of epidemiologic associations.

8.2 Differentiate between the terms effect measure modification, statistical interaction, and biologic interaction.

8.3 Describe how to assess whether there is evidence of effect measure modification.

8.4 Describe how to assess whether there is evidence of statistical interaction.

8.5 Calculate Breslow-Day test statistics using OpenEpi.

8.6 Describe what it means for effect measure modification to be scale-dependent.

8.7 Describe what it means for statistical interaction to be scale-dependent.

8.8 Understand the importance of effect measure modification in public health practice.

## THE IMPACT OF HISTORICAL POLICIES ON TODAY'S HEALTH

In the 1930s, the United States government established policies designed to increase housing options for lower- and middle-class White residents while intentionally forcing Black residents into urban housing projects.[1-3] These policies included a practice called "redlining" whereby mortgage lenders classified certain neighborhoods as being "hazardous" to investment. These neighborhoods were those with a high proportion of low-income residents and racial and ethnic minorities. The practice of redlining intentionally created segregated neighborhoods and led to differences in economic opportunities that have had a lasting impact on the health of those who have lived in redlined communities.[4,5] As we'll see in this chapter, the impact of redlining has not had the same impact on everyone, contributing to racial and ethnic health inequities.

Now that you know the basics of the four main analytic epidemiologic study designs, we will learn about more nuanced considerations that are relevant to all analytic designs. The first of these considerations is a phenomenon called **effect measure modification (EMM)**. This is an important concept that may arise in analytic epidemiologic studies when there are some subgroups of the sample population for whom the exposure has a different effect on the outcome than in other subgroups. For example, some prescription medications may be associated with different side effects in individuals who smoke versus those who do not smoke. In this case, we would say that smoking is an **effect modifier**, meaning that it *modifies the effect* of the medication on side effects. When effect measure modification happens, we must report multiple measures of association: one for each relevant subset of the sample population. In our example, we would need to report a measure of association for the effect of the medication on side effects in smokers, and another (different!) measure of association for the effect of the medication on side effects in nonsmokers.

The concept of effect measure modification is incredibly important for public health practice as it helps quantify how different groups of individuals are impacted by the exposures that we study.

## EFFECT MEASURE MODIFICATION BASICS (LEARNING OBJECTIVE 8.1)

Perhaps the most relatable way to think about effect measure modification is through the phrase "one size *doesn't* fit all." When we report a single measure of association for an analytic epidemiologic study, we are taking a "one size fits all" approach—meaning that we assume that the impact of the exposure on the outcome is the same for the entire sample population and thus does not differ by subgroup (e.g., the risk ratio that describes the association between red meat consumption and coronary heart disease is the same for men who exercise three times a week as it is for men who exercise less often).

However, when there is effect measure modification, the "one size fits all" approach fails because we need more than one measure of association to describe how the exposure impacts the outcome in different subgroups. These subgroups are formally referred to as **strata**, which are mutually exclusive categories of individuals in the sample population. For example, in the United States, geography of residence might be **stratified** into five regions: Midwest, Northeast, Southeast, Southwest, and West. Alternatively, a sample population of babies might be stratified by age with the following categories: younger than 3 months, 3 to 5 months, 6 to 8 months, and 9 to 12 months. When creating these strata, all individuals in the sample population should be included in one stratum and one stratum only.

Formally, effect measure modification (sometimes referred to as **effect heterogeneity** or **stratum-specific heterogeneity**) is defined as occurring when the measure of association differs across values of a third variable. This third variable is often described as an **effect modifier**. Some examples of effect measure modification are described in the text that follows and summarized in **Table 8.1**.

For example, while hormonal contraceptives can be used for pregnancy prevention, they are also prescribed for a variety of noncontraceptive indications including for menstrual cycle regularity, improved bone mineral density, treatment of pelvic pain due to endometriosis, and many other uses.[6] When oral contraceptives were introduced in the 1960s, they were found to be associated with an increased risk of myocardial infarction (commonly known as heart attack), particularly among smokers.[7] Over time, oral contraceptives with lower doses

**TABLE 8.1 EXAMPLES OF EFFECT MEASURE MODIFICATION: ASSOCIATIONS FOR WHICH "ONE SIZE DOESN'T FIT ALL"**

| Exposure | Outcome | Effect Modifier | Explanation | Impact on Measures of Association |
|---|---|---|---|---|
| Low-dose estrogen oral contraceptives | MI | Smoking status | Low-dose estrogen oral contraceptives are not associated with MI among nonsmokers. However, smokers who take low-dose estrogen oral contraceptives *do* have an increased risk of MI compared to smokers who do not take low-dose estrogen oral contraceptives. | $RR_{nonsmokers} = 1$ $RR_{smokers} > 1$ |
| Quadrivalent HPV vaccine | Cervical cancer | Age at first vaccination | While the quadrivalent HPV vaccine is effective at preventing cervical cancer among those who received their first vaccine before age 30, it is *most* effective for those who initiated their HPV vaccines before age 17. | $RR_{overall} < 1$ $RR_{vax\ before\ age\ 17} < RR_{vax\ after\ age\ 17}$ |
| Historical redlining | Breast cancer stage at diagnosis | Race and ethnicity | Living in a nonredlined neighborhood has no impact on breast cancer stage at diagnosis for non-Latina Black women. However, non-Latina White women who lived in nonredlined neighborhoods had a decreased likelihood of late-stage breast cancer diagnosis than non-Latina White women who lived in redlined neighborhoods. | $OR_{non\text{-}Latina\ Black\ women} = 1$ $OR_{non\text{-}Latina\ White\ women} < 1$ |

HPV, human papillomavirus; MI, myocardial infarction; OR, odds ratio; RR, risk ratio.

of estrogen were introduced. Subsequent studies found that even at low doses, smokers taking estrogen-containing oral contraceptives had an increased risk of myocardial infarction; however, there was no association between taking estrogen-containing oral contraceptives and myocardial infarction among nonsmokers.[8] For this reason, the American College of Obstetricians and Gynecologists tailored their recommendations for prescribing oral contraceptives to include detailed information about risks and options for smokers.[9]

Another example of effect measure modification occurs in the context of exploring the effectiveness of the human papillomavirus (HPV) vaccine across different age groups. Two types of HPV (HPV16 and HPV18) are responsible for the majority of cervical cancer cases.[10] HPV vaccination prevents *new* infections but does not treat *existing* HPV infections or HPV-related diseases.[11] Given that HPV incidence increases soon after first sexual intercourse,[12] it is important to evaluate the effectiveness of the HPV vaccine at preventing high-grade cervical lesions across different age groups. Investigators used healthcare registers in Sweden to determine whether quadrivalent HPV vaccination (a vaccine that targets four HPV types, including HPV16 and HPV18) was effective at preventing cervical dysplasia (abnormal cells on the cervix, which can lead to cervical cancer), and whether the effectiveness differed depending on how old the girls and young women were when they received their first HPV vaccine.[13] This study found that the quadrivalent HPV vaccine was effective in preventing moderate cervical dysplasia among all girls and women who were vaccinated before age 30; however, the vaccine was *most* effective for those who initiated their vaccines before age 17. For this reason, Sweden initiated a school-based HPV vaccination program for girls in fifth and sixth grade to maximize protection from the vaccine.[14]

A final example of effect measure modification is an exploration of how the legacy of historical redlining on breast cancer stage at diagnosis differs by racial and ethnic groups in the United States.[15] The stage at which cancer is diagnosed is an important factor when studying health inequities, because the earlier breast cancer is detected, the better chance that treatment will be successful. Investigators used data from a state cancer registry to identify individuals diagnosed with breast cancer from 2008 to 2017. The registry contained information about whether breast cancer cases were detected early or late, as well as the individuals' race and ethnicity, and their residential address. These addresses were compared against the 1930s Home Owners' Loan Corporation mortgage security redlining maps to determine whether an individual lived in an area that was redlined or not. Investigators found that for non-Latina White women, living in a nonredlined neighborhood (versus a redlined neighborhood) was associated with a decreased likelihood of having a late-stage breast cancer diagnosis (versus an early-stage diagnosis); however, non-Latina Black women did not have this same advantage—in this subgroup, those who lived in a nonredlined neighborhood were just as likely to have a late-stage breast cancer diagnosis as those who lived in a redlined neighborhood. This finding is an example of how structural racism impacts different groups in different ways: non-Latina White women had better outcomes when they did not live in redlined neighborhoods (compared to those who did live in redlined neighborhoods); however, non-Latina Black women had the same health outcomes, regardless of where they lived.

## Linking Effect Measure Modification to the Development of Epidemiologic Study Hypotheses

In **Chapter 3, "Introduction to Analytic Epidemiologic Study Designs and Measures of Association,"** we introduced this example of a structure that can be used to formulate a study hypothesis for an analytic epidemiologic study:

> In a **population**, those who are **exposed** have a **<different/higher/lower/not different> frequency** of the outcome compared to those who are **unexposed**.

Investigators can adapt this structure if they are interested in assessing whether there is evidence of effect measure modification to indicate that the association between the exposure and outcome might be different for different subgroups of the sample population:

> The association between an **exposure** and a **health outcome** in a **subgroup of a population** is **different** from the association between the **exposure** and **health outcome** in a *different* **subgroup of the population**.

Another way to structure an analytic epidemiologic study hypothesis that incorporates effect measure modification is:

> The association between an **exposure** and a **health outcome** in a **population** is **modified** by a **third variable** (i.e., the **effect modifier**).

### Why Is It Called "Effect Measure Modification"?

Recall that the measures that quantify the relationship between an exposure and a health outcome are called **measures of association**. This terminology signals that we may have observed an association between the exposure and outcome in our study; however, we have not yet established whether the exposure *caused* the outcome.

If we go one step further to assume that the exposure–outcome relationship is *causal*, we instead refer to measures of association as **measures of effect** (i.e., they quantify the *effect* [cause] of the exposure on the outcome).

When considering effect measure modification, we assume that the measure of association is a good estimate of the measure of effect, meaning that there is minimal impact of error, both systematic (**Chapter 9, "Error in Epidemiologic Research and Fundamentals of Confounding"; Chapter 10, "Selection Bias"; Chapter 11, "Information Bias and Screening and Diagnostic Tests"**) and random (**Chapter 12, "Random Error in Epidemiologic Research"**). Additionally, when there is evidence of effect measure modification, this means that the measure of effect is *modified* (i.e., changed) by some third variable. That is, the appropriate measure of effect to report *depends* on which group we're talking about.

## FIGURE 8.1 DIFFERENT CONCEPTS OF INTERACTION IN ANALYTIC EPIDEMIOLOGIC RESEARCH

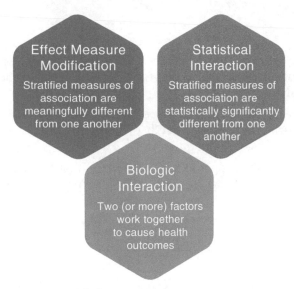

## Related Terminology (LEARNING OBJECTIVE 8.2)

Sometimes effect measure modification is referred to as **interaction**. While these terms are often used interchangeably, are differentiated in more advanced epidemiology.[16] To avoid confusion, we have chosen to strictly use the term effect measure modification to refer to the situation when an exposure has a different effect on the outcome in different subgroups of the sample population.

While the primary focus of this chapter is on effect measure modification, there are two other types of interaction: statistical and biologic interaction, which are described in the text that follows and summarized in **Figure 8.1**.

**Statistical interaction.** A statistical test can be used to determine whether the **stratum-specific measures of association** (i.e., the measures of association that describe the relationship between the exposure and the outcome for the different subgroups of the sample population) are *statistically* different from one another. We will explore this phenomenon in greater detail later in this chapter and will also describe statistical testing in **Chapter 12, "Random Error in Epidemiologic Research."**

**Biologic interaction**. This concept is related to what actually *causes* an outcome to occur. Biologic interaction is said to occur when there are two (or more) factors that must be present for an outcome to occur. For example, phenylketonuria (PKU) is a rare genetic disorder that prevents the body from producing an enzyme that is needed to break down phenylalanine.[17] People with PKU must follow diets that limit phenylalanine; if they don't, serious conditions may arise including significant brain damage. In this example, we would say that there is evidence of biologic interaction between PKU and diets containing phenylalanine.

- Among people who follow diets that limit phenylalanine, there is no association between PKU and significant brain damage; however,

- Among people who *don't* follow diets that limit phenylalanine, there is a strong positive association between PKU and significant brain damage.

This biologic interaction is why babies are screened for PKU at birth. PKU screening allows parents and their healthcare team to work together to identify appropriate diets to prevent any negative effects of this rare inherited disorder.[17]

## Concepts of Interaction

There are three concepts of interaction:

- Effect measure modification is a phenomenon that occurs when the measure of association between the exposure and outcome of interest differs for different subgroups of the sample population, called **strata**.
  - When effect measure modification is present, investigators should report multiple measures of association to appropriately describe the impacts of the exposure within subgroups of their sample population.
- **Statistical interaction**—Investigators can conduct statistical tests to evaluate whether the stratified measures of association are different from one another from a statistical perspective.
- **Biologic interaction**—Occurs when two or more factors must be present for an outcome to occur.

## EFFECT MEASURE MODIFICATION ASSESSMENT (LEARNING OBJECTIVE 8.3)

To assess whether there is evidence of effect measure modification, we must calculate **stratified** (also called **stratum-specific**) **measures of association** and determine whether they are different from one another. To do this, we begin by stratifying our data by the **potential effect modifier**. This means that we will have separate tables that show the distribution of our exposure and outcome for each of the different levels of the potential effect modifier. Figure 8.2 presents data adapted from the previously described case-control study that evaluated whether the association between low-dose oral contraceptives and myocardial infarction differed for heavy smokers and nonsmokers.[8]

## FIGURE 8.2 ASSOCIATION BETWEEN LOW-DOSE ORAL CONTRACEPTIVE USE AND MYOCARDIAL INFARCTION, STRATIFIED BY SMOKING STATUS

| Stratum 1 Heavy Smokers | Currently using low-dose oral contraceptives (E+) | Not using low-dose oral contraceptives (E−) |
| --- | --- | --- |
| Cases of Myocardial Infarction | 17 | 215 |
| Controls | 13 | 265 |

| Stratum 2 Nonsmokers | Currently using low-dose oral contraceptives (E+) | Not using low-dose oral contraceptives (E−) |
| --- | --- | --- |
| Cases of Myocardial Infarction | 11 | 138 |
| Controls | 158 | 1,662 |

*Source*: Data from Rosenberg L, Palmer JR, Rao RS, Shapiro S. Low-dose oral contraceptive use and the risk of myocardial infarction. *Arch Intern Med.* 2001;161(8):1065–1070. https://doi.org/10.1001/archinte.161.8.1065

Once the data have been stratified, we calculate stratum-specific measures of association. Since these investigators used a case-control design, we will calculate odds ratios (ORs) to obtain separate estimates of the associations between low-dose oral contraceptives and myocardial infarction for heavy smokers and nonsmokers.

# FIGURE 8.3 VISUALIZING ASSESSMENT OF EFFECT MEASURE MODIFICATION

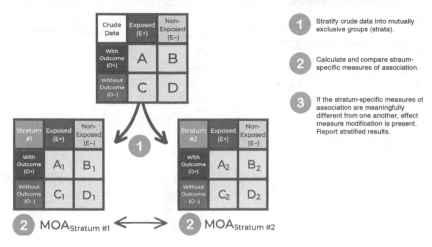

MOA, measure of association.

$$OR_{\text{heavy smokers}} = \frac{17 \times 265}{215 \times 13} = 1.61 \qquad OR_{\text{nonsmokers}} = \frac{11 \times 1{,}662}{138 \times 158} = 0.84$$

Once we have calculated our stratum-specific measures of association, we compare them to determine whether the association between our exposure and outcome *differs* for the different subgroups. The association between low-dose oral contraceptives and myocardial infarction is not the same for heavy smokers and nonsmokers (ORs of 1.61 and 0.84, respectively). Later in this chapter, we will explore a more formal way to make this assessment, but at this stage, we see that there is a *positive* association (OR greater than 1) between low-dose oral contraceptives and myocardial infarction among *heavy smokers*, while there is a *negative* association (OR less than 1) between low-dose oral contraceptives and myocardial infarction among *nonsmokers*. This information tells us that the impact of low-dose oral contraceptives on heart health is different depending on an individual's smoking status. We describe this by saying that the association between low-dose oral contraceptives and myocardial infarction is *modified* by smoking status. Since we've learned that heavy smokers have an increased likelihood of having myocardial infarction when taking low-dose oral contraceptives and that there is no relationship between low-dose oral contraceptives and myocardial infarction among nonsmokers, we should report the two stratum-specific ORs that we calculated previously, rather than a single OR that combines data for heavy smokers and nonsmokers.

While we see effect measure modification of the association between low-dose oral contraceptives and myocardial infarction by smoking status, this example also points to likely biologic (i.e., causal) interaction. Studies suggest that it is the combination of contraceptive hormones with the cardiovascular effects of smoking that causes an individual to have an increased risk of myocardial infarction.[18]

The process of assessing whether there is evidence of effect measure modification is summarized in **Figure 8.3** where we first stratify the overall study data into mutually exclusive groups (strata) and calculate stratum-specific measures of association. If the stratum-specific measures of association are *meaningfully* different from one another, then we say that there is effect measure modification and we must report the stratum-specific measures, rather than reporting the crude measure of association (i.e., the measure that would be calculated using the overall study data where everyone was included in the same R×C table). We will discuss how to determine whether the stratified measures of association are different from one another later in this chapter.

## Pause to Practice 8.1

### Effect Measure Modification Assessment Using Stratified Measures of Association

Figure 8.4 shows data adapted from the cohort study described previously which evaluated the effectiveness of the HPV vaccine depending on the age at which an individual initiated their vaccine series.[13]

### FIGURE 8.4 ASSOCIATION BETWEEN HUMAN PAPILLOMAVIRUS VACCINATION AND CERVICAL DYSPLASIA, STRATIFIED BY AGE AT HUMAN PAPILLOMAVIRUS VACCINATION INITIATION

| Stratum 1 Initiated HPV vaccine between the ages of 17 and 19 years | | | | Stratum 2 Initiated HPV vaccine between the ages of 20 and 29 years | | | |
|---|---|---|---|---|---|---|---|
| | Received HPV Vaccine (E+) | Did Not Receive HPV Vaccine (E−) | TOTAL | | Received HPV Vaccine (E+) | Did Not Receive HPV Vaccine (E−) | TOTAL |
| Cases of Cervical Dysplasia | 11 | 2,927 | 2,938 | Cases of Cervical Dysplasia | 27 | 6,691 | 6,718 |
| Person-Years | 8,153 | 559,553 | 567,706 | Person-Years | 3,651 | 540,008 | 543,659 |

HPV, human papillomavirus.
*Source:* Herweijer E, Sundström K, Ploner A, Uhnoo I, Sparén P, Arnheim-Dahlström L. Quadrivalent HPV vaccine effectiveness against high-grade cervical lesions by age at vaccination: a population-based study. *Int J Cancer.* 2016;138(12):2867–2874. https://doi .org/10.1002/ijc.30035

1. Using those who were unvaccinated as the reference group, name and calculate the appropriate ratio measure of association that describes the association between HPV vaccination and the incidence of cervical dysplasia *among those who initiated their HPV vaccination series between the ages of 17 and 19.* Provide a one-sentence interpretation of this measure.

2. Using those who were unvaccinated as the reference group, name and calculate the appropriate ratio measure of association that describes the association between HPV vaccination initiation and the incidence of cervical dysplasia *among those who initiated their HPV vaccination series between the ages of 20 and 29.* Provide a one-sentence interpretation of this measure.

3. Compare your answers to Questions 1 and 2. Does there appear to be a positive or negative association between HPV vaccination and cervical dysplasia? Does this association appear to be modified by the age at which an individual initiated their HPV vaccine series?

4. Do you think that this example could also represent biological (i.e., causal) interaction? Why or why not?

## STATISTICAL INTERACTION ASSESSMENT (LEARNING OBJECTIVE 8.4)

As previously noted, statistical interaction is assessed using statistical tests to determine whether the stratified measures of association are **statistically significantly** different from one another. This statistical assessment is one consideration that investigators may use to determine whether it is most appropriate to report stratified measures of association, or if a summary (i.e., single) measure of association is sufficient.

# Basic Principles of Statistical Inference

At this stage we will provide a brief overview of statistical inference as it applies to assessing statistical interaction. Statistical inference is addressed in greater detail in **Chapter 12, "Random Error in Epidemiologic Research."**

We use statistical tests as a quantitative assessment of whether our stratified measures of association are statistically different from one another. To do this, we need three related components which are described in the text that follows: **null and alternative hypotheses,** a **statistical test**, and an **alpha level**.

**Null and alternative hypotheses.** As noted in **Chapter 3, "Introduction to Analytic Epidemiologic Study Designs and Measures of Association,"** etiologic hypotheses—statements that describe the research questions at hand—are foundational to analytic epidemiology. When considering hypotheses for statistical inference, we distinguish between two types of hypotheses: the **null hypothesis** (denoted $H_0$) and the **alternative hypothesis** (denoted $H_A$). In **Chapter 3, "Introduction to Analytic Epidemiologic Study Designs and Measures of Association,"** we introduced the term **null value** to describe the value of a measure of association when there is no relationship between an exposure and an outcome (i.e., 0 for difference measures, and 1 for ratio measures). A null hypothesis follows this same logic—it is a hypothesis that posits that there is truly no difference between two measures that are being compared.

As its name suggests, the alternative hypothesis provides an alternative to the null hypothesis, positing that there truly *is* a difference between two measures that are being compared.

When assessing whether there is evidence of statistical interaction, our null hypothesis and alternative hypothesis are given as follows:

**Null hypothesis:** There is *no* evidence of statistically significant interaction between the exposure and potential effect modifier.

**Alternative hypothesis:** There *is* evidence of statistically significant interaction between the exposure and potential effect modifier.

Alternatively, we could write our null hypothesis and alternative hypothesis in terms of our stratified measures of association:

**Null hypothesis:** The associations between the exposure and outcome are *not* statistically significantly different from one another across different levels of the potential effect modifier.

**Alternative hypothesis:** The associations between the exposure and outcome *are* statistically significantly different from one another across different levels of the potential effect modifier.

Returning to the case-control study of the association between low-dose oral contraceptive use and myocardial infarction is different for heavy smokers versus nonsmokers, our null hypothesis and alternative hypothesis could be written as follows:

**Null hypothesis:** There is *no* evidence of statistically significant interaction between low-dose oral contraceptive use and smoking.

**Alternative hypothesis:** There *is* evidence of statistically significant interaction between low-dose oral contraceptive use and smoking.

Or...

**Null hypothesis:** The odds ratio that describes the association between low-dose oral contraceptive use and myocardial infarction among heavy smokers is *not* statistically significantly different from the OR that describes the association between low-dose oral contraceptive use and myocardial infarction among nonsmokers.

**Alternative hypothesis:** The odds ratio that describes the association between low-dose oral contraceptive use and myocardial infarction among heavy smokers *is* statistically significantly different from the odds ratio that describes the association between low-dose oral contraceptive use and myocardial infarction among nonsmokers.

**Breslow-Day test for statistical interaction.** Once we have constructed our null hypothesis and alternative hypothesis and have calculated our stratified measures of association, we need to conduct a statistical test to determine whether the stratum-specific measures of association are different from one another from a statistical perspective. For a stratified analysis (i.e., the types of analyses shown here, where data are stratified by the potential effect modifier), the **Breslow-Day test for interaction** is one statistical test that can be used to assess whether there is evidence of statistical interaction.

Each statistical test yields a **test statistic** and a corresponding **p-value**. The formulas for these differ depending on the situation; fortunately, online calculators, such as OpenEpi (openepi.com),[19] can help determine whether there is evidence of statistically significant interaction.

**Alpha level.** To decide whether there is evidence of statistically significant interaction, we compare the p-value for the Breslow-Day test to a threshold that we set for statistical significance. This threshold is called **alpha**, and is typically set at 0.05. Alpha and p-values are described in detail in **Chapter 12, "Random Error in Epidemiologic Research."** For now, we want to know how the p-value for the Breslow-Day test compares to alpha = 0.05.

- If p-value is 0.05 or greater:
  - Do not reject the null hypothesis.
  - This means that there is *no* evidence of statistically significant interaction.
- If p-value is less than 0.05:
  - Reject the null hypothesis.
  - This means that there *is* evidence of statistically significant interaction.

## Using OpenEpi for Statistical Assessment of Effect Measure Modification
(LEARNING OBJECTIVE 8.5)

Online calculators, such as OpenEpi,[19] can be very useful for conducting some epidemiologic analyses, including assessing whether stratified measures of association are statistically significantly different from one another. Before using OpenEpi for statistical assessment of effect measure modification, we will walk you through a brief orientation to this open-source tool.

Begin by visiting openepi.com. For analyses that use a traditional 2×2 data layout, select "Two by Two Table" from the main menu, and then click to enter your study data (**Figure 8.5A**).

Notice that the default data layout in OpenEpi orients the exposure and the outcome differently than the convention that we have used in this textbook. You need to pay attention to which values you are inputting to calculate your measures based on the table orientation to avoid incorrectly calculated measures. Instructions for how to change the data table to

## FIGURE 8.5A INTRODUCTION TO OPENEPI – HOMEPAGE

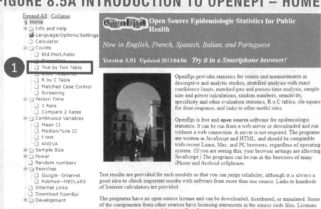
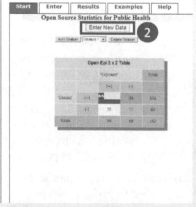

For risk-, prevalence-, and odds-based data, select "Two by Two Table." Then click "Enter New Data."
*Source*: https://openepi.com. Copyright (c) 2003, 2008 Andrew G. Dean et al., Atlanta, GA, USA

the orientation we have used in this textbook are shown in **Figure 8.5B**. To change the table orientation, click on "Settings" just above the data table, and select "Exposure" from the dropdown menu so that the exposure will be represented in the columns and the outcome will be represented in the rows. You must then return to the main menu, and select "Two by Two Table" again. Once you click "Enter New Data" you will see that your 2×2 table has been reoriented to follow the convention that we've used in this text, with the exposure of interest presented in the columns and the outcome of interest presented in the rows.

Since we will use OpenEpi to assess whether our stratified measures of association are statistically significantly different from one another, we will need to enter the data separately for each subgroup of our sample population. Begin by entering the data for the first stratum, then click "Add Stratum," and a blank data table will appear where you can enter the data for the second stratum. Continue until a 2×2 table has been generated for each level of your potential effect modifier. If you need to go back to edit data that you have already entered, select the appropriate stratum from the dropdown menu.

As you will see, OpenEpi returns a lot of output, separated into four distinct sections.

The first section includes your 2×2 tables—one for each stratum, and a crude table that combines all your strata. It is helpful to review the data that appear in this section to be sure that you haven't made any errors when entering your data.

The second section is labeled "Chi Square and Exact Measures of Association," which we can bypass for now but will come back to in **Chapter 13, "Introduction to Epidemiologic Data Analysis."**

The third and fourth sections are labeled "Risk-Based Estimates and 95% Confidence Intervals" and "Odds-Based Estimates and Confidence Limits," respectively.

- Notice that when you entered your data, you did not specify the study design that was used to generate the data. For this reason, you must be familiar with the study design that was used, and select the appropriate output for your analysis.

- Although the output doesn't specify where to look for information related to a cross-sectional study, investigators can use the information included in the "Risk-Based Estimates and 95% Confidence Intervals" since the underlying statistical formulae are the same for risk- and prevalence-based measures (all that differs is our interpretation depending on the study design!).

## FIGURE 8.5B INTRODUCTION TO OpenEpi—CHANGING THE 2×2 TABLE ORIENTATION

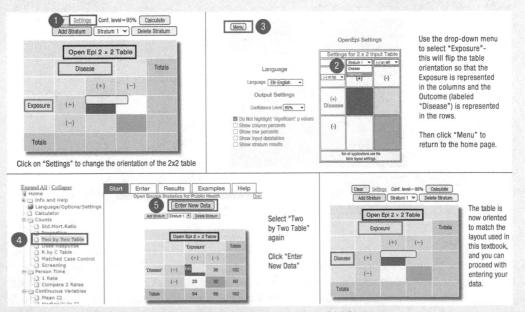

*Source*: https://openepi.com. Copyright (c) 2003, 2008 Andrew G. Dean et al., Atlanta, GA, USA

In the case-control study of oral contraceptive use, recall that we observed the following relationships between low-dose oral contraceptives and myocardial infarction:

$$OR_{\text{heavy smokers}} = \frac{17 \times 265}{215 \times 13} = 1.61$$

$$OR_{\text{nonsmokers}} = \frac{11 \times 1{,}662}{138 \times 158} = 0.84$$

While 1.61 and 0.84 seem like very different measures of association, we may want to test whether they are *statistically* different from one another. After entering the stratified data in OpenEpi (**Figure 8.6**),[19] we find that the *p*-value associated with the Breslow-Day test statistic is 0.19 (labeled "Breslow-Day test for interaction of odds ratio over strata" in OpenEpi), which is greater than the alpha threshold of 0.05. This means that the stratified ORs are *not* statistically significantly different from one another. Note that the term *statistically significant* simply refers to whether there are differences from a *statistical* perspective—it does *not* imply that the difference is meaningful from a public health perspective. We will revisit how to report these study findings in the next section where we consider whether the stratified measures of association are meaningfully and/or statistically different from one another.

**FIGURE 8.6 USING OpenEpi TO ASSESS WHETHER THE ODDS RATIOS FOR THE ASSOCIATION BETWEEN LOW-DOSE ORAL CONTRACEPTIVE USE AND MYOCARDIAL INFARCTION ARE STATISTICALLY DIFFERENT FOR SMOKERS AND NONSMOKERS**

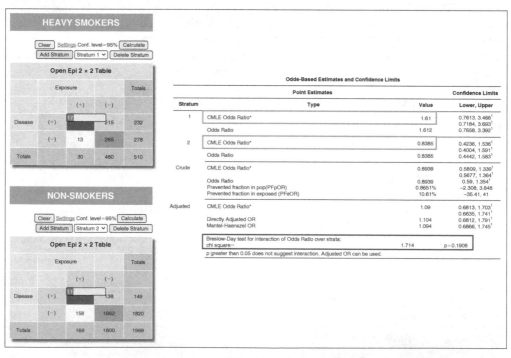

*Source*: https://openepi.com. Copyright (c) 2003, 2008 Andrew G. Dean et al., Atlanta, GA, USA

Next, consider the example of the impact of historical redlining on health described earlier in the chapter. Recall that investigators conducted a study among women recently diagnosed with breast cancer to explore the association between historical redlining and breast cancer stage at diagnosis (late vs. early), and whether this association differed for non-Latina Black and non-Latina White women.[15] These study findings are summarized in **Figure 8.7**.

# FIGURE 8.7 ASSOCIATION BETWEEN NOT LIVING IN A REDLINED NEIGHBORHOOD AND HAVING A LATE-STAGE BREAST CANCER DIAGNOSIS, STRATIFIED BY RACE

| Stratum 1 Non-Latina Black Women | Living in a neighborhood that was NOT redlined (E+) | Living in a neighborhood that WAS redlined (E−) |
|---|---|---|
| Breast cancer diagnosed at a late stage | 21 | 84 |
| Breast cancer diagnosed at an early stage | 190 | 793 |
| TOTAL | 211 | 877 |

| Stratum 2 Non-Latina White Women | Living in a neighborhood that was NOT redlined (E+) | Living in a neighborhood that WAS redlined (E−) |
|---|---|---|
| Breast cancer diagnosed at a late stage | 29 | 98 |
| Breast cancer diagnosed at an early stage | 761 | 832 |
| TOTAL | 790 | 930 |

$$RR_{\text{non-Latina Black}} = \frac{21/211}{84/877} = 1.04 \qquad RR_{\text{non-Latina White}} = \frac{29/790}{98/930} = 0.35$$

*Source*: Data from Plascak JJ, Beyer K, Xu X, Stroup AM, Jacob G, Llanos AAM. Association between residence in historically redlined districts indicative of structural racism and racial and ethnic disparities in breast cancer outcomes. *JAMA Netw Open*. 2022;5(7):e2220908. https://doi.org/10.1001/jamanetworkopen.2022.20908

In this study, investigators found that there was no association between historical redlining and breast cancer stage at diagnosis among non-Latina Black women (RR = 1.04); however, the risk of a late stage cancer diagnosis among non-Latina White women who lived in nonredlined areas was much lower than the risk of a late stage cancer diagnosis among non-Latina White women who lived in redlined areas (RR = 0.35). After entering the stratified data in OpenEpi (Figure 8.8), we find that the *p*-value for the Breslow-Day test is 0.0004

# FIGURE 8.8 USING OpenEpi TO ASSESS WHETHER THE ASSOCIATIONS BETWEEN REDLINING AND BREAST CANCER STAGES AT DIAGNOSIS ARE STATISTICALLY DIFFERENT FOR NON-LATINA BLACK AND NON-LATINA WHITE WOMEN

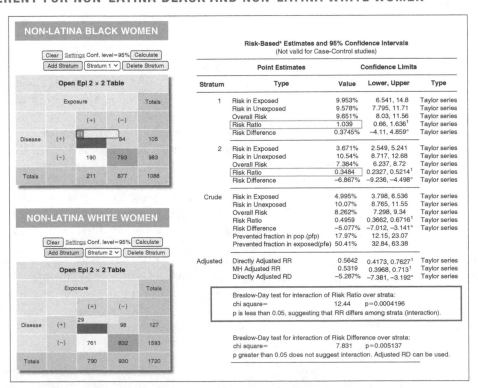

*Source*: https://openepi.com. Copyright (c) 2003, 2008 Andrew G. Dean et al., Atlanta, GA, USA

(labeled "Breslow-Day test for interaction of risk ratio over strata" in OpenEpi), which is less than the alpha threshold of 0.05. This suggests that the risk ratio for the association between historical redlining and breast cancer stage at diagnosis among non-Latina Black women (RR = 1.04) was statistically significantly different from the risk ratio for the association between historical redlining and breast cancer stage at diagnosis among non-Latina White women (RR = 0.35).

In plain language, living in a nonredlined area (relative to a redlined area) did not improve early detection of breast cancer for non-Latina Black women; however, it *did* improve early detection of breast cancer for non-Latina White women. This finding is an example of the impact of historical structural racism on modern day health.

## HOW DIFFERENT IS DIFFERENT?

Recall that effect measure modification and statistical interaction are related concepts, each evaluating differences in stratum-specific measures of association from different perspectives. Whether there is evidence of measure modification depends on whether the stratified measures of association are *meaningfully* different from one another. On the other hand, whether there is evidence of statistical interaction depends on whether the stratified measures of association are *statistically significantly* different from one another. When stratified measures of association are meaningfully different from one another, investigators should report the stratified measures of association, regardless of statistical significance.

What constitutes a meaningful difference depends on a number of factors including potential impact on health policy or clinical decision-making, and potential to reduce health inequities. For example, it is possible that stratum-specific risk ratios of 2.2 and 2.4 are statistically significantly different from one another. However, practically speaking, they may not be different enough to warrant different public health recommendations or interventions.

If the measures of association are *meaningfully* different from one another, one should report the stratified measures of association, even if they are not *statistically* different from one another. This was the case for the study of the association between low-dose oral contraceptives and myocardial infarction. Although the stratified measures of association weren't *statistically* different from one another using an alpha of 0.05, the implications of a positive association among smokers warranted reporting of the results separately for heavy smokers and nonsmokers. In fact, findings from this and other studies were enough of a concern that organizations such as the U.S. Centers for Disease Control and Prevention,[20] the American College of Obstetricians and Gynecologists,[9] and the World Health Organization[21] provided guidelines related to the risks associated with smoking while taking oral contraceptives, particularly for those aged 35 years and older. Stratified measures of association that are meaningfully but not statistically different from one another can arise when there is a small number of individuals in one or more of the strata. We'll discuss the impact of sample size on statistical testing further in **Chapter 12, "Random Error in Epidemiologic Research."**

If the stratified measures of association are *not* meaningfully different from one another, regardless of statistical significance, then it may not be necessary to report stratified measures of association. An important exception is in cases where effect measure modification was central to the research question, it may be useful to report the stratified measures to show that the exposure didn't have a different effect on the outcome across the strata.

## Pause to Practice 8.2

### Assessing Whether Stratified Measures of Association Are Statistically Significantly Different From One Another

The following questions consider a statistical assessment of effect measure modification in the HPV vaccine study described previously,[13] the data for which are shown in Figure 8.4, reproduced below.

| Stratum 1<br>Initiated HPV vaccine between the<br>ages of 17 and 19 years | | | | Stratum 2<br>Initiated HPV vaccine between the<br>ages of 20 and 29 years | | | |
|---|---|---|---|---|---|---|---|
| | Received HPV Vaccine (E+) | Did Not Receive HPV Vaccine (E−) | TOTAL | | Received HPV Vaccine (E+) | Did Not Receive HPV Vaccine (E−) | TOTAL |
| Cases of Cervical Dysplasia | 11 | 2,927 | 2,938 | Cases of Cervical Dysplasia | 27 | 6,691 | 6,718 |
| Person-Years | 8,153 | 559,553 | 567,706 | Person-Years | 3,651 | 540,008 | 543,659 |

1. What are the $H_0$ and $H_A$ for testing the presence of statistical interaction for this research question?

2. Enter these data in OpenEpi,[19] using the "Compare 2 Rates" option under "Person Time." Find the $p$-value for the Breslow-Day test that compares the rate ratios for those who initiated vaccines between the ages of 17 and 19 and those who initiated their vaccines between the ages of 20 and 29.

3. Compare your $p$-value against an alpha level of 0.05. Do you reject the $H_0$?

4. Provide a two- to three-sentence summary of the study findings.

### Understanding the Relationship Between Effect Measure Modification, Statistical Interaction, and Biological Interaction

Let's consider some possible combinations of the three concepts that we've discussed:

#### Effect measure modification and no statistical interaction

Stratified measures of association may be meaningfully different from one another; however, they may not be statistically significantly different from one another. This is a common occurrence when there are not enough participants within each stratum (you'll find more details on statistical testing and sample size in Chapter 12, "Random Error in Epidemiologic Research," and Chapter 13, "Introduction to Epidemiologic Data Analysis").

#### Statistical interaction and no effect measure modification

Stratified measures of association may be statistically significantly different from one another, but the differences might not be of public health importance. This is particularly common when the stratified sample sizes are quite large.

#### Statistical interaction and no biological interaction

Stratified measures of association may be statistically significantly different from one another, but the stratified measure may not actually be the factor that is *causing* the difference. For example, this is often the case when investigators find that race and ethnicity are effect modifiers. Race, a social construct, is not what *causes* the difference; rather, it is most often a marker for the effects of racism.

### Effect Measure Modification Assessment

- To determine whether there is evidence of effect measure modification in a particular sample population, investigators begin by stratifying the data by the potential effect modifier. **Stratification** is the process by which data are split into mutually exclusive groups.

- Investigators then calculate **stratum-specific measures of association** to obtain separate measures of association for each of the different levels of the potential effect modifier.

- Finally, the stratum-specific measures of association are compared to determine whether they are meaningfully different from one another.

- Statistical tests, such as the Breslow-Day test for interaction, can be used to determine whether the stratified measures of association are different from one another from a *statistical* perspective. For an alpha cutoff of 0.05:

  - *p*-values less than 0.05 suggest that there is evidence that the stratified measures of association are statistically significantly different from one another.

  - *p*-values of 0.05 or more suggest that there is no evidence that the stratified measures of association are statistically significantly different from one another.

- When stratified measures of association are meaningfully different from one another, regardless of whether they are statistically different from one another, one should report the stratified measures of association. Whether an observed difference is meaningful depends on the research question and potential public health implications of the findings.

## EFFECT MEASURE MODIFICATION AND STATISTICAL INTERACTION ARE SCALE-DEPENDENT

An oddity of interaction assessment is that whether we find evidence of effect measure modification or statistical interaction depends upon the so-called "scale" that we are using. If there is evidence of effect measure modification or statistical interaction, it can be present on the **multiplicative scale**, **additive scale**, both scales, or neither scale.

### Scale Dependency of Effect Measure Modification (LEARNING OBJECTIVE 8.6)

- **Effect measure modification on the multiplicative scale** occurs when the stratum-specific *ratio* measures of association (e.g., risk ratio [RR], rate [incidence density] ratio [IDR], prevalence ratio [PR], and odds ratio [OR]) are meaningfully different from one another.

- **Effect measure modification on the additive scale** occurs when the stratum-specific *difference* measures of association (e.g., risk difference [RD], rate [incidence density] difference [IDD], and prevalence difference [PD]) are meaningfully different from one another.

### Scale Dependency of Statistical Interaction (LEARNING OBJECTIVE 8.7)

- **Statistical interaction on the multiplicative scale** occurs when the stratum-specific *ratio* measures of association (e.g., RR, IDR, PR, and OR) are statistically significantly different from one another.

- **Statistical interaction on the additive scale** occurs when the stratum-specific *difference* measures of association (e.g., RD, IDD, and PD) are statistically significantly different from one another.

In the examples presented thus far in this chapter, the measures of association that we have compared across strata have been *ratio* measures of association. Thus, in these instances, we were considering effect measure modification and statistical interaction on the *multiplicative* scale.

In the case of the association between low-dose oral contraceptives and myocardial infarction, we found evidence of effect measure modification on the multiplicative scale ($OR_{nonsmokers}$ = 0.84, $OR_{heavy\ smokers}$ = 1.61), but no evidence of statistical interaction on the multiplicative scale (*p*-value for Breslow-Day test comparing stratum-specific odds ratios = 0.19).

To determine whether there is evidence of effect measure modification on the additive scale, we would need to compare *difference* measures of association. Recall that the study of low-dose oral contraceptives and myocardial infarction was a case-control study, so the only measure of association is the exposure odds ratio. While there are formulae that can be used to assess whether there is evidence of effect measure modification on the additive scale for a case-control study,[22] this is beyond the scope of this text. Instead, we will return to the study of historical redlining and breast cancer stage at diagnosis, the data for which appear in **Figure 8.7**.[15]

Recall that the stratum-specific risk ratios for non-Latina Black and non-Latina White women were 1.04 and 0.35, respectively. Not only are these measures of association meaningfully different from one another, but we also found that they are statistically different from each other (*p*-value for Breslow-Day test comparing stratum-specific risk ratios = 0.00042). Thus, we can conclude that there is evidence of both effect measure modification and statistical interaction on the multiplicative scale.

We can now compare the stratum-specific risk differences to see whether there is evidence of effect measure modification or statistical interaction on the *additive* scale.

$$RD_{non-Latina\ Black} = \frac{21}{211} - \frac{84}{877} = 0.0037$$

$$RD_{non-Latina\ White} = \frac{29}{790} - \frac{98}{930} = -0.069$$

The stratum-specific risk differences are on opposite sides of the null value and suggest a near null association between historical redlining and breast cancer stage at diagnosis for non-Latina Black women and a small negative association between historical redlining and breast cancer stage at diagnosis for non-Latina White women. Whether these values are meaningfully different from one another (and thus if there is evidence of effect measure modification on the additive scale) is up to interpretation. The decision about whether there is evidence of statistical interaction on the additive scale is less ambiguous: The *p*-value for the Breslow-Day test comparing the stratum-specific risk differences (called "interaction of risk difference over strata" in OpenEpi is 0.005 (which you can see in **Figure 8.8**),[19] which is also less than the alpha value of 0.05. This suggests that the stratified risk differences are statistically significantly different from one another, meaning that there is also evidence of statistical interaction on the additive scale. These results are summarized in **Table 8.2** and indicate that there is evidence of effect measure modification and statistical interaction on both the multiplicative and additive scales.

**TABLE 8.2 SUMMARY OF ASSESSMENT OF EFFECT MEASURE MODIFICATION AND STATISTICAL INTERACTION BETWEEN REDLINING AND RACE ON THE MULTIPLICATIVE AND ADDITIVE SCALES**

| Scale | Comparison of the stratified measures of association allows for an assessment effect measure modification on the relevant scale. | | Comparison of *p*-values to alpha (0.05) allows for an assessment of statistical interaction on the relevant scale. |
|---|---|---|---|
| | Measure of Association for Non-Latina Black Women | Measure of Association for Non-Latina White Women | Breslow-Day *p*-value |
| Additive *Compare RDs* | $RD = \frac{21}{211} - \frac{84}{877} = 0.0037$ | $RD = \frac{29}{790} - \frac{98}{930} = -0.069$ | $p_{additive} = 0.005$ |
| Multiplicative *Compare RRs* | $RR = \frac{21/211}{84/877} = 1.04$ | $RR = \frac{29/790}{98/930} = 0.35$ | $p_{multiplicative} = 0.0004$ |

RD, risk difference; RR, risk ratio.

## Pause to Practice 8.3

### Assessing Whether There Is Evidence of Effect Measure Modification on the Additive Scale, Multiplicative Scale, or Both Scales

Let's return to the study that evaluated the efficacy of the HPV vaccine depending on the age at which an individual initiated their vaccine series,[13] the data for which were presented in Figure 8.4.

1. Calculate the stratum-specific rate differences.

2. What are the null and alternative hypotheses for testing the presence of effect measure modification on the additive scale in this data set?

3. Enter these data at OpenEpi.com, using the "Compare 2 Rates" option under "Person Time." Find the $p$-value for the Breslow-Day test that compares the rate differences for those who initiated vaccines between the ages of 17 and 19 and those who initiated their vaccines between the ages of 20 and 29.

4. Compare your $p$-value against an alpha level of 0.05. Do you reject the null hypothesis?

5. Using your previous answers and those from **Pause to Practice 8.2,** is there evidence of statistical interaction on the multiplicative scale, additive scale, or both scales?

6. Using your previous answers and those from **Pause to Practice 8.2,** is there evidence of effect measure modification on the multiplicative scale, additive scale, or both scales?

## Which Scale to Choose and How to Report Study Findings

Since effect measure modification and/or statistical interaction can be present on one, both, or neither scale, how do investigators know which measures of association, ratio or difference measures, to calculate and report? Typically, investigators decide which measure of association they will use first, which then determines whether they will report the presence of effect measure modification and statistical interaction on the multiplicative or the additive scale. However, many analytic techniques used in epidemiology (e.g., logistic regression and survival analyses) are inherently multiplicative meaning that they yield ratio measures of association. For this reason, most analyses unfortunately default to only evaluating the presence of effect measure modification and interaction on the multiplicative scale. Unless investigators explicitly look for effect measure modification and interaction on the additive scale, these potentially important differences are often missed.

## Highlights

### Scale Dependency

- Effect measure modification and statistical interaction have **scale dependence**, meaning that they may be present when calculating ratio or difference measures of association.
- Scale dependency of effect measure modification
  - If there are meaningful differences in stratum-specific ratio measures of association, this is indicative of effect measure modification on the **multiplicative scale**.
  - If there are meaningful differences in stratum-specific difference measures of association, this is indicative of effect measure modification on the **additive scale**.

- Scale dependency of statistical interaction
  - If there are statistically significant differences between stratum-specific **ratio measures of association**, this is indicative of statistical interaction on the **multiplicative scale**.
  - If there are statistically significant differences between stratum-specific **difference measures of association**, this is indicative of statistical interaction on the **additive scale**.
- It is possible to have evidence of effect measure modification or statistical interaction on either the additive or the multiplicative scale, to have evidence of these on both scales, or to have no evidence on either scale.

## SELECTING VARIABLES TO CONSIDER AS POTENTIAL EFFECT MODIFIERS

Before beginning a data analysis, you should have an idea of which variables (if any!) you plan to consider as potential effect modifiers. To decide which variables to consider, it is important to look to previous literature to generate a list of variables that could plausibly impact the association between your exposure and outcome. This approach helps avoid a practice that is sometimes described as a "fishing expedition" where all possible variables in a data set are evaluated as potential effect modifiers. As with all epidemiologic research, your analysis should be hypothesis driven and grounded in previous literature. Effect measure modification is not relevant for all research questions, and so it may not be considered at all.

There may be times when you would like to consider a variable as an effect modifier, but the size of your sample population is too small to test whether there are any statistically significant differences accross strata. As we previously described, and will discuss further in **Chapter 12, "Random Error in Epidemiologic Research,"** statistical testing is heavily impacted by a study's sample size. If the sample is too small, you can still calculate and compare stratified measures of association; however, you may not be able to detect whether they are statistically significantly different from one another.

## THE PUBLIC HEALTH IMPORTANCE OF UNDERSTANDING EFFECT MEASURE MODIFICATION (LEARNING OBJECTIVE 8.8)

Effect measure modification is an important concept for public health because it helps investigators better understand the nuances of how various exposures impact health *differently* for different subgroups of a population. It's important to recognize that certain exposures, like low-dose oral contraceptives, aren't *similarly* harmful for all groups; rather, there is a segment of the population who might be at greater risk of negative health consequences if they are exposed. We will discuss three ways in which effect measure modification is important from a public health perspective.

### Using Effect Measure Modification to Identify "High Risk" Groups

It is important to know whether certain groups have an increased risk of a negative health outcome when they are exposed, such as smokers who use low-dose oral contraceptives. In this case, pharmaceutical companies include information about the increased risks associated with smoking while using oral contraceptives in their package inserts, and healthcare providers make decisions about contraceptive counseling and prescriptions based on a patient's smoking status.

## Targeting Interventions to Particular Subgroups of a Population

Through effect modification assessment, investigators may learn that a particular exposure is more effective in a particular population. This was the case in the study of HPV vaccination where the vaccine was associated with a decreased incidence of cervical dysplasia in those who received the vaccine at both younger and older ages; however, the effect was *strongest* for those who were vaccinated at younger ages. For this reason, HPV vaccination is routinely recommended for administration at age 11 or 12 years.[23]

## Obtaining a Better Understanding of Causation

By observing differences in the effect of an exposure for different subgroups, investigators may gain some insight into how different factors work together to influence health outcomes. They can use this information to explore the biological mechanisms that might be responsible for the observed results. In the case of low-dose oral contraceptives, investigators were able to learn that smokers who use oral contraceptives had faster nicotine metabolism and a heighted physiologic stress response, which may explain the impact on cardiovascular health seen among smokers who use oral contraceptives.[18]

## WHERE WE'VE BEEN AND WHAT'S UP NEXT

In this chapter, we hope to have convinced you that a "one size fits all" approach doesn't always work when it comes to reporting the association between an exposure and a health outcome. An exposure could have no effect on one group but might be harmful (or protective) for another; alternatively, the exposure could be associated with the outcome among everyone, but the association could be stronger for a subgroup of the population. When stratified measures of association are meaningfully different from one another, it's important to report the results separately for the different groups to best tell the story that your data have revealed. Note that effect measure modification is not any sort of error; rather, it is something that is of scientific interest and can better help describe the nuances of how exposures impact health in populations.

There are times, however, when we *are* concerned about third variables introducing error in our results, which is what we will discuss next in **Chapter 9, "Error in Epidemiologic Research and Fundamentals of Confounding."** Our transition to confounding marks an important step in your journey to learn the fundamentals of epidemiology. We are moving from learning about study designs and reporting measures of association, to considering **systematic error**, or ways in which our study results may be flawed. In the coming chapters we will describe how to limit, detect, and address systematic error due to confounding (**Chapter 9**), selection bias (**Chapter 10**), and information bias (**Chapter 11**).

---

## END OF CHAPTER PROBLEM SET

### Questions 1 to 7 are adapted from:

Cheng ZH, Wei YM, Li HT, Yu HZ, Liu JM, Zhou YB. Gestational diabetes mellitus as an effect modifier of the association of gestational weight gain with perinatal outcomes: a prospective cohort study in China. *Int J Environ Res Public Health*. 2022;19(9):5615. https://doi.org/10.3390/ijerph19095615. PMID: 35565005; PMCID: PMC9101455.

**Gestational weight gain (GWG),** defined as the amount of weight that a person gains during their pregnancy, is an important factor that healthcare providers monitor during the course of pregnancy. Both too little and too much weight gain during pregnancy are associated with adverse pregnancy outcomes.

**Gestational diabetes** is a condition that can develop during pregnancy, whereby a pregnant person is unable to make and use insulin properly. Gestational diabetes is a concern for both the pregnant person and their developing baby.

Finally, there are other factors that healthcare providers monitor to assess the health of developing and newborn babies, one of which is the *baby's weight relative to their gestational age*. Being either small or large for gestational age (SGA or LGA, respectively) is associated with complications among newborn babies.

Investigators undertook a cohort study of 9,838 pregnancies to evaluate the association between GWG and several adverse pregnancy outcomes. They specifically wanted to know *whether GWG had a different effect on these outcomes for those who had gestational diabetes compared to those who did not have gestational diabetes.* The data for the association between GWG (comparing those in the highest quartile of GWG to those in the first three quartiles of GWG) and delivering a baby who was LGA are shown in the table that follows, stratified by gestational diabetes status (**Table 8.3**).

**TABLE 8.3 ASSOCIATION BETWEEN GESTATIONAL WEIGHT GAIN AND LARGE FOR THEIR GESTATIONAL AGE, STRATIFIED BY GESTATIONAL DIABETES STATUS**

|  | Gestational Diabetes (*N* = 2,611) | | No Gestational Diabetes (*N* = 7,227) | |
| --- | --- | --- | --- | --- |
|  | **Fourth Quartile of GWG** | **Quartiles 1–3 of GWG** | **Fourth Quartile of GWG** | **Quartiles 1–3 of GWG** |
| **LGA** | 130 | 257 | 180 | 495 |
| **Not LGA** | 522 | 1,702 | 1,626 | 4,926 |
| **TOTAL** | 652 | 1,959 | 1,806 | 5,421 |

GWG, gestational weight gain; LGA, large for gestational age.

*Source*: Data from Cheng ZH, Wei YM, Li HT, Yu HZ, Liu JM, Zhou YB. Gestational Diabetes Mellitus as an Effect Modifier of the Association of Gestational Weight Gain with Perinatal Outcomes: A Prospective Cohort Study in China. *Int J Environ Res Public Health*. 2022;19(9):5615. https://doi.org/10.3390/ijerph19095615

1. Given the research question noted in italics in the previous text, "gestational diabetes" is being considered as which type of variable in this study?

2. *Name, calculate,* and *interpret* the appropriate stratum-specific *ratio* measure of association that describes the relationship between GWG (fourth quartile vs. quartiles 1–3) and LGA for *those who had gestational diabetes.*

3. *Name, calculate,* and *interpret* the appropriate stratum-specific *ratio* measure of association that describes the relationship between GWG (fourth quartile vs. quartiles 1–3) and LGA for *those who did NOT have gestational diabetes.*

4. Enter these data in OpenEpi and find the *p*-value for the Breslow-Day test that compares the measures that you calculated in Questions 2 and 3.

   Given your answers to Questions 2 through 4, indicate which of the following statements are true. For statements that are false, indicate what would need to be changed in order for the statement to be true.

5. The association between GWG and LGA is strongest among those who had gestational diabetes.

6. At an alpha level of 0.05, there is evidence of statistically significant interaction between GWG and gestational diabetes on the additive scale.

7. Assume that the difference between the stratum-specific RRs is clinically important. Investigators should only report the findings that show the relationship between GWG and LGA overall (i.e., ignoring gestational diabetes status).

**Question 8 refers to the following scenario. Use Table 8.4 to complete the sentence that describes how the scenario maps to the potential study results.**

You have conducted a cohort study of the relationship between air pollution and respiratory symptoms in children, and found that there is significant interaction according to whether or not the child had been breastfed.

**TABLE 8.4 WORD BANK**

| the same | different | the cohort | air pollution | respiratory symptoms |
|---|---|---|---|---|
| breastfed | not breastfed | exposed to air pollution | not exposed to air pollution | confounded |

8. The rate ratio that describes the relationship between _____ and _____ is _____ for children who were _____ compared to the rate ratio that describes this relationship for children who were _____.

**Questions 9 to 12 describe different study findings. After reading each study description, explain whether the study found evidence of effect measure modification. Provide an explanation to support your answer.**

9. Among a population of Hispanic adults, those residing in neighborhoods with high segregation had a higher risk of incident metabolic syndrome compared to those residing in neighborhoods with low segregation.[24]

10. Investigators found that oral contraceptives are less effective for preventing unintended pregnancy when taken with rifampin, an antibiotic.[25]

11. A study conducted in Argentina found that women with higher levels of education had better health outcomes than those with lower levels of education. This association was stronger for women living in more urban areas compared to those living in less urban areas.[26]

12. A cohort study to assess the association between smoking cessation during pregnancy and preterm birth found that those who quit earlier in pregnancy had a preterm birth rate that was similar to that of nonsmokers. This association was the same for non-Hispanic White and non-Hispanic Black women.[27]

# REFERENCES

1. Hillier AE. Redlining and the home owners' loan corporation. *J Urban Hist*. 2003;29(4):394–420. https://doi.org/10.1177/0096144203029004002

2. Winling LC, Michney TM. The roots of redlining: academic, governmental, and professional networks in the making of the new deal lending regime. *J Am Hist*. 2021;108(1):42–69. https://doi.org/10.1093/jahist/jaab066

3. Zenou Y, Boccard N. Racial discrimination and redlining in cities. *J Urban Econ*. 2000;48(2):260–285. https://doi.org/10.1006/juec.1999.2166

4. Lee EK, Donley G, Ciesielski TH, et al. Health outcomes in redlined versus non-redlined neighborhoods: a systematic review and meta-analysis. *Soc Sci Med*. 2022;294:114696. https://doi.org/10.1016/j.socscimed.2021.114696

5. Swope CB, Hernández D, Cushing LJ. The relationship of historical redlining with present-day neighborhood environmental and health outcomes: a scoping review and conceptual model. *J Urban Health*. 2022;99(6):959–983. https://doi.org/10.1007/s11524-022-00665-z

6. ACOG practice bulletin no. 110: noncontraceptive uses of hormonal contraceptives. *Obstet Gynecol*. 2010;115(1):206–218. https://doi.org/10.1097/AOG.0b013e3181cb50b5

7.  Jain AK. Cigarette smoking, use of oral contraceptives, and myocardial infarction. *Am J Obstet Gynecol*. 1976;126(3):301–307. https://doi.org/10.1016/0002-9378(76)90539-1

8.  Rosenberg L, Palmer JR, Rao RS, Shapiro S. Low-dose oral contraceptive use and the risk of myocardial infarction. *Arch Intern Med*. 2001;161(8):1065–1070. https://doi.org/10.1001/archinte.161.8.1065

9.  American College of Obstetricians and Gynecologists. ACOG Practice Bulletin No. 206: use of hormonal contraception in women with coexisting medical conditions. *Obstet Gynecol*. 2019;133(2):e128–e150. https://doi.org/10.1097/AOG.0000000000003072

10. Burd EM. Human papillomavirus and cervical cancer. *Clin Microbiol Rev*. 2003;16(1):1–17. https://doi.org/10.1128/CMR.16.1.1-17.2003

11. Harper DM, DeMars LR. HPV vaccines—a review of the first decade. *Gynecol Oncol*. 2017;146(1):196–204. https://doi.org/10.1016/j.ygyno.2017.04.004

12. Winer RL, Feng Q, Hughes JP, O'Reilly S, Kiviat NB, Koutsky LA. Risk of female human papillomavirus acquisition associated with first male sex partner. *J Infect Dis*. 2008;197(2):279–282. https://doi.org/10.1086/524875

13. Herweijer E, Sundström K, Ploner A, Uhnoo I, Sparén P, Arnheim-Dahlström L. Quadrivalent HPV vaccine effectiveness against high-grade cervical lesions by age at vaccination: a population-based study. *Int J Cancer*. 2016;138(12):2867–2874. https://doi.org/10.1002/ijc.30035

14. Folkhälsomyndigheten. HPV-vaccinuppföljning [HPV vaccine follow-up]. Updated December 16, 2022. https://www.folkhalsomyndigheten.se/smittskydd-beredskap/vaccinationer/nationella-vaccinationsprogram/uppfoljning-av-vaccinationsprogram/hpv-vaccinuppfoljning

15. Plascak JJ, Beyer K, Xu X, Stroup AM, Jacob G, Llanos AAM. Association between residence in historically redlined districts indicative of structural racism and racial and ethnic disparities in breast cancer outcomes. *JAMA Netw Open*. 2022;5(7):e2220908. https://doi.org/10.1001/jamanetworkopen.2022.20908

16. VanderWeele TJ. On the distinction between interaction and effect modification. *Epidemiology*. 2009;20(6):863–871. https://doi.org/10.1097/EDE.0b013e3181ba333c

17. Blau N, van Spronsen FJ, Levy HL. Phenylketonuria. *Lancet*. 2010;376(9750):1417–1427. https://doi.org/10.1016/S0140-6736(10)60961-0

18. Allen AM, Weinberger AH, Wetherill RR, Howe CL, McKee SA. Oral contraceptives and cigarette smoking: a review of the literature and future directions. *Nicotine Tob Res*. 2019;21(5):592–601. https://doi.org/10.1093/ntr/ntx258

19. Dean AG, et al. OpenEpi: open source epidemiologic statistics for public health. 2013. http://www.openepi.com/SampleSize/SSPropor.htm

20. Curtis KM, Tepper NK, Jatlaoui TC, et al. U.S. medical eligibility criteria for contraceptive use, 2016. *MMWR Recomm Rep*. 2016;65(3):1–103. https://doi.org/10.15585/mmwr.rr6503a1

21. World Health Organization. *Improving Access to Quality Care in Family Planning: Medical Eligibility Criteria for Contraceptive Use*. 2nd ed. World Health Organization; 2000

22. Starr JR, McKnight B. Assessing interaction in case-control studies: type I errors when using both additive and multiplicative scales. *Epidemiology*. 2004;15(4):422–427. https://pubmed.ncbi.nlm.nih.gov/15232402/

23. Centers for Disease Control and Prevention. HPV vaccination recommendations. 2021. https://www.cdc.gov/vaccines/vpd/hpv/hcp/recommendations.html

24. Pichardo CM, Pichardo MS, Gallo LC, et al. Association of neighborhood segregation with 6-year incidence of metabolic syndrome in the Hispanic community health study/study of Latinos. *Ann Epidemiol*. 2023;78:1–8. https://doi.org/10.1016/j.annepidem.2022.11.003

25. Dickinson BD, Altman RD, Nielsen NH, Sterling ML; Council on Scientific Affairs, American Medical Association. Drug interactions between oral contraceptives and antibiotics. *Obstet Gynecol*. 2001;98(5 Pt 1):853–860. https://doi.org/10.1016/s0029-7844(01)01532-0

26. Fleischer NL, Diez Roux AV, Alazraqui M, Spinelli H, De Maio F. Socioeconomic gradients in chronic disease risk factors in middle-income countries: evidence of effect modification by urbanicity in Argentina. *Am J Public Health*. 2011;101(2):294–301. https://doi.org/10.2105/AJPH.2009.190165

27. Moore E, Blatt K, Chen A, Van Hook J, DeFranco EA. Relationship of trimester-specific smoking patterns and risk of preterm birth. *Am J Obstet Gynecol*. 2016;215(1):109.E1–109.E6. https://doi.org/10.1016/j.ajog.2016.01.167

# FIGURE M.1 COLOR-CODING APPLIED TO EPIDEMIOLOGIC STUDY DESCRIPTIONS

## PANEL A. COLOR-CODING KEY FOR EXPOSURE AND OUTCOME (ALL CHAPTERS)

- Exposure variables appear in dark blue. When referring to the exposed and non-exposed groups separately, they appear in dark blue and light blue, respectively.

- Outcome variables appear in dark red. When referring to those with and without the outcome separately, they appear in dark red and gray, respectively.

| Crude Data | Exposed (E+) | Non-Exposed (E−) |
|---|---|---|
| With Outcome (O+) | A | B |
| Without Outcome (O−) | C | D |

Research question: What is the association between smoking and lung cancer?

Example study findings: During a 15-year follow-up period, those who smoked at least one pack of cigarettes per day were three times as likely to develop lung cancer as those who did not smoke at all.

## PANEL B. COLOR-CODING KEY FOR EFFECT MODIFIERS

- Effect measure modifiers appear in dark green.

Research question: Does the association between smoking and lung cancer differ by occupation?

Example study findings: During a 15-year follow-up period, those who worked in construction who smoked at least one pack of cigarettes per day were four times as likely to develop lung cancer as those who worked in construction who did not smoke at all.

However, during the same 15-year follow-up period, those who worked in office settings who smoked at least one pack of cigarettes per day were two times as likely to develop lung cancer as those who worked in office settings who did not smoke at all.

## PANEL C. COLOR-CODING KEY FOR CONFOUNDERS

- Confounders appear in orange.

Research question: Is the association between smoking and lung cancer confounded by cannabis use?

Example study findings: After controlling for cannabis use, the 15-year risk of lung cancer among those who smoked at least one pack of cigarettes per day was 2.8 times that of those who did not smoke at all.

## PANEL D. COLOR-CODING KEY FOR SOURCE & SAMPLE POPULATIONS

- Source population appears in pink and sample population appears in lime green.

Example study description: Our study was comprised of 150 students from a public university in New York that has a total of 20,000 enrolled students.

## TABLE M.1 CALCULATIONS AND KEY FEATURES OF COMMON MEASURES OF OUTCOME FREQUENCY

| Measure of Frequency | Interpretation | Units | Range of Possible Values | Calculation |
|---|---|---|---|---|
| **Risk**<br>*"Cumulative incidence"* | Proportion of at-risk individuals who develop a newly occurring outcome during a specified time-period | Expressed as a decimal or percentage | 0.0 – 1.0<br>or<br>0% – 100% | $$\frac{\text{\# of outcomes newly occurring during a follow-up period}}{\text{Total number of at-risk people observed during a follow-up period}}$$ |
| **Rate**<br>*"Incidence density"* | Measure of how quickly new outcomes occur in at-risk persons during a follow-up period | Expressed per unit of person-time | ≥ 0 | $$\frac{\text{\# of outcomes newly occurring during a follow-up period}}{\text{Total at-risk person-time}}$$ |
| **Prevalence**<br>*"Point prevalence"* | Proportion of a population that has an existing outcome at a particular point in time | Expressed as a decimal or percentage | 0.0 – 1.0<br>or<br>0% – 100% | $$\frac{\text{\# of existing outcomes observed at a point in time}}{\text{Total population at a point in time}}$$ |

## TABLE M.2 DEFINING FEATURES OF FOUR COMMON ANALYTIC EPIDEMIOLOGIC STUDY DESIGNS

| | Study Design | Participants Initially Classified by... | Follow-Up of an At-Risk Population? | Measure(s) of Outcome Frequency | Measure(s) of Association[a] |
|---|---|---|---|---|---|
| **Experimental** | Controlled Trials | Exposure | Yes | Risk[b] and/or rate | Risk ratio and risk difference[b] <br><br> Rate ratio and rate difference |
| **Observational** | Cohort | Exposure | Yes | Risk[b] and/or rate | Risk ratio and risk difference[b] <br><br> Rate ratio and rate difference |
| | Case-Control | Outcome | No | None | Exposure odds ratio |
| | Cross-Sectional | Exposure and Outcome | No | Prevalence | Prevalence ratio and prevalence difference |

[a]This list is not exhaustive, but encompasses the measures described in detail in this text.
[b]Recall that it is only appropriate to calculate risk if everyone in a population is followed until they either get the outcome or complete the same duration of study follow-up time.

## TABLE M.3 STRENGTHS AND LIMITATIONS OF FOUR MAJOR ANALYTIC EPIDEMIOLOGIC STUDY DESIGNS

| | Study Design | | Temporality Established by Design? | Efficient for Study of Rare Exposures? | Efficient for Study of Rare Outcomes?[a] |
|---|---|---|---|---|---|
| **Experimental** | Controlled Trials | | Yes | Yes | No |
| **Observational** | Cohort | Conducted in Real Time | Yes | Yes | No |
| | | Conducted Using Historical Records | Yes | Yes | Potentially[b] |
| | Case-Control | | Yes | No | Yes |
| | Cross-Sectional | | No[c] | No | No |

[a]Or outcomes with long latency periods or for exposure-outcome relationships with long induction periods.
[b]If ample data are available, a cohort study conducted using historical data could be efficient for the study of rare outcomes.
[c]While temporality is not established by design, temporality may be inferred depending on how the questions are asked.

# TABLE M.4 FORMULAE AND KEY FEATURES OF COMMON MEASURES OF ASSOCIATION

| Measure of Association[a] | Interpretation | Study Design(s) | Units | Range | Calculation |
|---|---|---|---|---|---|
| Risk ratio (RR) | The [length of follow-up] risk of the outcome in the exposed is RR times the risk of the outcome in the unexposed. | Controlled trials and cohort designs | None | $[0, \infty)$ | $\dfrac{(A/N_1)}{(B/N_0)}$ |
| Risk difference (RD) | The difference in the [length of follow-up] risk of the outcome in the exposed versus the unexposed is RD. | Controlled trials and cohort designs | Expressed as a decimal or percentage | $[-1, 1]$ | $\left(\dfrac{A}{N_1}\right) - \left(\dfrac{B}{N_0}\right)$ |
| Prevalence ratio (PR) | The prevalence of the outcome in the exposed is PR times the prevalence of the outcome in the unexposed. | Cross-sectional designs | None | $[0, \infty)$ | $\dfrac{(A/N_1)}{(B/N_0)}$ |
| Prevalence difference (PD) | The difference in the prevalence of the outcome in the exposed versus the unexposed is PD. | Cross-sectional designs | Expressed as a decimal or percentage | $[-1, 1]$ | $\left(\dfrac{A}{N_1}\right) - \left(\dfrac{B}{N_0}\right)$ |
| Exposure odds ratio (EOR) | The odds of the exposure among the cases is EOR times the odds of exposure among the controls. | Case-control designs | None | $[0, \infty)$ | $\dfrac{(A \times D)}{(B \times C)}$ |
| Rate (incidence density) ratio (IDR) | The rate of the outcome in the exposed is IDR times the rate of the outcome in the unexposed. | Controlled trials and cohort designs | None | $[0, \infty)$ | $\dfrac{(A/PT_1)}{(B/PT_0)}$ |
| Rate (incidence density) difference (IDD) | The difference in the rate of the outcome in the exposed versus the unexposed is IDD. | Controlled trials and cohort designs | Expressed per unit of person-time | $(-\infty, \infty)$ | $\left(\dfrac{A}{PT_1}\right) - \left(\dfrac{B}{PT_0}\right)$ |

**2x2 Data Layout**

|  | Exposed (E+) | Unexposed (E−) | TOTAL |
|---|---|---|---|
| Outcome (O+) | A | B | $M_1$ (A+B) |
| No Outcome (O−) | C | D | $M_0$ (C+D) |
| TOTAL | $N_1$ (A+C) | $N_0$ (B+D) | N |

|  | Exposed (E+) | Unexposed (E−) | TOTAL |
|---|---|---|---|
| Outcome (O+) | A | B | $M_1$ (A+B) |
| Person-Time | $PT_1$ | $PT_0$ | $PT_{total}$ ($PT_1 + PT_0$) |

aThis list is not exhaustive, but encompasses the measures described in detail in this text.

## FIGURE M.2. SUMMARY OF EFFECT MEASURE MODIFICATION ASSESSMENT

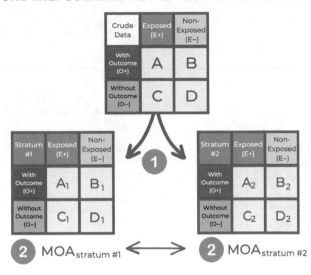

1. Stratify crude data into mutually exclusive groups (strata).

2. Calculate and compare stratum-specific measures of association (MOA).

3. If the stratum-specific measures of association are meaningfully different from one another, effect measure modification is present. Report stratified results.

## FIGURE M.3 CLASSIFICATION OF ERROR IN EPIDEMIOLOGIC RESEARCH

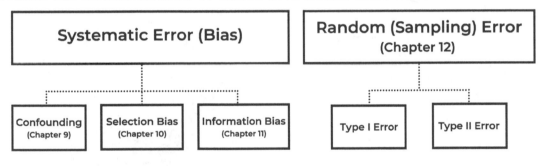

## FIGURE M.4 DISTINGUISHING BETWEEN RANDOM AND SYSTEMATIC ERROR

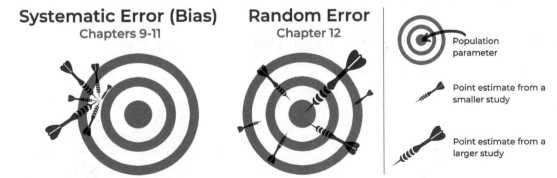

## FIGURE M.5 SUMMARY OF CONFOUNDING ASSESSMENT USING STRATIFIED ANALYSIS

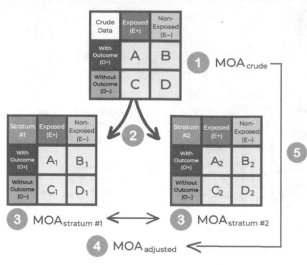

1. Calculate the crude measure of association (MOA).

2. Stratify crude data into mutually exclusive groups (strata).

3. Calculate and compare stratum-specific measures of association.

4. If the stratum-specific measures of association are not meaningfully different from each other, calculate an adjusted measure of association.

5. Compare the crude measure to the adjusted measure—if they are meaningfully different, confounding is present. The analysis must adjust for this variable.

## FIGURE M.6 CONCEPTUALIZING SELECTION BIAS

**Selection bias** occurs when...
the <u>measure of association</u> calculated in the sample population is... meaningfully different form the <u>measure of effect</u> in the **source population**.

Potential sources of selection bias:

- Loss to follow-up
- Flawed selection processes
- Low participation
- Participation non-response

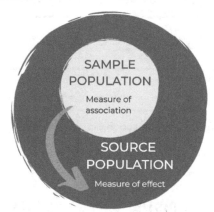

SAMPLE POPULATION

Measure of association

SOURCE POPULATION

Measure of effect

## FIGURE M.7 CONCEPTUALIZING INFORMATION BIAS

**Information bias** occurs when...

there is error in the measurement of the **exposure** or **outcome**...

that leads to a measure of association that is meaningfully different form what would have been obtained if all variables had been measured correctly.

Potential sources of information bias:

- Faulty measurement devices
- Poorly written questionnaires
- Incorrect self-report
- Data entry errors

# CHAPTER 9

# ERROR IN EPIDEMIOLOGIC RESEARCH AND FUNDAMENTALS OF CONFOUNDING

## KEY TERMS

adjusted measures of association

bias

confounder

confounding

crude measures of association

external validity

internal validity

point estimate

population parameter

random error

stratified analysis

systematic error

## LEARNING OBJECTIVES

9.1 Differentiate between the two types of error in epidemiology: systematic error and random error.

9.2 Define and distinguish between population parameters and point estimates.

9.3 Define and distinguish between internal validity and external validity.

9.4 Identify the direction of bias.

9.5 Define confounding.

9.6 Assess for confounding using a priori criteria.

9.7 Illustrate confounding using the confounding triangle.

9.8 Assess for confounding using a data-based method.

9.9 Interpret an adjusted measure of association.

9.10 Describe three strategies for controlling for confounding during the design stage of a study, and describe how each of these break the link(s) between the confounder and the exposure and/or outcome.

9.11 Use stratified analysis to control for confounding.

9.12 Distinguish between effect measure modification and confounding.

## DISENTANGLING INFLUENCES OF EARLY LIFE EXPERIENCES AND BEHAVIORS LATER IN LIFE

Prevention of traumatic events is important during any life stage, but it is particularly critical to prevent these events among children. Adverse childhood experiences (ACEs), such as experiencing or witnessing violence or household instability due to substance use or incarceration, have been studied extensively and been found to be associated with a range of poor health outcomes.[1] Research suggests that prevention of ACEs is crucial not just for the health of the those who experience them, but also for their future children: children of adults who experienced ACEs may be more likely to be subject to ACEs themselves.[2]

Given the wide-reaching impact of ACEs, investigators have explored their relationship with a number of outcomes including posttraumatic stress disorder, obesity, and cardiovascular health. In some cases, it is important to consider whether ACEs may help explain the associations that we see in other exposure–outcome relationships.

This chapter explores the phenomenon of confounding through an adapted view of a study evaluating the association between lower educational attainment and marijuana use during pregnancy, with a focus on whether considering the role of ACEs changes our understanding of this relationship.[3] This is an important topic because marijuana use during pregnancy is on the rise,[4] and some studies have found that marijuana use during pregnancy is associated with both short- and long-term risks for the baby, including preterm birth and developmental delays.[5]

You may wonder, if we are interested in learning about the relationship between lower educational attainment and marijuana use during pregnancy, why do we need to worry about ACEs? The reason is because it is plausible that those who experienced ACEs may be less likely to graduate from college, *and* these individuals may also be at an increased risk for marijuana use during pregnancy. In this chapter, we will walk you through the puzzle that is confounding, and illustrate why it is important to consider the role of ACEs in the context of a study of the relationship between lower educational attainment and marijuana use during pregnancy.

## INTRODUCTION TO ERROR (LEARNING OBJECTIVE 9.1)

We are now transitioning from our presentation of epidemiologic study designs to address the reality that epidemiologic studies are not error-free. This chapter begins a four-chapter series on the impact of error in epidemiologic research, which is split into two distinct categories: systematic error (**Chapter 9, "Error in Epidemiologic Research and Fundamentals of Confounding"; Chapter 10, "Selection Bias"; and Chapter 11, "Information Bias and Screening and Diagnostic Tests"**) and random error (**Chapter 12, "Random Error in Epidemiologic Research"**). The classification of error in epidemiologic research is described in the text that follows and illustrated in **Figure 9.1**.

**Systematic error**, also called **bias**, results from a flaw in the design, conduct, or analysis of a study that leads to incorrect conclusions. Questions about the **internal validity** (i.e., accuracy) of the study results arise when a study has been influenced by systematic error. Broadly, there are three main sources of bias in epidemiologic research: confounding, information bias, and selection bias. Each of these are defined briefly in the following list, and described in detail in **Chapter 9, "Error in Epidemiologic Research and Fundamentals of Confounding"; Chapter 10, "Selection Bias"; and Chapter 11, "Information Bias and Screening and Diagnostic Tests,"** respectively.

## FIGURE 9.1 CLASSIFICATION OF ERROR IN EPIDEMIOLOGIC RESEARCH

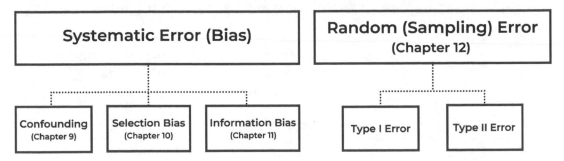

- **Confounding** is an error that occurs when the association of interest is mixed with the effect of an extraneous factor (a **confounder**) that is not balanced across comparison groups.
- **Selection bias** is an error that occurs when results obtained from the sample population are meaningfully different from what would have been obtained from the source population.
- **Information bias** is an error that occurs when there is inaccurate measurement of the exposure, outcome, and/or other variables of interest.

**Random error**, also called **sampling error**, occurs because we typically make inferences about a population using an estimate obtained from a **sample** of that population. Just by chance, we might calculate different estimates if we were to conduct the same study on different individuals selected from the same population. As the sample size increases (and thus gets closer to the size of the population that we sampled from), random error decreases. The presence of random error is inversely related to the concept of **precision.** Measures that are subject to less random error are said to be more precise, while those that are subject to more random error are said to be less precise. There are two types of random error (type I and type II errors), which are described in **Chapter 12, "Random Error in Epidemiologic Research."**

## Populations, Parameters, and Point Estimates
### (LEARNING OBJECTIVE 9.2)

Before further distinguishing between systematic and random error, it is important to think about how close our study results are to the true values in the population that we sample from. As introduced in **Chapter 4, "Randomized Controlled Trial Designs,"** investigators begin their epidemiologic studies by identifying a group of individuals who are *eligible* to be recruited for their study. This group comprises the **source population**. Participants who are ultimately *selected* from the source population for inclusion in the study comprise the **sample population**. As previously noted, we use information from our sample population to make inference (i.e., draw conclusions) about the source population. A schematic of the source and sample populations is shown in **Figure 9.2**.

Ultimately, we want the study results calculated from our sample population to be close to what we would have calculated if we had been able to study everyone in the source population. Unfortunately, we do not have access to these true values from the source population (if we did, we wouldn't need to do the study!). To conceptualize error in epidemiologic research, we distinguish between our study results calculated from the sample population, called **point estimates**, and the unobserved true values in the source population, called **population parameters**. Returning to our discussion of internal validity, we would say that studies with good internal validity yield point estimates that are close to the population parameter.

## FIGURE 9.2 SOURCE AND SAMPLE POPULATIONS IN EPIDEMIOLOGIC RESEARCH AND THEIR RELATIONSHIP TO POPULATION PARAMETERS AND POINT ESTIMATES

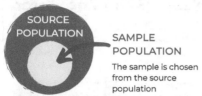

SAMPLE POPULATION

The sample is chosen from the source population

Epidemiologists make inferences about the source population using data obtained from the sample population

| SOURCE POPULATION | SAMPLE POPULATION |
|---|---|
| **Population Parameter**  Unobserved truth | **Point Estimate**  Calculated using study data |
| True Frequency<br>• *How common is the* exposure or outcome *in the source population?*<br>• e.g., The true prevalence of marijuana use during pregnancy among pregnant people in North and South Dakota from 2017-2019 | Measure of Frequency<br>• *How common is the* exposure or outcome *in the sample population?*<br>• e.g., Prevalence of marijuana use during pregnancy calculated using the 2017-2019 North and South Dakota PRAMS data |
| Measure of Effect<br>• *What is the true association between the* exposure and outcome *in the source population?*<br>• e.g., The true prevalence ratio that quantifies the association between lower education and marijuana use during pregnancy among pregnant people in North and South Dakota from 2017-2019 | Measure of Association<br>• *What is the association between the* exposure and outcome *obtained using data from the sample population?*<br>• e.g., Prevalence ratio that quantifies the association between lower education and marijuana use during pregnancy calculated using the 2017-2019 North and South Dakota PRAMS data |

We can further distinguish between the point estimate and population parameter when thinking about the relationship between an exposure and outcome of interest. The point estimate calculated using data from a sample population is called the **measure of association**, which is used to estimate the population parameter, called the **measure of effect**.

Let's revisit the cross-sectional study described at the beginning of this chapter which explored the role of education in marijuana use during pregnancy.[3] The study data came from the North and South Dakota Pregnancy Risk Assessment Monitoring System (PRAMS) sites, which recruited residents of North and South Dakota who had delivered a liveborn baby between 2017 and 2019. We can consider two different sets of population parameters and point estimates for this study:

**Frequency of marijuana use during pregnancy**

- **Population parameter**: the true proportion of pregnant individuals who used marijuana during pregnancy in North and South Dakota between 2017 and 2019.
- **Point estimate**: the prevalence of marijuana use calculated using the North and South Dakota 2017 to 2019 PRAMS data.

**Association between lower educational attainment and marijuana use during pregnancy**

- **Population parameter**: the true prevalence ratio that describes the association between not having graduated from college and marijuana use during pregnancy among all individuals who delivered a liveborn infant in North and South Dakota between 2017 and 2019. *This is an example of a measure of effect.*
- **Point estimate**: the prevalence ratio for the association between not having graduated from college and marijuana use during pregnancy calculated using the North and South Dakota 2017 to 2019 PRAMS data. *This is an example of a measure of association.*

## Distinguishing Between Internal and External Validity
### (LEARNING OBJECTIVE 9.3)

**Validity** is a term used in epidemiologic research to describe the accuracy of study results when compared with some other population. We distinguish between two types of validity: internal and external validity.

**Internal validity** is inversely associated with the influence of systematic error (or bias; Figure 9.3). Studies with good internal validity yield point estimates that are close to their corresponding population parameters in the source population. The more systematic error there is, the less valid the results are, and vice versa.

## FIGURE 9.3 RELATIONSHIP BETWEEN SYSTEMATIC ERROR AND INTERNAL VALIDITY

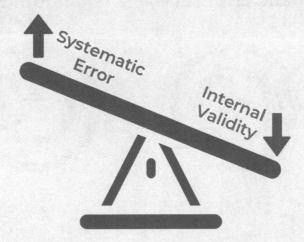

**External validity**, on the other hand, refers to whether results from a study are applicable to the target population(s). This relates to the concept of **generalizability**, which is discussed in **Chapter 10, "Selection Bias."**

Studies lacking internal validity also lack external validity (we would not want to apply incorrect results to another population!). Another way to think about this is that internal validity is a prerequisite for external validity.

For example, consider a study to estimate the prevalence of chicken pox vaccination status among children in Poland. If the study collected vaccination status by asking the children whether they had received a chicken pox vaccine, it is likely that we would get erroneous information since children might not know exactly which vaccines they have received. Such a study would lack internal validity because our point estimate of the prevalence of chicken pox vaccination would be quite different from the true prevalence (the population parameter) among children in Poland. The study would *also* lack external validity, because we wouldn't want to use these incorrect results to try to understand something about the prevalence of chicken pox vaccination in other populations, such as children in a neighboring country.

While a study cannot have external validity without internal validity, it is important to note that a study *can* have internal validity without external validity. For example, suppose we had accurately estimated the prevalence of chicken pox vaccination among children in Poland. This means that our point estimate approximated the population parameter, and thus the results are internally valid. However, it may not be appropriate to assume that the prevalence of chicken pox vaccination among children in Poland is the same as that of neighboring countries. For example, such countries may have important differences in healthcare systems or cultural norms around vaccination, which could lead to a very different prevalence of chicken pox vaccination. Thus, our internally valid findings may not be externally valid.

## Distinguishing Between Systematic and Random Error

A graphical representation of the difference between systematic and random error is shown in **Figure 9.4**. The centers of the targets represent the population parameter that we wish to make inferences about, and each dart represents the point estimate from a study that was conducted with the goal of estimating that population parameter. It is important to note that study results can be (and most often are!) affected by *both* random and systematic error; however, we are considering these errors separately for illustrative purposes.

**FIGURE 9.4 DISTINGUISHING BETWEEN SYSTEMATIC ERROR (BIAS) AND RANDOM ERROR**

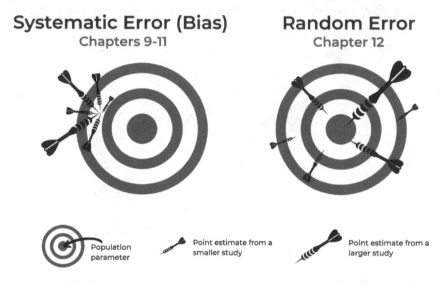

The target on the left depicts how the point estimates relate to the population parameter in the presence of systematic error only (i.e., no random error). No matter how many darts we throw, our point estimates consistently miss the center of the target. As previously described, systematic error is a flaw in the study that leads to incorrect conclusions. Without addressing the underlying flaw, we will continue to obtain the same (incorrect!) estimate of the population parameter. Notice that these darts have varying sizes, which represent studies with larger and smaller sample sizes. Whether a study is influenced by systematic error does not depend on sample size, and we cannot reduce systematic error by increasing the sample size.

In contrast, the target on the right depicts how the point estimates relate to the population parameter in the presence of random error only (i.e., no systematic error). Not only are the darts no longer landing in a predictable location, but we notice that the larger the darts are, the closer they are to the population parameter at the center of the target. As the size of the sample population increases, the less random error there is, and the closer the point estimate will be to the population parameter.

The role of statistical testing is another important feature that distinguishes random error from systematic error. Statistical testing is only used to quantify the impact of random error on study results (**Chapter 12, "Random Error in Epidemiologic Research"**). As you will see, statistical tests are *not* used to quantify the impact of systematic error on study results. Instead, we will consider whether our study results are likely meaningfully different from the population parameter in the presence of systematic error.

A summary of the differences between random error and systematic error is shown in **Table 9.1**.

**TABLE 9.1 DISTINGUISHING BETWEEN RANDOM ERROR AND SYSTEMATIC ERROR**

| | Systematic Error (Bias) | Random Error |
|---|---|---|
| Brief definition | A flaw in the study that leads to incorrect conclusions<br><br>A lack of systematic error leads to a measure that is <u>valid</u> | Sampling error<br><br>A lack of random error leads to a measure that is <u>precise</u> |
| Impact of changes in sample size | Systematic error is not affected by study sample size | Random error decreases as study sample size increases |
| Role of statistical testing | Not assessed using statistical tests | Can be quantified using statistical tests |

## DIRECTION OF BIAS (LEARNING OBJECTIVE 9.4)

Before transitioning to a deep dive into confounding, we will explore an important concept relevant for all types of systematic error, which is the **direction of bias**. We often want to provide more information than just noting whether a measure of association is likely to be biased. It can be helpful to additionally indicate whether the observed measure of association suggests a stronger or weaker association between the exposure and outcome of interest than what would be indicated by the population parameter.

Bias can operate in three possible directions: toward the null, away from the null, and across the null. Each of these are described in the text that follows and summarized in **Figure 9.5**. To determine the direction of bias, we evaluate whether the point estimate is closer to, further away from, or on the other side of the null value relative to the population parameter.

## FIGURE 9.5 IDENTIFYING THE DIRECTION OF BIAS

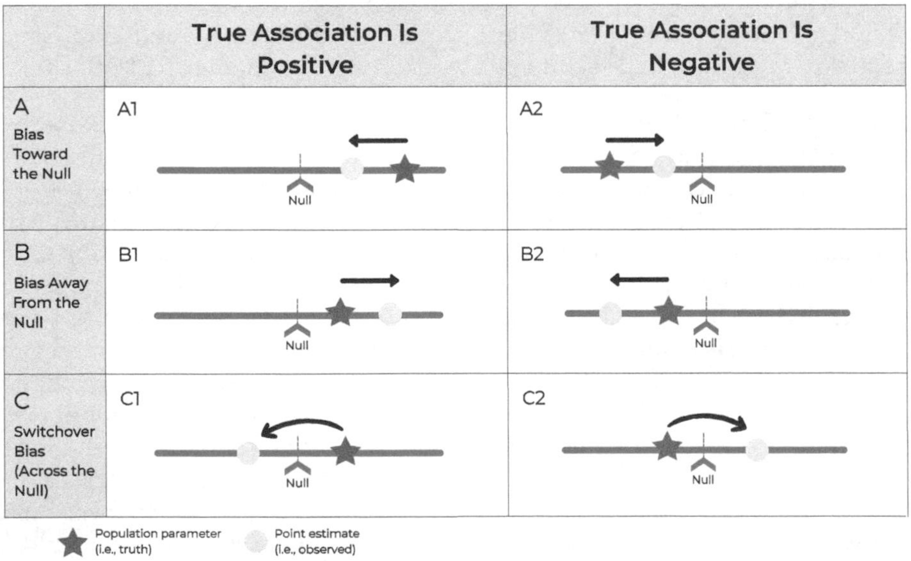

A description of the three possible directions of bias is given in the text that follows, each of which includes an example related to one of the three main types of systematic error: confounding, selection bias, and information bias.

**Bias toward the null** (**Figure 9.5–Panel A**) occurs when the observed association suggests that the relationship between the exposure and outcome of interest is weaker than it truly is (i.e., the point estimate is closer to the null than the population parameter). This means that the point estimate for a positive association will be *smaller* than the corresponding population parameter (**Figure 9.5–Panel A1**), and that the point estimate for a negative association will be *larger* than the corresponding population parameter (**Figure 9.5–Panel A2**). An example of bias toward the null occurred in a study that explored whether severe maternal morbidity was associated with adverse cardiovascular events in mothers up to 2 years postpartum.[6] Prior to considering the impact of other factors, investigators found that there were 19.7 excess adverse cardiovascular events per 1,000 deliveries among those who experienced severe maternal morbidity compared to those who did not (i.e., risk difference = 0.0197) over 2 years of follow-up. However, after accounting for the influence of several confounders (e.g., age, substance use disorder, asthma, etc.), investigators found that this measure rose to 27.9 excess adverse cardiovascular events per 1,000 deliveries (i.e., risk difference = 0.0279) over 2 years of follow-up. In this example, the biased comparison that ignored the influence of these other factors *underestimated* the association that accounted for confounding by these factors.

**Bias away from the null** (**Figure 9.5–Panel B**) occurs when the observed association suggests that the relationship between the exposure and outcome of interest is stronger than it truly is (i.e., the point estimate is further from the null than the population parameter). This means that the point estimate for a positive association will be *larger* than the corresponding population parameter (**Figure 9.5–Panel B1**), and that the point estimate for a negative association will be *smaller* than the corresponding population parameter (**Figure 9.5–Panel B2**). Suppose investigators were interested in studying the association between stress and irritable bowel syndrome (IBS) and shared this information with potential participants during study recruitment. Individuals with IBS who experience high levels of stress may be more motivated than others to participate in such a study, given their personal connection to both of these factors. There is a known positive association between stress and IBS[7]; however, given this imbalance in participation, we would likely observe a higher prevalence of IBS among those experiencing high stress than if the investigators had not shared information about the study goals with potential participants. In this example, the biased measure of association that ignores imbalanced participation would lead to an *overestimate* of the association between stress and IBS that accounted for differential participation (i.e., selection bias—described in **Chapter 10, "Selection Bias"**).

**Switchover bias** (**Figure 9.5–Panel C**) occurs when a truly positive association appears negative, or vice versa (i.e., the point estimate is on the opposite side of the null relative to the population parameter). This means that the point estimate for a truly positive association will appear to the left of the null (**Figure 9.5–Panel C1**), and that the point estimate for a truly negative association will appear to the right of the null (**Figure 9.5–Panel C2**). Consider an example of a study to evaluate the association between self-reported condom use and incidence of sexually transmitted infections (STIs). If used consistently and correctly, we expect that the incidence of STIs would be lower among those who report using condoms compared to those who report not using condoms (i.e., there should be a negative association between regular condom use and STIs). However, suppose that several individuals did not want to disclose not using condoms, and thus reported regularly using condoms when they truly did not. These individuals are also more likely to have incident STIs, due to their lack of condom use. In this situation, the risk of STIs will be higher among those reporting regular condom use than if we had correct condom use data for all study participants. This could lead to a situation where condom use appears to have a *positive* association with incident STIs due to errors in the reporting of the exposure (i.e., misclassification of the exposure—described in **Chapter 11, "Information Bias and Screening and Diagnostic Tests"**).

## Conceptualizing the Population Parameter and the Unknown Truth

A common question among learners of epidemiology is "How can we know the direction of the bias if we do not know what the truth is?" This question makes a lot of sense, because if we knew what the truth is, we would not need to conduct our study!

The idea behind evaluating the direction of bias is to consider whether a given measure of association is more or less likely to be internally valid than another measure. Measures of association that fail to account for systematic errors (confounding, selection bias, or information bias) will likely be less internally valid than those that do account for these errors.

When illustrating examples of systematic error, instructors often provide learners with examples where both the true and biased data are given. Although hypothetical, these examples are crucial to understanding the underlying concepts. As you continue in your epidemiologic studies, you will find that, given some context about a particular research question, you will be able to think through how various errors are likely to impact the R×C table and thus predict the likely direction of the bias. Don't worry if this feels confusing at this stage—it will become more intuitive as you get more practice!

## Highlights

### Overview of Error in Epidemiologic Research

There are two types of error in epidemiologic research:

- **Systematic error** (also called **bias**)—flaws in the design, conduct, or analysis of a study that lead to incorrect conclusions. There are three main types of systematic error:
  - confounding (**this chapter**)
  - selection bias (**Chapter 10**)
  - information bias (**Chapter 11**)

- **Random error** (also called **sampling error**)—occurs because epidemiologists often study a sample, rather than an entire source population (**Chapter 12**)

- Random, but not systematic, error can be reduced by increasing the size of the sample population. To reduce systematic error, investigators must address the underlying cause that is leading to bias.

- The **source population** is the group of individuals who are eligible to be selected for participation in a given epidemiologic study.

- The **sample population** is the group of individuals who are ultimately selected for participation in a given epidemiologic study.

- The **population parameter** is the unobserved true value in the source population. Investigators use a **point estimate** calculated using data from their sample population to estimate the population parameter.

Epidemiologists distinguish between two types of **validity**:

- **Internal validity** is an indication of the extent to which the study results have been influenced by systematic error (bias).

- **External validity** is the extent to which the study results can be applied to an external population (also called **generalizability**, which is discussed further in **Chapter 10**).

- Internal validity is a prerequisite for external validity.

The **direction of bias** is determined by comparing the point estimate to the population parameter, relative to the null value. Bias can operate in one of three directions:

- **Bias toward the null**—An observed association suggests that the relationship between the exposure and outcome of interest is weaker than it really is (i.e., the point estimate is closer to the null than the population parameter).

- **Bias away from the null**—An observed association suggests that the relationship between the exposure and outcome of interest is stronger than it really is (i.e., the point estimate is further from the null than the population parameter).

- **Switchover bias**—A true positive association appears negative, or vice versa (i.e., the point estimate is on the opposite side of the null from the population parameter).

## CONFOUNDING BASICS (LEARNING OBJECTIVE 9.5)

Confounding is the first type of systematic error that we will discuss in detail in this textbook. **Confounding** occurs when the measure of association that describes the relationship between the exposure and outcome of interest is incorrect (i.e., too big, too small, or on the other side of the null) because the association is "mixed" with one or more extraneous variables that are imbalanced across the comparison groups. Ignoring the influence of these extraneous variables, called **confounders**, leads to an unfair comparison and a biased (i.e., invalid) measure of association. The familiar phrase "correlation does not imply causation" can be helpful to begin to understand confounding. It reminds us that two things may be associated with one another, but that one doesn't necessarily *cause* the other; sometimes, noncausal associations can be explained (all or in part) by confounding.

Let's begin by considering the association between alcohol consumption and lung cancer, shown using simulated data in **Figure 9.6–Panel A**. The frequency of lung cancer increases as alcohol consumption increases; however, after accounting for confounding, this association is not quite as strong as it appears. This relationship can be partially explained by confounding due to smoking. On average, those who consume more alcoholic beverages are more likely to smoke (**Figure 9.6–Panel B**), *and* there is a strong association between smoking and lung cancer (**Figure 9.6–Panel C**). In this example, we would say that smoking *confounds* the association between alcohol consumption and lung cancer.

When we ignore the influence of smoking, as shown in **Figure 9.6–Panel A**, we are making an unfair comparison because nondrinkers, on average, smoke fewer cigarettes than those who drink more. **Figure 9.6–Panel D** provides a complete picture to understand

## FIGURE 9.6 ILLUSTRATING CONFOUNDING OF THE ASSOCIATION BETWEEN ALCOHOL CONSUMPTION AND LUNG CANCER BY SMOKING STATUS

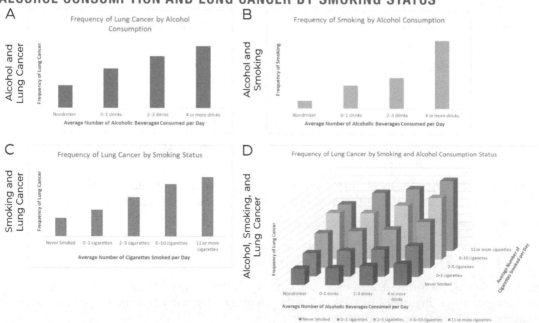

what is happening. To understand the effect of drinking accounting for (or *controlling for*) smoking, we can look *within* strata of smoking (i.e., examine the sets of bars that are all the same color), which allows us to understand the influence of alcohol consumption on lung cancer while holding smoking constant. We see that the occurrence of lung cancer is nearly the same regardless of the average number of alcoholic drinks consumed (meaning that, with some exceptions, the bars that are all the same color are nearly identical in height). Once we control for smoking status, the association between alcohol consumption and lung cancer is attenuated compared to the data in Panel A. Notice that a strong positive association remains between lung cancer occurrence and increasing average number of cigarettes smoked, even after controlling for alcohol consumption. To see this, compare the dark blue, orange, grey, yellow, and light blue bars within strata of (i.e., controlling for) alcohol consumption.

In this example, prior to controlling for smoking frequency, we observed a strong positive association between alcohol consumption and lung cancer. After controlling for smoking frequency, this association is not quite as strong as it once appeared, which is an example of bias away from the null.

The following list offers two additional examples that can be used to illustrate confounding:

- Increases in ice cream sales are associated with decreases in influenza cases.
    - This is an example of confounding by temperature. Ice cream sales increase as the temperature increases, *and* influenza cases decrease as the temperature increases.
- Birth order is associated with Down syndrome (i.e., babies who are the third born, for example, are more likely to have Down syndrome than babies who are the first born).[8]
    - This is an example of confounding by age of the birthing parent. On average, children with higher birth orders are born to older parents, *and* older birthing parents are at greater risk for having a baby with Down syndrome due to an increased likelihood of having a fertilized egg that has an extra copy of chromosome 21.

Both examples illustrate bias away from the null due to confounding. In both cases, there is no true (i.e., causal) relationship between the exposures and outcomes. In the case of ice cream sales and influenza cases, there appears to be a *negative* association before accounting for confounding by temperature (i.e., as ice cream sales increase, influenza cases decrease). In the case of birth order and Down syndrome, there appears to be a *positive* association before accounting for confounding by age of the birthing parent (i.e., increases in birth order are associated with increases in the frequency of Down syndrome).

## Confounding Terminology

Confounding is sometimes described as a "confusion or mixing of effects" because the effect of the third (i.e., extraneous) variable is mistaken as part of the effect of the exposure. The resulting distortion in the measure of association is described as **confounding**, and the extraneous variable that is responsible for that distortion is called a **confounder**.

The **crude measure of association** is the measure calculated using the entire sample population and only considers the relationship between the exposure and the outcome. In the context of confounding, crude measures of association are also called **unadjusted measures of association**. All the measures of association that were calculated previously in this textbook were crude (i.e., unadjusted) measures of association.

As we move through this chapter, we will discuss how to calculate measures of association that aim to address confounding—these are called **adjusted measures of association**, and are measures that *adjust* or *control for* confounding.

To distinguish adjusted measures of association from crude measures of association, investigators will often use a lowercase "a" in front of the abbreviation for the adjusted measure of association (e.g., an adjusted odds ratio may be written as "aOR"). Occasionally, investigators will distinguish crude measures of association by adding a lowercase "c" in front of the abbreviation for the crude measure of association (e.g., a crude odds ratio may be written as "cOR"). We will use this notation moving forward for clarity. However, note that you may see variations in formatting when reading the epidemiologic literature.

The remainder of this chapter will be devoted to three main topics: assessing confounding, addressing confounding, and distinguishing confounding from effect measure modification. Before proceeding, it may be helpful to understand the difference between assessing and addressing confounding:

- **Confounding assessment** refers to the identification of variables that confound the exposure–outcome association.

- **Addressing confounding** involves employing strategies that attempt to reduce confounding by variables identified in the assessment stage.

We describe assessing and addressing confounding, and their related strategies, in the text that follows. A summary of these strategies is shown in **Figure 9.7**, which you may wish to revisit upon completion of this chapter.

## FIGURE 9.7 SUMMARY OF METHODS FOR ASSESSING AND ADDRESSING CONFOUNDING

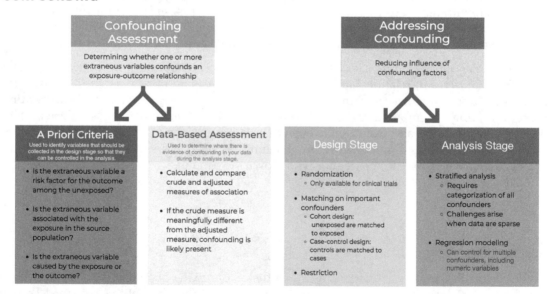

## Examples of Confounding in Everyday Life

The term *confounding* is not typically used in conversation, but the concept is something that can intuitively arise as we consider whether the associations that we observe in everyday life are real (i.e., causal), or whether they could be explained (either entirely, or partially) by something else. What are some examples that you can think of where confounding might explain associations observed in everyday life?

## Confounding Basics

- **Confounding** occurs when the measure of association that describes the relationship between the exposure and outcome of interest is distorted by the influence of an extraneous variable (called a **confounder**).

- In the presence of confounding, the association between the exposure and outcome can be entirely or partially explained by the confounder.

- Measures of association calculated using the entire sample population that do not account for confounders are called **crude** or **unadjusted measures of association**. Measures of association that **adjust** or **control** for confounders are called **adjusted measures of association**.

## CONFOUNDING ASSESSMENT

Confounding assessment is the process by which investigators determine whether one or more extraneous variables confound an exposure–outcome relationship, and typically takes place at two distinct points in the research process: when the study is being designed and when the data are being analyzed. During the study design stage, we assess which variables are likely to be confounders of our exposure–outcome relationship to ensure that we collect information on these variables. As you'll see shortly, we can't adjust for confounding during the analysis if we haven't collected data on the possible confounders! Once the data have been collected, we can then determine whether there is evidence of confounding in our study that must be addressed during the analysis. We will describe two methods of confounding assessment that map to each of these stages: a priori criteria for confounding assessment during the study design stage and a data-based method for confounding assessment during the data analysis stage.

### A Priori Criteria for Confounding Assessment During the Study Design Stage (LEARNING OBJECTIVE 9.6)

The **a priori criteria** are a set of three criteria that must hold for a variable to be considered a possible confounder in our analysis. A priori is a Latin phrase that means "from the earlier" and is used to describe information that investigators deduce using knowledge that they already have, rather than through empirical observation. Extraneous variables that are eligible to be considered as potential confounders must meet each of these three criteria:

1. The extraneous variable must be a risk factor for the outcome in the unexposed.

2. The extraneous variable must be associated with the exposure in the source population.

3. The extraneous variable cannot be caused by the exposure or the outcome.

These criteria are often illustrated using a **confounding triangle**, which is shown in **Figure 9.8–Panel A** (Learning Objective 9.7). Pay close attention to the direction of the arrows in **Figure 9.8**: for a variable to meet the a priori criteria, there must be arrows that connect the potential confounder to *both* the exposure and the outcome *and* both arrows must be pointing *away* from the confounder. These arrows represent causal relationships between the variables of interest, and their direction is an indication of temporality (i.e., which variable came first). Note that these associations could be positive or negative, and that this strategy is a thought experiment employed when designing an epidemiologic study to ensure that data are collected for all potential confounders of interest. When assessing which variables are likely to meet the a priori criteria and possibly confound the exposure–outcome relationship, we consider what information is already known about the relationships between the exposure, outcome,

**FIGURE 9.8 USING THE CONFOUNDING TRIANGLE TO ILLUSTRATE THE A PRIORI CRITERIA FOR CONFOUNDING**

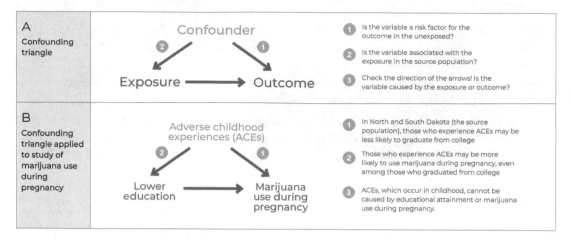

and other related factors. Consultation with subject matter experts and reviewing relevant literature are two helpful strategies to help determine whether the a priori criteria are likely to be met.

## A Closer Look at the a Priori Criteria

There are two elements of the first two a priori criteria that warrant some additional discussion:

1. The extraneous variable must be a risk factor for the outcome in the unexposed.
2. The extraneous variable must be associated with the exposure in the source population.

Broadly speaking, we know that in order for an extraneous variable to confound an exposure–outcome relationship, it must be associated with both the exposure and outcome. The idea behind the details underlined in the previous list is that we want to be sure that we are isolating the influence of this extraneous variable on the outcome (criterion 1) and on the exposure (criterion 2). That is, we want to be sure that the extraneous variable is associated with both the exposure independent of the outcome, *and* associated with the outcome independent of the exposure.

Returning to the study of marijuana use during pregnancy in North and South Dakota, let's consider the association between lower education (not having graduated from college vs. having graduated from college) and marijuana use during pregnancy (yes vs. no). Let's use the a priori criteria to assess whether ACEs could possibly confound the exposure–outcome relationship (**Figure 9.8–Panel B**):

1. Are ACEs a risk factor for marijuana use during pregnancy in those who graduated from college?

   *Yes, a review of the existing literature indicates that those who have experienced ACEs are more likely to use marijuana during pregnancy, even if they graduated from college.*[9] *This means that the first criterion is satisfied.*

2. Are ACEs associated with being a college graduate in North and South Dakota?

   *A UK study found that those who experienced four or more ACEs were less likely to have graduated from college than those who experienced three or fewer ACEs.*[10] *Although these data are from the UK, we may hypothesize that the same relationship is likely to hold in other populations, and suspect that the second criterion is likely satisfied.*

3. Are ACEs caused by being a college graduate or by marijuana use during pregnancy? *Given that ACEs would have occurred earlier in life, it is impossible for college graduation to cause adverse events that occurred in childhood. Similarly, it is impossible for marijuana use during pregnancy to cause adverse events that occurred in childhood. This means that the third criterion is satisfied.*

Given that all three a priori criteria are met, we conclude that ACEs should be considered as a potential confounder of the association between lower education and marijuana use during pregnancy.

## Pause to Practice 9.2

### Evaluation of the a Priori Criteria in Epidemiologic Studies

1. Let's revisit the association between birth order and Down syndrome that was introduced earlier in this chapter. Does age of the birthing parent meet the a priori criteria to be a confounder of this association? Write out the a priori criteria using the same structure used in the example about marijuana use during pregnancy and indicate whether you think each of the criteria hold, and why.

2. Consider another example adapted from a cross-sectional study designed to understand the factors associated with housing conditions that could increase the risk of death.[11] Since living in an extremely cold home is a risk factor for death among older individuals, investigators wanted to identify which factors were associated with having difficulties paying heating bills among older men in the UK with the goal of identifying areas for targeted prevention. One of the factors considered was whether the individual reported feeling isolated from others. Investigators considered several potential confounders; however, for our purposes, we will only explore the potential confounding effect of having chronic health conditions. Does having chronic health conditions (yes vs. no) meet the a priori criteria to be a confounder of the association between feeling isolated from others (sometimes/often vs. rarely/never) and having difficulty paying for heating bills (yes vs. no)?

## Data-Based Method for Confounding Assessment During the Analysis Stage (LEARNING OBJECTIVE 9.8)

The **data-based method for confounding assessment** provides a quantitative assessment strategy that is used during the data analysis stage, as opposed to the a priori criteria which are used during the study design stage. The data-based method allows investigators to determine whether there is evidence of confounding in their data and involves a comparison of crude and adjusted measures of association. If the crude measure of association is *meaningfully different* from the measure of association that is calculated after adjusting for the confounder, we conclude that confounding is present by this variable and it should be adjusted for in the analysis. What constitutes a meaningful difference may depend on the specific research question and context; however, more than a ±10% difference between the crude and adjusted measures of association is often considered an indication of meaningful confounding. Since we have given some thought about which variables are likely to confound the exposure–outcome relationship, we consider the adjusted measure of association to have greater internal validity than the crude measure of association.

Let's revisit the cross-sectional study of the association between education and marijuana use during pregnancy. The prevalence ratio that describes the unadjusted association between lower education and marijuana use during pregnancy can be calculated using the data shown in **Figure 9.9**:

## FIGURE 9.9 CRUDE DATA ADAPTED FROM THE CROSS-SECTIONAL STUDY OF MARIJUANA USE DURING PREGNANCY

|  | Not College Graduate (E+) | College Graduate (E−) | TOTAL |
|---|---|---|---|
| Marijuana Use During Pregnancy (O+) | 275 | 7 | 282 |
| No Marijuana Use During Pregnancy (O−) | 3,536 | 1,581 | 5,117 |
| TOTAL | 3,811 | 1,588 | 5,399 |

$$cPR = \frac{\text{Prevalence of outcome among exposed}}{\text{Prevalence of outcome among unexposed}} = \frac{275/3,811}{7/1,588} = 16.4$$

The adjusted prevalence ratio that describes the association between lower education and marijuana use during pregnancy that controls for the experience of ACEs is 12.4. We will explain how to calculate this adjusted measure later in the chapter. For now, let's focus on comparing the crude and confounder-adjusted measures of association to determine whether there is evidence of meaningful confounding.

When using the data-based method for confounding assessment, investigators can calculate the percent difference between the crude and adjusted measures of association as shown in **Equation 9.1**:

$$\text{Percent difference} = \left( \frac{\text{Crude measure} - \text{Adjusted measure}}{\text{Adjusted measure}} \right) \times 100\% \tag{9.1}$$

Let's compare the crude and adjusted measures of association from the cross-sectional study of marijuana use during pregnancy:

$$\text{Percent difference} = \left( \frac{16.4 - 12.4}{12.4} \right) \times 100\% = 32\%$$

There is a 32% difference between the crude and adjusted measures of association, which is substantial. Using a ±10% difference as a cutoff for whether a crude measure of association is meaningfully different from an adjusted measure of association, we would conclude that there is evidence of a meaningful difference, and thus that the experience of ACEs does confound the association between lower education and marijuana use during pregnancy in this study.

Another way to think about this is that there is an important difference in our understanding of the relationship between lower education and marijuana use during pregnancy once we account for the experience of ACEs. Both the crude and adjusted prevalence ratios suggest a positive association between lower education and marijuana use during pregnancy; however, this association is attenuated (i.e., not as strong) once we account for the influence of the experience of ACEs. This is an example of bias away from the null, which is illustrated in **Figure 9.10**. The blue circle represents the adjusted measure of association, and the orange open circle represents the crude measure of association.

## FIGURE 9.10 DIRECTION OF BIAS IN THE STUDY OF MARIJUANA USE DURING PREGNANCY

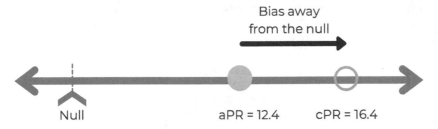

aPR, adjusted prevalence ratio; cPR, crude prevalence ratio

*Source:* Testa A, Jackson DB, Boccio C, Ganson KT, Nagata JM. Adverse childhood experiences and marijuana use during pregnancy: findings from the North Dakota and South Dakota PRAMS, 2017–2019. *Drug Alcohol Depend.* 2022;230:109197. https://doi.org/10.1016/j .drugalcdep.2021.109197

When assessing the direction of bias between crude and adjusted measures, we begin by orienting the crude and adjusted measures on a number line relative to their null value and then we draw an arrow *from* the adjusted measure *toward* the crude measure. The direction of the arrow may be toward, away from, or crossing the null. This aligns with what we previously described when we found the direction of bias by drawing arrows from the population parameter to the point estimate. Our assumption is that the adjusted measure of association is closer to the population parameter (i.e., the true value in the source population) because we have controlled for a confounder. In our example, we see that the crude prevalence ratio is further from the null than the adjusted prevalence ratio, thus illustrating that failure to control for the experience of ACEs leads to bias away from the null.

A visual representation of what differences between the crude and adjusted measures of association would be suggestive of confounding is shown in **Figure 9.11**. In addition to calculating the percent difference between the crude and adjusted measures of association, we can also construct a "no confounding zone" around our adjusted measure of association, which is shaded in light blue. The width of this zone is determined by the percent change that was deemed meaningful for confounding assessment. If using a ±10% or greater change as a guideline, this zone would be calculated as shown in **Equation 9.2**.

Lower and upper bounds of the "no confounding zone"
$$= \text{Adjusted measure} \pm 0.1 \times \text{Adjusted measure} \tag{9.2}$$

If the crude measure of association falls inside of the "no confounding zone," this means that it is *not* meaningfully different from the adjusted measure of association, and we would conclude that there is no meaningful confounding by the variable of interest. If, however, the crude measure of association was to fall *outside* of the "no confounding zone," shaded in light orange in **Figure 9.11**, this means that the crude measure *is* meaningfully different from the adjusted measure of association, and we would conclude that there *is* evidence of confounding by the variable of interest.

## FIGURE 9.11 ILLUSTRATING THE "NO CONFOUNDING ZONE" AND DIRECTION OF BIAS

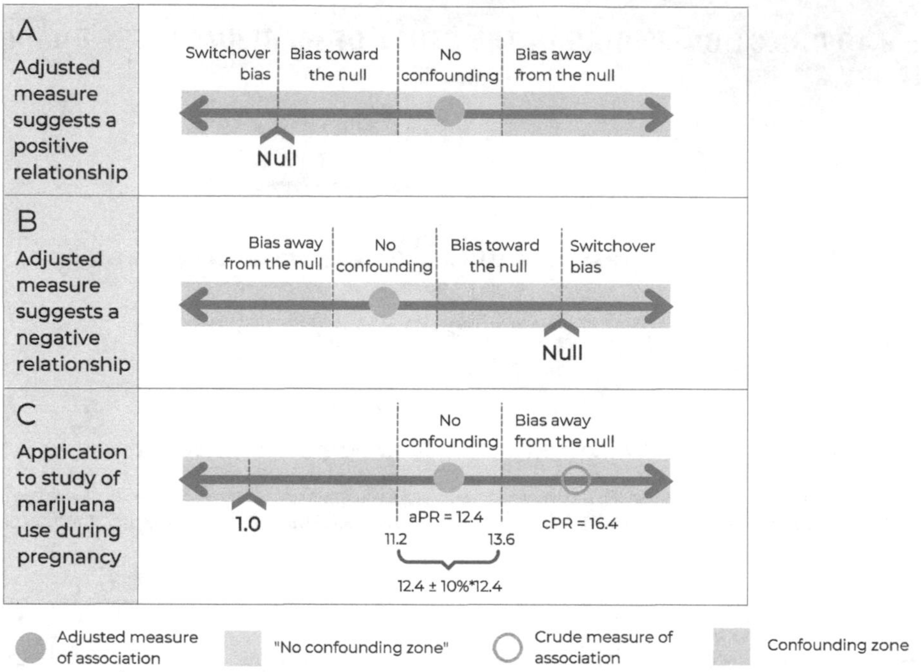

aPR, adjusted prevalence ratio; cPR, crude prevalence ratio

### An Important Note on Comparing Crude and Adjusted Measures of Association

It is important to remember that confounding assessment considers whether the crude measure of association is *meaningfully* different from the adjusted measure of association. While we typically use a ±10% or greater guideline to operationalize what we mean by "meaningful," we can think about this just as we did in **Chapter 8, "Effect Measure Modification and Statistical Interaction,"** when considering whether stratified measures of association were meaningfully different from one another. When a crude measure of association is ±10% or greater different from an adjusted measure, this means that our understanding of the relationship between the exposure and outcome of interest is quite different once we account for confounders of interest. This is of particular concern when the difference in our understanding would have different implications for public health action.

In the cross-sectional study of the relationship between lower education and marijuana use during pregnancy, the "no confounding zone" around the adjusted measure of association spans from 11.2 to 13.6 (calculated as $12.4 \pm 0.1 \times 12.4$). The crude prevalence ratio of 16.4 falls outside of this range, suggesting confounding by the experience of ACEs. This is consistent with our previous conclusion, where we found that the percent difference between the crude and adjusted measures of association was 32%, which indicates that these measures are meaningfully different from one another.

We can also use **Figure 9.11** to make an assessment about the direction of the bias by observing which segment of the orange "confounding zone" the crude measure of association falls in. **Figure 9.11–Panel A** illustrates the direction of bias for adjusted measures of association that suggest a positive relationship between the exposure and outcome (i.e., ratio measures greater than 1, and difference measures greater than 0). **Figure 9.11–Panel B** illustrates the direction of bias for adjusted measures of association that suggest a negative relationship between the exposure and outcome (i.e., ratio measures less than 1, and difference measures less than 0). Although we already showed that confounding by ACEs led to bias away from the null in **Figure 9.10**, **Figure 9.11–Panel C** shows what this looks like when employing the analogous "no confounding zone" technique.

## Interpreting and Reporting Adjusted Measures of Association
### (LEARNING OBJECTIVE 9.9)

### Interpreting Adjusted Measures of Association

In the cross-sectional study of marijuana use during pregnancy, the crude prevalence ratio for the association between lower education and marijuana use during pregnancy was 16.4. After controlling for the experience of ACEs, the adjusted prevalence ratio was 12.4. If we were preparing a written interpretation of these findings, we might say something like this:

> *After controlling for adverse childhood experiences (ACEs), the prevalence of marijuana use during pregnancy among those who didn't graduate from college was 12.4 times the prevalence of marijuana use during pregnancy among those who did graduate from college.*

When reporting an adjusted measure of association, it's important to include the variables that were controlled for in the interpretation, as shown.

### General Guidelines for Reporting Crude Versus Adjusted Measures of Association

When there is evidence of confounding by the extraneous variables under consideration, investigators should report the confounder-adjusted measures of association. You will often see investigators report both crude and adjusted measures of association. This is done to allow readers to compare the magnitudes of these measures to get an idea of how much confounding there was by the confounder(s) that were considered.

When the crude and adjusted measures of association are not meaningfully different from one another, there is no evidence of confounding by the extraneous variable(s) under consideration. Thus, it is not necessary to adjust for that variable in the analysis.

## Pause to Practice 9.3

### Data-Based Assessment of Confounding

Data adapted from the UK study described in **Pause to Practice 9.2** that identified factors associated with having difficulty paying heating bills are shown in **Table 9.2**.[11] Use these data to answer the questions that follow.

1.  Calculate the crude prevalence ratio that describes the association between reporting feeling isolated from others and having difficulty paying heating bills. Provide a one sentence interpretation of this finding.

2. The adjusted prevalence ratio that controls for confounding by chronic conditions is 2.27. Calculate the percent difference between the crude and adjusted measures of association.

3. Suppose, prior to data analysis, the investigators determined that a ±10% or greater difference in the crude and adjusted measures of association would be considered meaningful. What would they conclude about whether chronic health conditions confound the association between feeling isolated from others and having difficulty paying heating bills? If there is evidence of confounding, what is the direction of the bias?

TABLE 9.2 **CRUDE DATA FOR THE ASSOCIATION BETWEEN EXPERIENCING ISOLATION FROM OTHERS AND HAVING DIFFICULTY PAYING HEATING BILLS**

|  |  | Experiencing Isolation From Others | |
| --- | --- | --- | --- |
|  |  | Often or Sometimes (E+) | Rarely or Never (E–) |
| Difficulty Paying Heating Bills | Yes (O+) | 101 | 187 |
|  | No (O–) | 210 | 901 |
|  | TOTAL | 311 | 1,088 |

Digging Deeper

## Confounding Complications

### Directed Acyclic Graphs

When first learning about confounding, it is best to only consider one potential confounder at a time to lay a solid foundation for understanding the complex topic that is confounding. However, it is important to acknowledge that there are often a host of factors that may influence our exposure and outcome *and* that there are likely relationships between these other factors as well.

To determine which factors in this large web should be considered as confounders, epidemiologists use directed acyclic graphs (DAGs) to illustrate their assumptions about causal relationships between factors that could influence the exposure–outcome association.[12,13] DAGs can be used to identify variables that are likely to confound the exposure–outcome relationship. In fact, you've already seen a DAG in action: the confounding triangle described earlier (Figure 9.8A) is an example of a small DAG that considers the relationships between three variables of interest.

An example DAG that could be used in the study of marijuana use during pregnancy is shown in Figure 9.12 to illustrate the interconnectedness of several factors that might influence the exposure–outcome association. The arrows between variables indicate that two variables are causally associated, and the direction of the arrow indicates the temporality between the two variables (i.e., which variable came first?). Each DAG represents one set of assumptions about the many factors that may influence the exposure–outcome relationship; a different set of assumptions could lead to inclusion of additional variables, removal of some variables, or even changing the direction of some of the arrows. The beauty of DAGs is that investigators can construct multiple DAGs for the same research question to see whether making different assumptions would change their analytic plan.

### "Political" Variables

There are times when investigators are asked to control for extraneous variables for "political" reasons. These variables may not have been identified in a DAG as confounding the exposure–outcome relationship; however, a senior investigator, coauthor, or a peer reviewer

## FIGURE 9.12 EXAMPLE DIRECTED ACYCLIC GRAPH (DAG) FOR THE STUDY OF MARIJUANA USE DURING PREGNANCY

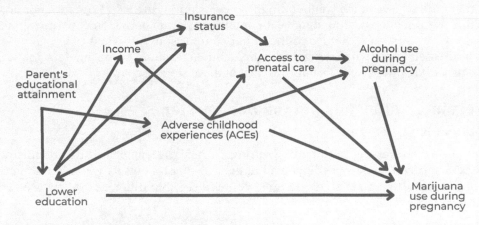

may request they be included in the analysis anyhow, often because other studies have controlled for these variables. When requests to control for these so-called "political variables" arise, investigators may choose to report results both with and without controlling for those variables. The best-case scenario is that these results are similar. When they are not, investigators may need to make the case to their coauthors and/or peer reviewers about why the variable(s) of concern should not be adjusted for in the analysis. This situation is more common than you might think and can be difficult to navigate.

## Highlights

### Confounding Assessment

There are two primary ways to assess whether a variable is likely to be a confounder in an epidemiologic study: the **a priori criteria** and the **data-based method**.

**A priori criteria** may be used to assess for confounding during the study design stage to determine which factors are likely to be confounders and thus should be included in the list of variables that will be collected as part of the study. These criteria are:

1. The confounder must be a risk factor for the outcome in the unexposed.
2. The confounder must be associated with the exposure in the source population.
3. The confounder cannot be caused by the exposure or the outcome.

The **data-based method** may be used to assess for confounding during the data analysis stage and involves comparing crude and adjusted measures of association to determine whether they are *meaningfully* different from one another. Evidence of more than a ±10% difference is generally considered suggestive of confounding; however, a decision about what will be considered meaningful for a given research question should be made by the investigative team prior to beginning the data analysis.

## ADDRESSING CONFOUNDING

Now that we know how to identify whether a variable confounds the exposure–outcome relationship, we are ready to think about ways that we can prevent and/or control for confounding in epidemiologic studies. For a variable to confound the exposure–outcome relationship, it must be associated with both the exposure *and* outcome of interest. The key to addressing confounding is to break at least one of these links (you can think about this as removing at least one of the arrows in the confounding triangle from Figure 9.8). When we eliminate the association between the confounding factor and the exposure or outcome, we are eliminating the underlying imbalance that led to the unfair comparison in the first place. Confounding can be addressed either when designing an epidemiologic study or during data analysis, and we will describe options available during each of these stages separately.

## Addressing Confounding in the Design Stage
### (LEARNING OBJECTIVE 9.10)

The options for addressing confounding during the design stage of a study are illustrated in Figure 9.13 and will be described in detail in the text that follows. Given the unique characteristics of each of the main study designs, you will see that different options are available depending on the design.

### FIGURE 9.13 ADDRESSING CONFOUNDING IN THE DESIGN STAGE

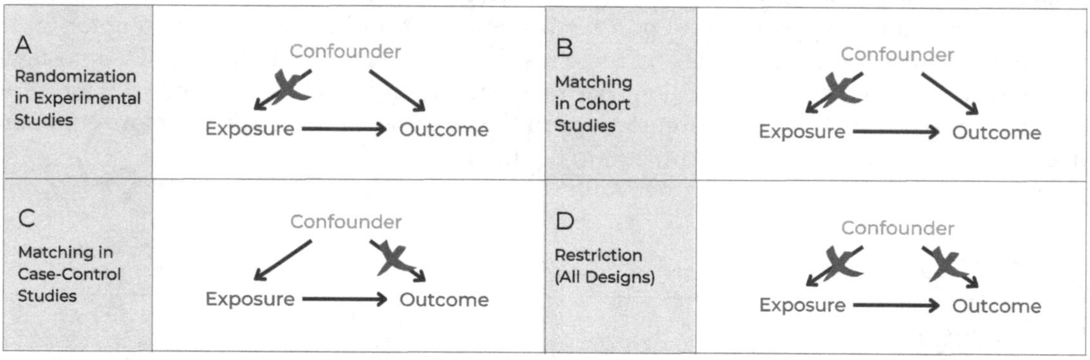

**Randomization.** As described in **Chapter 4, "Randomized Controlled Trial Designs,"** randomization is a technique used in experimental studies to assign participants to the different arms of a controlled trial. The goal of randomization is to obtain exposure groups that are as similar as possible, the only difference being which exposure condition they received. When randomization works, any differences in the frequency of the outcome between these groups can therefore be attributed to the exposure rather than confounding factors. Revisiting the example given in **Chapter 4, "Randomized Controlled Trial Designs,"** an observational study of the effect of a hypertension drug on mortality could have confounding by age if, on average, those who were taking the hypertension drug were older than those who were not. If it were ethical and feasible to conduct a randomized controlled trial to evaluate the effect of this hypertension drug, randomization would help balance the age distribution between the exposed and unexposed groups.

The primary benefit of randomization is that it breaks the link between the exposure and all potential factors that might confound the exposure–outcome relationship (Figure 9.13–Panel A). This means that investigators do not have to identify every single factor that might influence the exposure–outcome relationship, because randomization *should* yield exposure groups that are similar with respect to all confounders, even those that are not measured.

### MATCHING

Matching is a strategy that is available for addressing confounding when designing a cohort or case-control study; however, there are important differences in the logistics and implications of this strategy depending on which design is being used.

**Matching in cohort studies.** When matching is employed in cohort studies, investigators match one or more unexposed study participants to each exposed participant on one or more factors (for example, age, sex, race) that are thought to be confounders of the exposure–outcome relationship. Thus, matching in a cohort study breaks the link between the matched factors and the exposure of interest by forcing the distribution of the matched factors in the unexposed group to be the same as that of the exposed group (**Figure 9.13–Panel B**). For example, investigators wanted to learn whether the incidence of cancer among Canadian veterans was different from that of the general population.[14] Canadian veterans were matched to a group of non-veterans on age, sex, geography, and community-level income. The investigators suspected that the distribution of each of these factors might differ for veterans versus non-veterans *and* that these factors may also be related to cancer incidence. For example, on average, veterans may have been more likely to be male than non-veterans, *and* the incidence of cancer may be higher in males than females. By matching on these factors, investigators ensured that the non-veterans were as similar as possible to the veterans with respect to factors that might also influence their risk of cancer.

**Matching in case-control studies.** When matching is employed in case-control studies, investigators match one or more controls to each case on one or more factors that are thought to be confounders of the exposure–outcome relationship. Thus, matching in a case-control study breaks the link between the matched factors and the outcome of interest by forcing the distribution of the matched factors in the controls to be the same as that of the cases (**Figure 9.13–Panel C**). For example, investigators explored whether emergency department use differed for older adults experiencing elder mistreatment compared to older adults not experiencing elder mistreatment.[15] Cases were those who experienced elder mistreatment, and were identified using Medicare insurance claims. Controls who had not experienced elder mistreatment were matched to these cases on age, sex, race/ethnicity, and zip code. Investigators suspected that the distribution of these factors could be different for those experiencing elder mistreatment *and* for those who had multiple emergency department visits. For example, those who were older may unfortunately be more likely to experience elder mistreatment, *and* they may also be more likely to have multiple emergency department visits due to underlying health conditions. By matching on the selected factors, investigators ensured that older adults who did not experience elder mistreatment (the controls) were as similar as possible to those who *did* experience elder mistreatment (the cases) with respect to factors that could confound the association between emergency department use and elder mistreatment.

Investigators do need to be mindful about which factors are considered for matching—let's examine what might happen if we tried to evaluate the association between age (a matching factor) and elder mistreatment (the outcome). Suppose that 60% of the cases were aged 85 years or older. By matching on age, 60% of the controls would also be aged 85 years or older. Let's use this information to calculate the odds of being aged 85 years or older among cases and controls, and then find the odds ratio for the relationship between age and elder mistreatment.

$$\text{Odds of being aged} \geq 85 \text{ years among cases} = \frac{0.6}{1-0.6} = \frac{0.6}{0.4} = 1.5$$

$$\text{Odds of being aged} \geq 85 \text{ years among controls} = \frac{0.6}{1-0.6} = \frac{0.6}{0.4} = 1.5$$

$$\text{Odds ratio} = \frac{\text{Odds of being aged} \geq 85 \text{ years among cases}}{\text{Odds of being aged} \geq 85 \text{ years among controls}} = \frac{1.5}{1.5} = 1$$

By matching on age, we have forced the relationship between age (the confounder) and elder mistreatment (the outcome) to be null (thus breaking the link between this potential confounder and the outcome). This has important implications for the case-control design, where investigators are often interested in exploring the association between several exposures and the outcome of interest. Investigators should be judicious about which variables they decide to match on in a case-control study because these can no longer be considered as exposures of interest once the data are ready for analysis.

As we described in **Chapter 6, "Case-Control Designs,"** special considerations are required for the analysis of matched case-control data, and the specifics are beyond the scope of this text and are described elsewhere.[16,17]

**Additional matching-related considerations.** It is important to note that matching in an epidemiologic study is *directional*. In a matched cohort study, unexposed individuals are matched *to* exposed individuals, and in a matched case-control study, controls are matched *to* cases. Knowing that matching is directional can help you remember why and how it works: the **comparison group** (the unexposed in a cohort design, and the controls in a case-control design) is selected so that they have the same distribution of potential confounders as the **index group** (the exposed in a cohort design, and the cases in a case-control design).

Matching in both cohort and case-control studies can be done at either the individual or group levels. An illustration of individual- and group-level matching in case-control studies is shown in Figure 9.14. **Individual matching** may be what you first envisioned when thinking about matching in epidemiologic studies, where investigators identify one or more unique controls for each case in a case-control study (or unexposed individuals for each exposed individual in a cohort study) with similar attributes as the case with respect to the matching factors. Individual matching is illustrated in Figure 9.14–Panel A, where each control is matched to a case who shares the same smoking and occupational characteristics. In contrast, **group matching** (also called **frequency matching**) achieves a balance in the distribution of the matching factors across the comparison groups, but does not require exact matches for every case. Group, or frequency, matching is illustrated in Figure 9.14–Panel B. Although the controls are not matched individually to the cases, the overall distribution of smoking (50%) and construction work (67%) is the same for both cases and controls.

## FIGURE 9.14 ILLUSTRATION OF INDIVIDUAL AND GROUP (I.E., FREQUENCY) MATCHING

A. Cases and controls are individually matched on smoking and occupation

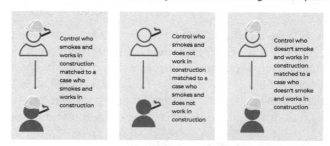

B. Cases and controls are frequency matched on smoking and occupation

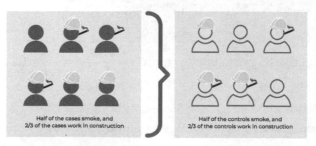

A benefit of matching is that it allows investigators to control for factors that could be difficult to otherwise account for in the analysis, such as neighborhood characteristics or genetics. Without intentional selection of individuals who reside in the same neighborhood, investigators might not have an adequate number of participants living in the same neighborhood to control for it using some of the analytic strategies that are described in the text that follows.

While matching has its benefits, it can complicate the process of identifying and enrolling participants in an epidemiologic study. Investigators must avoid matching on nonconfounders and consider that matching may require additional time and expense beyond what would be needed for other methods of confounding control.

**Restriction.** Restriction is a strategy that can be used when planning a study of any design and involves limiting enrollment of study participants to one level of a variable that is hypothesized to be a confounder of the exposure–outcome relationship. For example, if investigators were concerned about the likely confounding of smoking in the study of alcohol consumption and lung cancer, they might choose to only enroll nonsmokers in their study. Once enrollment has been restricted to nonsmokers, there is no longer an imbalance of smoking across those who drink alcohol *or* those who develop lung cancer, and thus smoking can no longer confound this association.

Restriction breaks the link between the confounder and *both* the exposure and outcome of interest (**Figure 9.13–Panel D**). While restriction can improve the internal validity of the study results by addressing confounding, it may reduce the external validity of the study results. A study of the impact of alcohol consumption on lung cancer conducted only among nonsmokers may not be **generalizable** (i.e., applicable) to smokers. Although this is a limitation of the use of restriction, recall that study results that lack internal validity also lack external validity.

## Pause to Practice 9.4

### Addressing Confounding When Designing an Epidemiologic Study

The scenarios provided in the text that follows are examples of studies that have used the previously described methods for confounding control in the design stage. For each scenario, identify the exposure(s), outcome(s), and potential confounder(s). Then, indicate which method of confounding control has been employed, and describe how it has broken one or more of the links in the confounding triangle.

1.  A study of total calcium intake and colorectal cancer was conducted only among women enrolled in the Nurses' Health Study.[18]

2.  A smoking cessation intervention may be administered in one of two ways: opt-in, where participants have to actively sign up to receive the intervention, or opt-out, where participants are enrolled in the intervention by default and can decline to participate. Investigators tested whether an opt-out smoking cessation counseling strategy was more effective than an opt-in strategy by randomly assigning smokers to one of these two groups.[19] They found much better outcomes among those in the opt-out group, including medication and counseling use, quit attempts, and patients' sense of control over quitting.

3.  In response to an observed increase in basal cell carcinoma diagnoses, particularly at younger ages, investigators conducted a case-control study to explore whether there was an association between cosmetic tattoos and basal cell carcinoma.[20] Controls were selected to have the same distribution of sex and age groups as those with a basal cell carcinoma diagnosis. Those with basal cell carcinoma were more likely to have had cosmetic tattoos than the controls, and the association between cosmetic tattoos and basal cell carcinoma was strongest for green and yellow tattoo colors.

## Addressing Confounding in the Analysis Stage

Confounding can be addressed during the analysis stage of a study by calculating measures of association that *adjust*, or *control for*, one or more confounders of interest. Adjusted measures of association can be obtained using **stratified analysis** (introduced in **Chapter 8, "Effect Measure Modification and Statistical Interaction,"**) or **regression modeling** (**Chapter 13, "Introduction to Epidemiologic Data Analysis"**). We describe both of these in the text that follows, with a greater emphasis on stratified analysis as it helps visualize what is happening in the data.

## Restriction Can Also Be Used in the Analysis Stage of a Study to Control for Confounding

Although we described the use of **restriction** earlier as a decision occurring during the design stage of a study, it can also be used during the analysis stage. The underlying idea is the same: the analysis (rather than enrollment) is limited to individuals who share the same value for a confounder of interest. In this way, we break the link between the confounder and the exposure as well as between the confounder and the outcome.

Note that the use of restriction for control of confounding is less common than other methods described in this text. However, it is a useful method to describe for those first learning about different methods of confounding control because it helps illustrate what we are trying to accomplish, which is reducing or eliminating variation in an extraneous variable that could bias our study results.

## Adjusting for Confounding Using Stratified Analysis
### (LEARNING OBJECTIVE 9.11)

A stratified analysis can be used to calculate an adjusted measure of association. The steps for calculating an adjusted measure of association using a stratified analysis are described in the text that follows and shown in **Figure 9.15**.

## FIGURE 9.15 CALCULATING ADJUSTED MEASURES OF ASSOCIATION USING STRATIFIED ANALYSIS

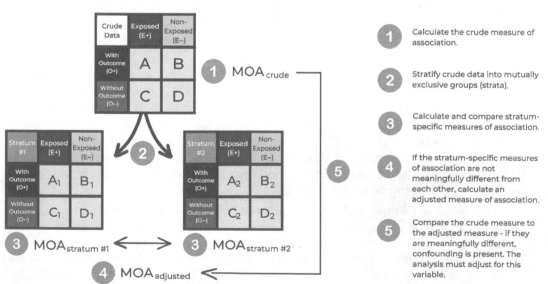

MOA, measure of association.

1. Calculate the crude measure of association that describes the unadjusted relationship between the exposure and outcome of interest.

2. Stratify data into mutually exclusive groups (strata) that correspond to the different levels of the suspected confounder.

3. Calculate and compare the stratum-specific measures of association.

4. If the stratum-specific measures of association are not meaningfully different from each other, calculate an adjusted measure of association.

   *Recall that if the stratum-specific measures of association are meaningfully different from each other, this is evidence of **effect measure modification (Chapter 8, "Effect Measure Modification and Statistical Interaction")**, and the stratified measures should be reported. We will discuss the difference between effect measure modification and confounding later in the chapter.*

5. Compare the crude measure of association to the adjusted measure of association to look for meaningful differences. If there is a *meaningful* difference between crude and adjusted measures of association, then there is confounding, and the adjusted measure of association must be reported.

   *Note that what is considered a **meaningful difference** should be decided before the analysis. Often, more than a 10% difference calculated using the percent difference formula (**Equation 9.1**) is used as a guideline.*

Let's work through this process using data adapted from the cross-sectional study of marijuana use during pregnancy, shown in **Figure 9.16**.

## FIGURE 9.16 CRUDE AND STRATIFIED DATA ADAPTED FROM THE CROSS-SECTIONAL STUDY OF MARIJUANA USE DURING PREGNANCY

|  | Not College Graduate (E+) | College Graduate (E−) | TOTAL |
|---|---|---|---|
| Marijuana Use During Pregnancy (O+) | 275 | 7 | 282 |
| No Marijuana Use During Pregnancy (O−) | 3,536 | 1,581 | 5,117 |
| TOTAL | 3,811 | 1,588 | 5,399 |

| Stratum 1 (C+): Experienced 4 or more ACEs | | | |
|---|---|---|---|
|  | Not College Graduate (E+) | College Graduate (E−) | TOTAL |
| Marijuana Use During Pregnancy (O+) | 158 | 2 | 160 |
| No Marijuana Use During Pregnancy (O−) | 1,028 | 183 | 1,211 |
| TOTAL | 1,186 | 185 | 1,371 |

| Stratum 2 (C−): Experienced 3 or fewer ACEs | | | |
|---|---|---|---|
|  | Not College Graduate (E+) | College Graduate (E−) | TOTAL |
| Marijuana Use During Pregnancy (O+) | 117 | 5 | 122 |
| No Marijuana Use During Pregnancy (O−) | 2,508 | 1,398 | 3,906 |
| TOTAL | 2,625 | 1,403 | 4,028 |

1. Calculate the crude prevalence ratio for the association between lower education and marijuana use during pregnancy:

$$\text{cPR} = \frac{\text{Prevalence of outcome among exposed}}{\text{Prevalence of outcome among unexposed}} = \frac{275/3{,}811}{7/1{,}588} = 16.4$$

2. Stratify data into mutually exclusive groups (strata) that correspond to the different levels of experience of ACEs—*this is already done for us in the two tables at the bottom of Figure 9.16.*

3. Calculate and compare the stratum-specific measures of association:

$$\text{PR}_{4 \text{ or more ACEs}} = \frac{158/1{,}186}{2/185} = 12.3$$

$$\text{PR}_{3 \text{ or fewer ACEs}} = \frac{117/2{,}625}{5/1{,}403} = 12.5$$

The stratified measures of association are very close to one another, and we can conclude that this is *not* indicative of meaningful effect measure modification.

We now need to calculate an adjusted measure of association, which is typically done using statistical programming software. Some additional information related to calculating adjusted measures of association using stratified analysis is included in the "Calculating Adjusted Measures of Association Using Stratified Analysis" box that follows.

## Calculating Adjusted Measures of Association Using Stratified Analysis

When obtaining an adjusted measure of association, the most intuitive approach is to take the arithmetic mean (i.e., average) of the stratum-specific measures of association. For our example, it would look like this:

$$\text{aPR} = \frac{12.3 + 12.5}{2} = 12.4$$

While this approach is intuitive, it is too simplistic as it gives equal weight to each of the strata. Sometimes the strata are of different sizes, and as you will learn in **Chapter 12, "Random Error in Epidemiologic Research,"** there are reasons to feel more confident about results that are obtained from larger samples. Thus, you might want to give more weight to larger strata, or those that are less influenced by random error.

The preferred approach for calculating adjusted measures of association using a stratified analysis is to use a **Mantel-Haenszel adjusted** measure of association. This method gives different weights to different strata and is also useful because it can be calculated even when the data are sparse in some of the strata. The formulae for calculating Mantel-Haenszel adjusted measures of association differ depending on the measure and are beyond the scope of this text.[21] Fortunately, these measures can be calculated using OpenEpi, as we will show in the text that follows.

4. Since our stratified measures of association are not meaningfully different (12.3 and 12.5), we will calculate an adjusted measure of association using the Mantel-Haenszel method in OpenEpi. Highlights of the OpenEpi output are shown in **Figure 9.17**.

## FIGURE 9.17 OpenEpi OUTPUT FOR STRATIFIED ANALYSIS OF THE CROSS-SECTIONAL STUDY OF MARIJUANA USE DURING PREGNANCY

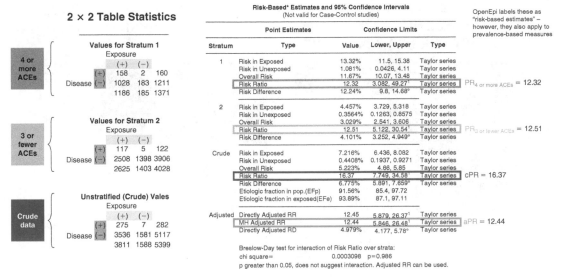

ACE, adverse childhood experience;    PR, prevalence ratio;    cPR, crude prevalence ratio;    aPR, adjusted prevalence ratio.

*Source*: Copyright © 2003, 2008 Andrew G. Dean et al., Atlanta, GA, USA.

5. Compare the crude prevalence ratio of 16.3 to the adjusted prevalence ratio of 12.4. As we previously showed, there is a 32% difference between these measures:

$$\text{Percent difference} = \left( \frac{16.4 - 12.4}{12.4} \right) \times 100\% = 32\%$$

Since there is a 32% difference between our crude and adjusted prevalence ratios, we conclude that they are meaningfully different from one another and that there is evidence of confounding of the association between lower education and marijuana use during pregnancy by ACEs.

## Pause to Practice 9.5

### Adjusting for Confounding Using Stratified Analysis

Let's return to the UK study described in **Pause to Practice 9.2** and **9.3** that identified factors associated with having difficulty paying heating bills.[11] You already evaluated whether the association between feeling isolated from others and having difficulty paying heating bills was confounded by chronic health conditions in **Pause to Practice 9.3**. In that problem set, you were given the adjusted measure of association. Now that you have learned about conducting stratified analysis to adjust for confounding, it is your turn to go through those steps to adjust for confounding by chronic health conditions in that study. Additional data adapted from this study are shown in **Figure 9.18** stratified by the presence of chronic health conditions. Note that these data were not available in the published manuscript, and the stratified data have been assumed for the purposes of this exercise and may not reflect the association that the investigators observed in their data.

1. Follow the previously outlined steps to conduct a stratified analysis to evaluate whether the association between feeling isolated from others and having difficulty paying heating bills is confounded by chronic health conditions.

2. Provide a one sentence interpretation of the study results. For this question, report the measure of association that has the best internal validity, given your previous findings.

**FIGURE 9.18 ADAPTED DATA FOR THE ASSOCIATION BETWEEN EXPERIENCING ISOLATION FROM OTHERS AND HAVING DIFFICULTY PAYING HEATING BILLS, STRATIFIED BY CHRONIC CONDITIONS**

| NO CHRONIC HEALTH CONDITIONS | | Experiencing Isolation From Others | |
| --- | --- | --- | --- |
| | | Often or Sometimes (E+) | Rarely or Never (E−) |
| Difficulty Paying Heating Bills | Yes (O+) | 56 | 43 |
| | No (O−) | 155 | 335 |
| | TOTAL | 211 | 378 |

| ONE OR MORE CHRONIC HEALTH CONDITIONS | | Experiencing Isolation From Others | |
| --- | --- | --- | --- |
| | | Often or Sometimes (E+) | Rarely or Never (E−) |
| Difficulty Paying Heating Bills | Yes (O+) | 45 | 144 |
| | No (O−) | 55 | 566 |
| | TOTAL | 100 | 710 |

## Digging Deeper

### Using Stratified Analysis to Control for More Than One Confounder

Although the previous examples illustrate the use of stratified analysis to control for one confounder of interest, this method can also be used to control for more than one confounder. To do this, investigators must create mutually exclusive strata of all possible combinations of the levels of these confounders.

For example, if we wanted to control for ACEs (four or more; three or fewer) and insurance status (public insurance; private insurance; no insurance) in our study of the association between lower education and marijuana use during pregnancy, we would need to create the following six mutually exclusive categories (two levels of ACEs × three levels of insurance):

- Four or more ACEs, public insurance
- Four or more ACEs, private insurance
- Four or more ACEs, no insurance
- Three or fewer ACEs, public insurance
- Three or fewer ACEs, private insurance
- Three or fewer ACEs, no insurance

Once these new strata have been created, the stratified analysis process moves forward just as previously described.

## Adjusting for Confounding Using Regression Modeling

While stratified analysis provides a useful visual representation to address confounding, it is less common than regression modeling, which uses mathematical formulas to describe the relationships of interest. Regression modeling can be used to assess for the presence of effect measure modification and to control for multiple confounders at once. It is described in greater detail in **Chapter 13, "Introduction to Epidemiologic Data Analysis."**

Regression modeling also provides a workaround for an important limitation of stratified analysis that we have yet to address, which is that stratified analysis cannot consider confounding by **numeric variables** such as age or annual household income. We discuss different types of variables in greater detail in **Chapter 13, "Introduction to Epidemiologic Data Analysis"**; however, in brief, numeric variables are those with numeric response options that can be either continuous (can take on an infinite set of values) or discrete (have a more limited set of response options). **Categorical variables**, on the other hand, have a more limited set of response options that fall into mutually exclusive categories (e.g., sex assigned at birth or highest level of educational attainment). Categorical variables lend themselves well to stratified analysis because the data are easily split across a limited number of categories (e.g., stratifying data by males and females). Numeric variables, however, would need to be collapsed (i.e., combined) into categories in order to be analyzed using stratified analysis. For example, it would not be feasible to have separate strata for every different dollar amount that corresponds to the annual household incomes of participants in a sample population. Instead, we would need to create categories where individuals with similar (but not identical) annual household incomes were grouped together. While categorizing annual household income would allow for confounding control using stratified analysis, it might not entirely control for confounding by household income due to **residual confounding**, which is described in the upcoming **Digging Deeper** segment.

When interpreting results from a published regression model, most epidemiologists will begin by closely reviewing the results tables included in a manuscript. It is helpful to closely review the tables' titles and footnotes to determine whether the investigators have reported crude and/or adjusted measures of association. Sometimes investigators will report results from several different models to illustrate whether, or how much, the results changed after including different sets of confounders in the model.

## Pause to Practice 9.6

### Interpreting Results From a Regression Model That Controls for Confounding

The following questions refer to the cross-sectional study of factors contributing to having difficulty paying heating bills that was previously described.[11] The questions specifically focus on a subset of the results presented by the study investigators. An adapted excerpt from the authors' findings is shown in **Table 9.3**, which includes results from both crude and adjusted analyses. These investigators used regression models (discussed in detail in **Chapter 13, "Introduction to Epidemiologic Data Analysis"**) for their analysis, which control for several confounders at once. The footnote of the table provides important information about which variables were considered as potential confounders for each analysis.

1. In the analysis of the association between age and having difficulty paying heating bills, which variables were considered as potential confounders? Using a ±10% or greater change as a guideline, is there evidence of confounding by these factors? If so, what is the direction of the bias?

2. The analysis of the association between occupation and having difficulty paying heating bills considered a three-level exposure: nonmanual, manual, and military. Individuals with military occupations or manual occupations were compared to those with nonmanual occupations. Which variables were considered as potential confounders in this analysis? Is there evidence of confounding by these factors when comparing those with manual occupations to those with nonmanual occupations? If so, what is the direction of the bias?

**TABLE 9.3 CRUDE AND ADJUSTED MEASURES OF ASSOCIATION FOR THE RELATIONSHIP BETWEEN SELECT CHARACTERISTICS AND HAVING DIFFICULTY PAYING HEATING BILLS**

| Characteristic | Unadjusted Model Prevalence Odds Ratio (cPOR) | Adjusted Model Prevalence Odds Ratio (aPOR) |
|---|---|---|
| Age (interpreted per 1-year increase in age) | 0.97 | 0.94[a] |
| Occupation | | |
| Nonmanual[b] | – | – |
| Manual | 2.57 | 1.66[c] |
| Military | 1.05 | 1.00[c] |
| Smoking | | |
| No[b] | – | – |
| Yes | 1.19 | 0.60[d] |

[a] Adjusted for occupation and smoking
[b] Reference group
[c] Adjusted for age and smoking
[d] Adjusted for age and occupation

*Source*: Adapted from Sartini C, Tammes P, Hay AD, et al. Can we identify older people most vulnerable to living in cold homes during winter? *Ann Epidemiol*. 2018;28(1):1–7.e3. https://doi.org/10.1016/j.annepidem.2017.11.008. Epub 2017 Dec 5. PMID: 29425531

3. In the analysis of the association between smoking status and having difficulty paying heating bills, which variables were considered as potential confounders? Using a ±10% or greater change as a guideline, is there evidence of confounding by these factors? If so, what is the direction of the bias?

4. After adjusting for potential confounders, which of the three characteristics has the strongest positive relationship with having trouble paying heating bills? How might public health and/or governmental officials use this information to address concerns related to the potential for cold-related deaths?

## Digging Deeper

## Residual Confounding

Residual confounding is described as confounding that remains, or is left over, even after attempting to control for it. There are three main causes of residual confounding:

- **Confounders that were not controlled for**. There are sometimes factors that confound the exposure–outcome association that we do not know about (e.g., genetic confounders that have not yet been discovered) and thus cannot control for. Other times there are factors that are likely to confound the exposure–outcome relationship that we know about, but we may not have collected data on and thus cannot control for them. Our inability to account for these factors may leave us with confounding that lingers, despite having controlled for other factors that we both knew about and measured.

- **Broad categorization of confounders.** The idea behind confounding control using stratified analysis is to examine the exposure–outcome relationship across groups that are as homogeneous as possible to break the link between the confounder(s) and the exposure and outcome. When we categorize a numeric confounder within broad categories, or when we define categories for a categorical confounder that are too broad, we may not achieve this goal since not everyone has the *exact* same values for the confounder(s) of interest.

- Returning to the example of annual household income, suppose investigators categorized the data into two groups:

  - those earning less than US$50,000 per year, and

  - those earning US$50,000 per year or more.

- While those earning less than US$50,000 per year might be more similar to each other compared to those earning US$50,000 or more per year, we might be concerned about lingering differences *within* each of these very broad groups. Recall that confounding results when there is an imbalance in the distribution of an extraneous variable that the related to both the exposure and outcome. With such a wide range of income levels within each of these two groups (e.g., those earning no income are included in the same category as those earning $49,999 per year), it could be that the income is distributed differently within exposure and outcome groups. In essence, these income categories may not be granular enough to fully address confounding by income. The groups can become more homogeneous as we create additional categories; however, this may not always fully address residual confounding.

- **Errors in measuring confounders of interest.** This is an interesting situation as it straddles two different types of systematic error: confounding *and* information bias. As was previously described briefly, and in detail in **Chapter 11, "Information Bias and Screening and Diagnostic Tests,"** information bias occurs when the measure of association is distorted due to errors in the measurement of the variables of interest. If our confounder is mis-measured, we may not adequately (i.e., fully) control for confounding by that variable.

---

## Highlights

## Addressing Confounding

There are opportunities to address confounding in both the design and data analysis stages of a study. The goal behind each of these methods is to break the link between the confounder and exposure and/or the confounder and the outcome.

Opportunities to address confounding when *designing* an epidemiologic study:

- **Randomization** breaks the link between confounders and the exposure. Randomization ideally achieves a balance between the exposure groups by all confounders, even those that were not measured. Randomization is limited to situations where it is both ethical and feasible to assign the exposure of interest.

- **Matching** can break the link between confounders and the exposure or the outcome depending on the study design.

  - In a cohort study, matching breaks the link between the matched factors and the exposure of interest. Unexposed individuals are matched to exposed individuals on important confounders.

  - In a case-control study, matching breaks the link between the matched factors and the outcome of interest. Controls are matched to cases on important confounders.

- Matching can occur at the **individual level** or at the group level (called **frequency matching**).

- **Restriction** addresses confounding by limiting study enrollment to individuals from only one stratum of a potential confounder, and thus breaks the links between the confounder and both the exposure and outcome. This may limit the study's generalizability (i.e., external validity).

Opportunities to address confounding when *analyzing* an epidemiologic study (i.e., the data-based method):

- **Stratified analysis**
  - Data are stratified into mutually exclusive categories of the confounder(s) of interest.
  - Investigators compute and compare **crude (unadjusted)** and **adjusted measures of association**.
  - If the unadjusted measure is meaningfully different from the adjusted measure, confounding is present and the adjusted measure of association should be reported.

- **Regression modeling**
  - Mathematical formulae are used to describe the relationship between variables of interest.
  - This is ideal for controlling for multiple confounders at once, including numeric variables.

## DISTINGUISHING BETWEEN EFFECT MEASURE MODIFICATION AND CONFOUNDING (LEARNING OBJECTIVE 9.12)

A very common question among new learners of epidemiology is, "What is the difference between effect measure modification and confounding?" This confusion is understandable because both concepts incorporate the influence of a third variable on the exposure–outcome relationship, and we can assess for both using stratified analyses or regression modeling. However, they differ in important ways, and it is critical to have a clear understanding of these distinctions. A side-by-side comparison of the definitions and differences between effect measure modification and confounding is described in **Table 9.4**.

Effect measure modification (**Chapter 8, "Effect Measure Modification and Statistical Interaction"**) occurs when the measure of association that describes the relationship between the exposure and the outcome is different for subgroups within the sample population. In other words, one size (meaning one measure of association) *doesn't* fit all—the impact of the exposure on the outcome *depends* on which group we're talking about. In the presence of effect measure modification, we must report multiple measures of association calculated within different subgroups of the sample population to adequately describe the different influences that the exposure has on the outcome.

Confounding occurs when the measure of association that describes the relationship between the exposure and outcome is *distorted* due to the presence of a third variable. This third variable is called a confounder and is associated with both the exposure and the outcome in the ways described in this chapter. In the presence of confounding, the crude measure of association is meaningfully different from the measure of association that adjusts for the confounder(s) of interest. Thus, to obtain a valid estimate of the association between the exposure and outcome, we must report an adjusted measure of association.

**TABLE 9.4 DISTINGUISHING BETWEEN EFFECT MEASURE MODIFICATION AND CONFOUNDING**

| | Effect Measure Modification (EMM) | Confounding |
|---|---|---|
| **Definition** | The relationship between the exposure and outcome is meaningfully different for different subgroups of the sample population. | The relationship between the exposure and outcome is distorted by the influence of an extraneous variable. |
| **Detection** | Stratified measures of association are meaningfully different from one another. | The crude measure of association is meaningfully different from the adjusted measure of association. |
| **Role of Statistical Tests in Detection** | Statistical tests cannot be used to determine whether there is evidence of effect measure modification. However, statistical tests can be used to determine whether the stratified measures of association are statistically significantly different from one another (i.e., if there is evidence of statistical interaction). | Statistical tests cannot be used to determine whether there is evidence of confounding. Instead, we look to see whether there are *meaningful* differences between crude (unadjusted) and adjusted measures of association. |
| **Variable Eligibility** | Any variables hypothesized to modify the association between the exposure and outcome are eligible to be considered as potential effect measure modifiers. | Only variables that meet the a priori criteria are eligible to be considered as potential confounders. |
| **Bias** | EMM is not a bias, and may or may not be of scientific interest. | Confounding is a bias that must be addressed to obtain valid results. |
| **Role of Stratified Analysis** | Stratified analysis is used to determine whether stratified measures of association are meaningfully different from one another across the levels of the potential effect modifier. | Stratified analysis can be used to calculate a measure of association that adjusts (controls) for the potential confounder. |
| **Scale Dependency** | Presence of EMM is scale-dependent. The presence of effect measure modification depends on the scale (additive vs. multiplicative) being considered, and there may be evidence of effect measure modification on the additive, multiplicative, or both scales, or no evidence of effect measure modification at all. | The presence of confounding is not scale dependent, and in the presence of confounding, both the crude ratio and difference measures of association will be distorted. |
| **What to Report** | If EMM is present, report multiple measures of association (one per stratum). | If confounding is present, report the adjusted measure of association that controls for the confounder(s) of interest. |

## Pause to Practice 9.7

### Discerning Whether a Third Variable Is an Effect Measure Modifier or Confounder

It is important to be able to identify whether a third variable is an effect measure modifier or a confounder when reading epidemiologic research, and this set of questions is intended to give you practice with this skill. For each study description, identify the exposure, outcome, and third variable of interest. Then indicate whether the third variable is being treated as an effect measure modifier or a confounder in that particular study and describe why you came to this conclusion.

1. A study from Denmark found that those who had a prior pregnancy loss were more likely to later deliver a child with congenital heart disease.[22] This association was notably stronger among those who had type 2 diabetes.

2. Investigators conducted a survey among Puerto Rican adults to determine whether the degree to which religion was important in someone's life influenced their intentions to receive a COVID-19 vaccine when one became available. Compared to those who said that religion was "less important" in their life, those who reported that religion was "very important" were less likely to report intentions to receive a COVID-19 vaccine (cPR = 1.55). This association remained very similar after adjusting for numerous variables, including education and perceived health (aPR = 1.51).[23]

3. There is a complicated relationship between breast cancer treatment and cardio-vascular health, and there are concerns that this may differ by race. To untangle this web, investigators used cancer registry data to evaluate the association between breast cancer treatments and cardiovascular disease mortality. They found no association between breast cancer hormone therapy and cardiovascular disease mortality among non-Hispanic White women; however, there was a positive association among non-Hispanic Black women.[24]

4. A study conducted among U.S. veterans found that those with latent tuberculosis had an increased rate of type 2 diabetes. This association remained after accounting for several demographic and health characteristics.[25]

## Stratified Analysis for Effect Measure Modification or Confounding Assessment

As previously described, stratified analysis can be used to evaluate whether there is evidence of effect measure modification or confounding in an epidemiologic study when the "third variable" can be categorized into mutually exclusive strata. The steps required when considering the impact that a third variable might have in an epidemiologic study are illustrated in Figure 9.19.

### FIGURE 9.19 FLOWCHART FOR ASSESSING THE IMPACT OF A THIRD VARIABLE IN AN EPIDEMIOLOGIC STUDY

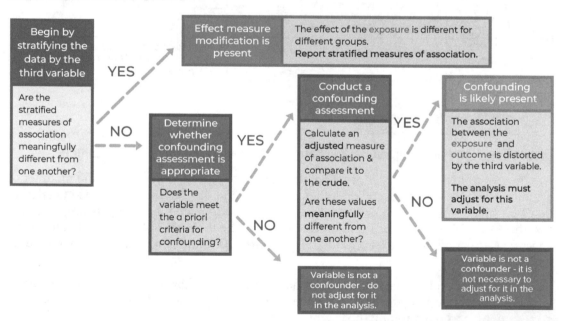

1. Stratify the data by the third variable.

2. If the stratified measures of association are meaningfully different from one another, effect measure modification is present by this variable → report stratified results.

3. If the stratified measures of association are not meaningfully different from one another (and the variable meets the a priori criteria), calculate an adjusted measure of association.

a. If the crude and adjusted measures of association are meaningfully different from one another, confounding is present by this variable → report adjusted results.

b. If the crude and adjusted measures of association are *not* meaningfully different from one another, variable is not a confounder → it is not necessary to adjust for it in the analysis.

Notice that effect measure modification is assessed prior to confounding—this is partly why we chose to present effect measure modification first (**Chapter 8, "Effect Measure Modification and Statistical Interaction"**) before introducing confounding.

<br>

**Digging Deeper**

### Can a Variable Be Both an Effect Measure Modifier and Meet the a Priori Criteria for Confounding?

Yes, a variable can be both an effect measure modifier and meet the a priori criteria for confounding! Although a variable meets the a priori criteria for confounding, investigators may find that when the data are stratified by that variable, the measure of association that describes the relationship between the exposure and outcome is *different* for the different groups.

Let's revisit the example described in **Chapter 8, "Effect Measure Modification and Statistical Interaction,"** where we explored the association between HPV vaccination and cervical dysplasia, and considered effect measure modification by age.[26] Recall that the HPV vaccine was effective at preventing cervical dysplasia for everyone in the sample population; however, the effect was strongest in those who initiated their HPV vaccines at an earlier age (i.e., rate ratios for those initiating between 17–19 years versus 20–29 years were 0.26 and 0.60, respectively). Thus, we concluded that age modified the association between HPV vaccination and cervical dysplasia.

Now let's consider whether age meets the a priori criteria:

- Age is associated with cervical dysplasia among those who didn't receive an HPV vaccine (i.e., a risk factor for the outcome among the unexposed)—*Meets criterion 1.*

- Age is also likely associated with HPV vaccination in the source population—those who are older have had more opportunity to get vaccinated—*Meets criterion 2.*

- Age is neither caused by HPV vaccination nor cervical dysplasia—*Meets criterion 3.*

What we see is that two things can be true: a variable can modify the association between the exposure and outcome, *and* it can also meet the a priori criteria for confounding. The presence of effect measure modification by a given variable supersedes confounding; thus, that factor is considered a modifier of the exposure–outcome relationship of interest, and investigators should report stratified results.

### How Reporting Stratified Results Addresses Potential Confounding

When reporting measures of association stratified by an effect modifier, we also account for potential confounding by that factor. We can think about this in relation to restriction as previously described. What is different here is that instead of restricting our entire analysis to one age group, we are restricting our analysis to the different levels of the effect modifier. In the HPV vaccination example, by stratifying on age, we eliminate the association between the age groups and HPV vaccination as well as the association between the age groups and cervical dysplasia.

## Effect Measure Modification Versus Confounding

- In the presence of effect measure modification, investigators must report *multiple* measures of association because the relationship between the exposure and outcome is different for the different levels of the effect modifier.

- In the presence of confounding, investigators must report an *adjusted* measure of association because the relationship between the exposure and outcome is distorted by the influence of this third variable.

- Similarities between effect measure modification and confounding:
  - Assessment for both considers the role that a third variable has in the relationship between an exposure and outcome of interest.
  - Both can be assessed using stratified analysis or regression modeling.

- Differences between effect measure modification and confounding:
  - Only confounding is a bias.
  - Effect measure modification may or may not be of scientific interest; confounding must be controlled.
  - Any variables hypothesized to modify the exposure–outcome relationship are eligible to be considered as potential effect modifiers; only variables that meet the a priori criteria are eligible to be considered potential confounders.
  - Only effect measure modification is scale-dependent.
  - Statistical tests can be used to consider whether stratified measures of association are statistically different from one another.
  - To assess for confounding, we assess whether crude and adjusted measures of association are *meaningfully* different from one another, and statistical tests should not be used.

## WHERE WE'VE BEEN AND WHAT'S UP NEXT

In this chapter, you have learned about the two broad categories of error in epidemiologic research, systematic error (also called bias) and random error, as well as how to evaluate the direction of bias.

We have taken a deep dive into confounding, which is the first of the three main types of systematic error. You now know that confounding arises when there is an imbalance in a third variable that distorts the relationship between the exposure and outcome of interest. We have shown you how to assess whether there is likely confounding both using the a priori criteria as well as using a data-based method, and described a number of ways to address confounding in both the design and analysis stages of a study. Should you move forward in your epidemiologic studies, you will learn that there is a lot more than meets the eye when it comes to confounding, but we hope you will find that this introduction has laid a solid foundation for your future work.

Up next, we will continue exploring systematic error in epidemiologic research. You will learn about how the ways in which study participants enter and/or leave our study can lead to biased results (**Chapter 10, "Selection Bias"**), as well as how flawed measurement of our variables of interest can lead to biased results (**Chapter 11, "Information Bias and Screening and Diagnostic Tests"**).

Once we have finished our discussion of systematic error in epidemiologic research, we will turn our attention to random error (**Chapter 12, "Random Error in Epidemiologic**

**Research"**). Unlike systematic error, there is a straightforward way to reduce random error in an epidemiologic study, which is to increase the size of your sample population. We will explore two measures that quantify the impact of random error on epidemiologic study results, and we will discuss how sample size influences these measures.

## END OF CHAPTER PROBLEM SET

1. In your own words, describe the difference between random and systematic error.

2. In your own words, describe the relationship between the population parameter and the point estimate.

3. The point estimate is sometimes distinguished from the population parameter by putting a "hat (∧)" on top of the measure to note that it is an estimate. For example, a risk ratio estimated using data from a sample population might be abbreviated as $\widehat{RR}$, which would distinguish it from the population parameter abbreviated as RR. Indicate the direction of bias for each pair of population parameters and point estimates given in the following list, which are distinguished using this notation.

   a. RR = 1.25    $\widehat{RR}$ = 1.75    [RR: risk ratio]
   b. IDR = 0.23    $\widehat{IDR}$ = 0.56    [IDR: incidence density ratio]
   c. RD = 0.36    $\widehat{RD}$ = 0.75    [RD: risk difference]
   d. PD = -0.05    $\widehat{PD}$ = 0.08    [PD: prevalence difference]

4. Investigators undertook a cross-sectional study of mental health and well-being during the early months of the COVID-19 pandemic.[27] The crude prevalence ratio that described the association between vision impairment and loneliness was 1.74. After controlling for various factors like age, investigators found that the prevalence of loneliness among those with vision impairment was 1.65 times the corresponding prevalence among those without vision impairment.

   a. What is the exposure of interest?
   b. What is the outcome of interest?
   c. What extraneous variable is being considered a potential confounder?
   d. Is it plausible that the extraneous variable would meet the a priori criteria for a confounder? It not, explain why.
   e. Use the data-based method of confounding assessment to determine whether there is evidence of confounding using a ±10% or greater change as a guideline to indicate a meaningful difference between crude and adjusted measures of association. If there is evidence of confounding, what is the direction of the bias?

5. Investigators undertook a cohort study to evaluate whether smoking cessation would improve household food insecurity, with the hypothesis that money spent on cigarettes was constraining household food budgets.[28] The crude risk ratio for the association between smoking cessation and household food insecurity was 1.37. After controlling for several factors, including the sex of the participants, investigators found that the risk of food insecurity during the study period among those who continued smoking was 1.87 times the corresponding risk among those who quit smoking.

   a. What is the exposure of interest?
   b. What is the outcome of interest?

    c. What extraneous variable is being considered a potential confounder?

    d. Is it plausible that the extraneous variable would meet the a priori criteria? Explain why.

    e. Use the data-based method of confounding assessment to determine whether there is evidence of confounding using a ±10% or greater change as a guideline to indicate a meaningful difference between crude and adjusted measures of association. If there is evidence of confounding, what is the direction of the bias?

6. Let's consider the example of the association between alcohol consumption and lung cancer that was introduced in **Chapter 9, "Error in Epidemiologic Research and Fundamentals of Confounding."** In that example, both alcohol consumption and smoking status were included as ordinal variables, meaning that there were several different levels, each with increasing frequency of the relevant behavior. The data in Figure 9.20 consider the association between alcohol and lung cancer but categorize alcohol and smoking as dichotomous (two-level) variables. Assume the data come from a cohort study with no loss to follow-up or competing risks. Use the data that follow to conduct a stratified analysis to show that there is evidence of confounding by smoking in Figure 9.20, and indicate the direction of the bias.

## FIGURE 9.20 SAMPLE DATA OF THE ASSOCIATION BETWEEN ALCOHOL AND LUNG CANCER WHERE ALCOHOL AND SMOKING ARE DICHOTOMOUS

| CRUDE DATA | | | |
|---|---|---|---|
| | | Drinkers | Non drinkers |
| Lung | Yes | 75 | 25 | 100 |
| Cancer | No | 25 | 75 | 100 |
| | | 100 | 100 | |

| SMOKERS | | | |
|---|---|---|---|
| | | Drinkers | Non drinkers |
| Lung | Yes | 68 | 6 | 74 |
| Cancer | No | 7 | 4 | 11 |
| | | 75 | 10 | |

| NONSMOKERS | | | |
|---|---|---|---|
| | | Drinkers | Non drinkers |
| Lung | Yes | 7 | 19 | 26 |
| Cancer | No | 18 | 71 | 89 |
| | | 25 | 90 | |

**Questions 7 to 9 are designed to help you distinguish between effect measure modification and confounding.**

7. Given the popularity of e-cigarettes to assist in cigarette smoking cessation, investigators wanted to learn whether this method was effective long term.[29] After controlling for sociodemographic factors and a number of factors related to cigarette smoking history, they found that U.S. smokers who used e-cigarettes to quit smoking cigarettes were no more likely to have successfully abstained from cigarette use after 12 months than smokers who used other methods to quit smoking.
   a. What is the exposure of interest?
   b. What is the outcome of interest?
   c. What is/are the extraneous variable(s) considered?
   d. Does this study description illustrate considerations related to effect measure modification or confounding? Provide a brief explanation to support your answer.

8. Leprosy is a neglected tropical disease with consequences including skin lesions and nerve damage. Given that leprosy affects mostly poor and marginalized populations, investigators wanted to learn whether measures to address poverty could impact leprosy rates in a Brazilian cohort.[30] They compared the occurrence of new leprosy diagnoses among families who did and did not receive conditional cash transfers, which provided financial assistance so long as families maintained school attendance for their children and attended preventive health visits. Overall, they did not find that the conditional cash transfer program impacted leprosy rates. However, this program was associated with decreased leprosy rates among families living in areas with high leprosy burden.
   a. What is the exposure of interest?
   b. What is the outcome of interest?
   c. What is/are the extraneous variable(s) considered?
   d. Does this study description illustrate issues related to effect measure modification or confounding? Provide a brief explanation to support your answer.

9. Patients with coronary artery disease (CAD) may experience myocardial ischemia, which occurs when there is reduced blood flow to the heart. Two sources of myocardial ischemia among CAD patients have been identified: mental stress and conventional (i.e., physical exertion) stress. Investigators wanted to compare these two different sources of myocardial ischemia to evaluate their association with myocardial infarction (heart attack) and cardiovascular death.[31] The rate of these adverse heart conditions among those with mental stress-induced myocardial ischemia was 2.8 times the corresponding rate among those with conventional stress-induced myocardial ischemia. After accounting for the influences of medications, demographic factors, and clinical factors, the association was attenuated to a 2.5-fold difference.
   a. What is the exposure of interest?
   b. What is/are the outcome(s) of interest?
   c. What is/are the extraneous variable(s) considered?
   d. Does this study description illustrate issues related to effect measure modification or confounding? Provide a brief explanation to support your answer.

# REFERENCES

1. Petruccelli K, Davis J, Berman T. Adverse childhood experiences and associated health outcomes: a systematic review and meta-analysis. *Child Abuse Negl.* 2019;97:04127. https://doi.org/10.1016/j.chiabu.2019.104127

2. Narayan AJ, Lieberman AF, Masten AS. Intergenerational transmission and prevention of adverse childhood experiences (ACEs). *Clin Psychol Rev.* 2021;85:101997. https://doi.org/10.1016/j.cpr.2021.101997

3. Testa A, Jackson DB, Boccio C, Ganson KT, Nagata JM. Adverse childhood experiences and marijuana use during pregnancy: findings from the North Dakota and South Dakota PRAMS, 2017–2019. *Drug Alcohol Depend.* 2022;230:109197. https://doi.org/10.1016/j.drugalcdep.2021.109197

4. Hawkins SS, Hacker MR. Trends in use of conventional cigarettes, e-cigarettes, and marijuana in pregnancy and impact of health policy. *Clin Obstet Gynecol.* 2022;65(2):305–318. https://doi.org/10.1097/GRF.0000000000000690

5. Hurd YL, Manzoni OJ, Pletnikov MV, et al. Cannabis and the developing brain: insights into its long-lasting effects. *J Neurosci.* 2019;39(42):8250–8258. https://pubmed.ncbi.nlm.nih.gov/31619494/

6. Cartus AR, Jarlenski MP, Himes KP, et al. Adverse cardiovascular events following severe maternal morbidity. *Am J Epidemiol.* 2022;191(1):126–136. https://doi.org/10.1093/aje/kwab208

7. Qin HY, Cheng C-W, Tang X-D, et al. Impact of psychological stress on irritable bowel syndrome. *World J Gastroenterol.* 2014;20(39):14126–14131. https://doi.org/10.3748/wjg.v20.i39.14126

8. Rothman K. *Epidemiology: An Introduction.* 2nd ed. Oxford University Press; 2012.

9. Chung EK, Nurmohamed L, Mathew L, et al. Risky health behaviors among mothers-to-be: the impact of adverse childhood experiences. *Acad Pediatr.* 2010;10(4):245–251. https://doi.org/10.1016/j.acap.2010.04.003

10. Hardcastle K, Bellis MA, Ford K, et al. Measuring the relationships between adverse childhood experiences and educational and employment success in England and Wales: findings from a retrospective study. *Public Health.* 2018;165:106–116. https://doi.org/10.1016/j.puhe.2018.09.014

11. Sartini C, Tammes P, Hay AD, et al. Can we identify older people most vulnerable to living in cold homes during winter? *Ann Epidemiol.* 2018;28(1):1–7.e3. https://doi.org/10.1016/j.annepidem.2017.11.008

12. Lipsky AM, Greenland S. Causal directed acyclic graphs. *JAMA.* 2022;327(11):1083–1084. https://doi.org/10.1001/jama.2022.1816

13. Tennant PWG, Murray EJ, Arnold KF, et al. Use of directed acyclic graphs (DAGs) to identify confounders in applied health research: review and recommendations. *Int J Epidemiol.* 2021;50(2):620–632. https://doi.org/10.1093/ije/dyaa213

14. Mahar AL, Aiken AB, Cramm H, et al. Cancer incidence among Canadian veterans: a matched cohort study. *Cancer Epidemiol.* 2022;79:102199. https://doi.org/10.1016/j.canep.2022.102199

15. Rosen T, Zhang H, Wen K, et al. Emergency department and hospital utilization among older adults before and after identification of elder mistreatment. *JAMA Netw Open.* 2023;6(2):e2255853. https://doi.org/10.1001/jamanetworkopen.2022.55853

16. Mansournia MA, Jewell NP, Greenland S. Case-control matching: effects, misconceptions, and recommendations. *Eur J Epidemiol.* 2018;33(1):5–14. https://doi.org/10.1007/s10654-017-0325-0

17. Pearce N. Analysis of matched case-control studies. *BMJ.* 2016;352:i969. https://doi.org/10.1136/bmj.i969

18. Kim H, Hur J, Wu K, et al. Total calcium, dairy foods and risk of colorectal cancer: a prospective cohort study of younger US women. *Int J Epidemiol.* 2022;52(1):87–95. https://doi.org/10.1093/ije/dyac202

19. Richter KP, Catley D, Gajewski BJ, et al. The effects of opt-out vs opt-in tobacco treatment on engagement, cessation, and costs: a randomized clinical trial. *JAMA Intern Med.* 2023;183(4):331–339. https://doi.org/10.1001/jamainternmed.2022.7170

20. Barton DT, Zens MS, Marmarelis EL, et al. Cosmetic tattooing and early onset basal cell carcinoma: a population-based case–control study from New Hampshire. *Epidemiology.* 2020;31(3):448–450. https://doi.org/10.1097/EDE.0000000000001179

21. Lash TL, Haneuse S, Rothman KJ. *Modern Epidemiology.* 4th ed. Wolters Kluwer; 2021.

22. Ji H, Liang H, Yu Y, et al. Association of Maternal History of Spontaneous Abortion and Stillbirth with risk of congenital heart disease in offspring of women with vs without type 2 diabetes. *JAMA Netw Open*. 2021;4(11):e2133805. https://doi.org/10.1001/jamanetworkopen.2021.33805

23. López-Cepero A, Rodríguez M, Joseph V, et al. Religiosity and beliefs toward COVID-19 vaccination among adults in Puerto Rico. *Int J Environ Res Public Health*. 2022;19(18):11729. https://pubmed.ncbi.nlm.nih.gov/36141998/

24. Collin LJ, Troeschel AN, Liu Y, et al. A balancing act: Racial disparities in cardiovascular disease mortality among women diagnosed with breast cancer. *Ann Cancer Epidemiol*. 2020;4:4. https://pubmed.ncbi.nlm.nih.gov/32954254/

25. Magee MJ, Khakharia A, Gandhi NR, et al. Increased risk of incident diabetes among individuals with latent tuberculosis infection. *Diabetes Care*. 2022;45(4):880–887. https://pubmed.ncbi.nlm.nih.gov/35168250/

26. Herweijer E, Sundström K, Ploner A, et al. Quadrivalent HPV vaccine effectiveness against high-grade cervical lesions by age at vaccination: a population-based study. *Int J Cancer*. 2016;138(12):2867–2874. https://doi.org/10.1002/ijc.30035

27. Merten N, Schultz AA, Walsh MC, et al. Psychological distress and well-being among sensory impaired individuals during COVID-19 lockdown measures. *Ann Epidemiol*. 2023;79:19–23. https://doi.org/10.1016/j.annepidem.2023.01.002

28. Berry KM, Rivera Drew JA, Brady PJ, et al. Impact of smoking cessation on household food security. *Ann Epidemiol*. 2023;79:49–55.e3. https://doi.org/10.1016/j.annepidem.2023.01.007

29. Chen R, Pierce JP, Leas EC, et al. Use of electronic cigarettes to aid long-term smoking cessation in the United States: prospective evidence from the PATH cohort study. *Am J Epidemiol*. 2020;189(12):1529–1537. https://doi.org/10.1093/aje/kwaa161

30. Pescarini JM, Williamson E, Ichihara MY, et al. Conditional cash transfer program and leprosy incidence: analysis of 12.9 million families from the 100 million Brazilian cohort. *Am J Epidemiol*. 2020;189(12):1547–1558. https://doi.org/10.1093/aje/kwaa127

31. Vaccarino V, Almuwaqqat Z, Kim JH, et al. Association of mental stress-induced myocardial ischemia with cardiovascular events in patients with coronary heart disease. *JAMA*. 2021;326(18):1818–1828. https://doi.org/10.1001/jama.2021.17649

# CHAPTER 10

# SELECTION BIAS

## KEY TERMS

| | | |
|---|---|---|
| external validity | sample population | sensitivity analyses |
| generalizability | selection bias | source population |
| internal validity | selection probability | target population |

## LEARNING OBJECTIVES

10.1 Define the source and sample populations.
10.2 Define selection bias.
10.3 Describe reasons why selection bias may occur.
10.4 Describe how different study designs may be affected by selection bias.
10.5 Understand what the term differential means in the context of selection bias.
10.6 Understand how selection bias may affect an R×C table.
10.7 Understand strategies to reduce selection bias at the study design stage.
10.8 Correct for selection bias at the data analysis stage using selection probabilities.
10.9 Differentiate between internal and external validity.
10.10 Define the target population.
10.11 Differentiate between selection bias and lack of generalizability.

## UNDERSTANDING THE OPIOID CRISIS IN THE UNITED STATES

In the United States, the opioid epidemic has been deemed a public health emergency. The U.S. Centers for Disease Control and Prevention (CDC) estimates that the majority of drug overdose deaths are related to opioids,[1] with roughly 50,000 Americans dying from opioid-induced overdoses in 2019.[1] Deaths from the opioid crisis have increased markedly over the last few decades and are sometimes described as occurring in three "waves."[2] The first wave began in the 1990s and was linked to an increase in use of prescription opioid pain relievers after pharmaceutical representatives misled providers about the addictiveness of these medicines.[3] Before it became apparent that these medications are often highly addictive, misuse of prescription opioid pain relievers became rampant. The second wave began in 2010 and was linked to an increase in deaths related to heroin use. At the time of this writing in 2023, we are still in the third wave of the opioid epidemic, which began in 2013 and is linked to synthetic opioid use, such as fentanyl.[2]

Evidence-based prevention and treatment strategies are urgently needed to address the evolving opioid epidemic. However, opioid users and those at-risk of opioid-related overdoses can be a difficult population to study. Specifically, they may be hard to identify, recruit, and follow over the course of an epidemiologic study. For example, people who inject drugs (PWID) may be significantly less likely to join studies because of fear of legal repercussions related to illicit drug use,[4] and some opioid users may be difficult to enroll or follow in epidemiologic studies due to being unhoused or experiencing complex, compounding social and mental health factors. As we will discuss in this chapter, when epidemiologists encounter difficulty ensuring adequate participant selection, participation, follow-up, and response, **selection bias** may reduce the validity of our study results.

## INTRODUCTION TO SELECTION BIAS

Selection bias is the second of the three types of systematic error that we cover in this textbook. It is related to error caused by the way that participants either enter or leave your study. Before we discuss the details, it is important to revisit two key types of epidemiologic populations: the **source population** and the **sample population** (Learning Objective 10.1).

- The **source population** is the entire population of eligible individuals from which the study participants are sampled. In a cohort study, it is the population from which the cohort is selected based on the eligibility criteria defined by the investigators. In a case-control study, it is the population that gave rise to the cases.

- The **sample population** (also called the **study population**) is the subset of the source population that is enrolled in your study, and for whom exposure and outcome data are measured.

Selection bias occurs when the measure of association calculated from your sample population is *meaningfully different* from the measure of effect which *would have* been estimated if you had data from all eligible subjects in the source population (recall from **Chapter 8, "Effect Measure Modification and Statistical Interaction,"** that the **measure of effect** is defined as the true association between the exposure and outcome in the source population; Learning Objective 10.2). This concept is shown visually in **Figure 10.1**.

## FIGURE 10.1 CONCEPTUALIZING SELECTION BIAS

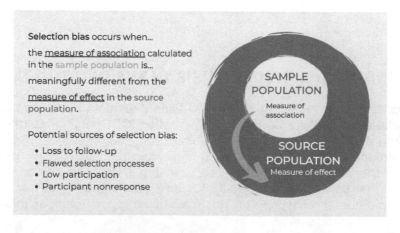

Selection bias occurs when...

the measure of association calculated in the sample population is...

meaningfully different from the measure of effect in the source population.

Potential sources of selection bias:
- Loss to follow-up
- Flawed selection processes
- Low participation
- Participant nonresponse

SAMPLE POPULATION
Measure of association

SOURCE POPULATION
Measure of effect

As also shown in **Figure 10.1**, selection bias can occur for different reasons including (Learning Objective 10.3):

1. **Participant loss to follow-up.** Loss to follow-up, which can occur in longitudinal studies (such as clinical trial or cohort designs), may result in selection bias if, for example, study participants are lost during the course of the study prior to data collection (e.g., subjects may relocate, die, lose interest in the study, or be unwilling to provide outcome data).

2. **Selection processes.** The manner in which participants are selected from the source population into the sample population may result in selection bias if, for example, some members of the source population are not considered for inclusion (e.g., because you didn't know they were in the source population or because of the sampling strategy used), or are unreachable (e.g., due to not having a phone or being highly mobile). A special type of selection bias arising from selection processes is called **survival bias,** which occurs when participants are not able to be selected and enrolled because they have died.

3. **Participation.** Even if subjects in the source population are reachable by study recruiters, they could refuse to participate in your study (e.g., due to lack of motivation to join a study), which may lead to selection bias.

4. **Participant nonresponse.** Selection bias may occur if participants refuse or are unable to provide either outcome and/or exposure data.

**Table 10.1** summarizes the sources of selection bias by the study designs that are most affected. Clinical trials and cohort studies are the only designs affected by loss to follow-up since they are the only designs that follow a group of individuals over time. Since the case-control and cross-sectional designs do not follow a group of individuals over time, they are only subject to selection bias due to errors in the selection process, participation, or participant nonresponse (Learning Objective 10.4).

**TABLE 10.1  SUMMARY OF SOURCES OF SELECTION BIAS BY STUDY DESIGNS MOST AFFECTED**

| Sources of Selection Bias | | Study Designs Affected |
|---|---|---|
| **Differential loss to follow-up in the** sample population | Occurs when outcome and exposure statuses influence the retention of participants in the sample population. | Can affect longitudinal designs like **cohort studies** and **controlled trials.** |
| **Differential subject selection from the source population** | Occurs when outcome and exposure statuses are different in the population selected into the sample population than in the source population. | Though differential selection processes can affect **any study design,** they are most problematic in **case-control** and **cross-sectional designs** since both outcome and exposure status are known, and can therefore influence subject selection.<br><br>**Survival bias** is a type of differential subject selection, and is particularly a concern in **case-control** designs using prevalent (rather than incident) cases and in **cross-sectional designs.** |
| **Differential subject participation from the source population** | Occurs when outcome and exposure statuses influence the participation of participants joining the sample population from the source population (e.g., self-selection bias). | Most problematic in **case-control** or **cross-sectional designs** since both outcome and exposure status are known and can therefore influence subject participation. |
| **Differential subject response in the** sample population | Occurs when outcome and exposure status are different in the **population providing data** in the sample population than in the **source population.** | Can affect **any study design.** |

Returning to the definition of selection bias, this phenomenon occurs when the measure of effect and measure of association are *meaningfully* different from one another due to selection processes, participation, loss to follow-up, or nonresponse. What constitutes a meaningful difference is study-specific and should be decided by the investigative team. For example, what difference would lead to different conclusions regarding whether the exposure and outcome are associated with one another? What difference would lead to different decisions about clinical practice or policies? As with confounding, there are no statistical tests or standard quantitative cutoffs to determine what difference in these measures indicates that selection is present in your study; this is a qualitative decision made by subject matter experts.

While investigators must be on the lookout for the four factors that can lead to selection bias, which were described earlier, it is important to note that these things won't *always* lead to selection bias. As an example, if all you know is that some study participants were lost to follow-up, this isn't enough information to determine whether the results are influenced by selection bias. For the possible sources of selection bias to lead to a biased measure of association, they must be **differential**, which means that these factors must be related to both exposure *and* outcome statuses (Learning Objective 10.5). We will explore this phenomenon in detail throughout the chapter; however, to get you started thinking about this issue, consider a cohort where 20% of the participants were lost to follow-up. If the loss to follow-up within each of the exposure/outcome groups in a 2x2 table (e.g., E+O+, E+O-, E-O+, E-O-) is also 20%, this will not introduce bias in the study. However, if those who were exposed and eventually develop the outcome of interest were *more* likely to be lost to follow-up than the other groups, then the study results are likely to be biased. Much of this chapter will be dedicated to understanding how such differential selection processes, participation, losses, or nonresponses can occur in epidemiologic studies, and how this can affect the calculated measures of association.

The main ways in which selection bias can influence an epidemiologic study are specific to the selected study design. This may not be surprising since a defining feature of the different study designs is *how* subjects are selected into the sample. Also consider that subjects may be lost over time only in study designs with longitudinal follow-up (i.e., controlled trials and cohorts). For that reason, we will first discuss the ways in which selection bias occurs within the context of each study design. Then, we will discuss ways to address the different sources of selection bias.

## SELECTION BIAS IN LONGITUDINAL DESIGNS

One key underlying reason for selection bias in studies with longitudinal follow-up (i.e., controlled trials and cohorts) is **differential loss to follow-up**. This means that the follow-up of the exposed and/or the unexposed study participants is different depending on their outcome status.

To see how this can happen, let's consider a study of medical cannabis use among individuals with opioid use disorder. Epidemiologic studies have hypothesized that cannabis use may improve pain management and therefore reduce opioid use and subsequent opioid-related harms, which has implications for policies related to legalization of medical marijuana.[5,6] However, concerns have been raised about the impact of selection bias in some cohort studies exploring this topic due to the potential for differential loss to follow-up.[5]

Consider the hypothetical data from a cohort of opioid users requiring pain management exploring the association between medical cannabis use and opioid overdose shown in **Figure 10.2**. In this example, we are assuming that everyone in the source population was selected and agreed to participate, and that the main source of selection bias for this study would be from loss to follow-up. To illustrate the impact of selection bias, we are comparing data from the source population to the sample population. As indicated in **Figure 10.2**, during the follow-up period, 10% of all medical cannabis users (both those who experienced an opioid overdose and those who did not experience an opioid overdose) and 10% of non-cannabis users who did not experience an opioid overdose were lost to follow-up. However, 30% of non-cannabis users who eventually experienced an opioid overdose were lost to follow-up, making the loss to follow-up *differential*.

## FIGURE 10.2 HYPOTHETICAL COHORT STUDY OF MEDICAL CANNABIS USE AND OPIOID OVERDOSE WITH DIFFERENTIAL LOSS TO FOLLOW-UP

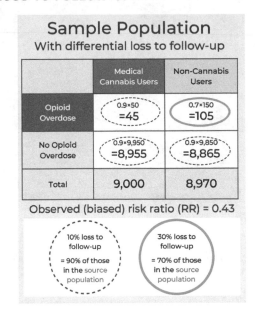

Since selection bias occurs when the measure of association calculated from the sample population is meaningfully different from what would have been observed if we had complete follow-up for all 20,000 individuals in the source population, we will calculate and compare the unbiased risk ratio (RR) in the source population and the estimated (biased) risk ratio from the sample population. Since this is a cohort study and given that we know there is loss to follow-up, it would be preferable to calculate rates and rate-based measures of association in the sample population. However, we will use risks in this example as it is easier to demonstrate the concepts and allows for a direct comparison with the unbiased measure calculated from the source population.

When we compare the risk ratios from the source (RR = 0.33) and sample (RR = 0.43) populations, we observe selection bias *toward the null*, which is due to differential loss to follow-up. Thus, while medical cannabis use was found to be protective against opioid overdose in our sample, its true effect in the source population was actually stronger than what we estimated using data from the sample population.

While we have compared the measures of association calculated in both the source and sample populations, **Figure 10.3** helps us to think about the impact of the selection bias more generally on our 2×2 table (Learning Objective 10.6).

Let's begin by calculating the risk in the *exposed* in both the source and sample populations:

$$\text{Risk}_{\text{exposed-source}} = \frac{A}{(A+C)}$$

$$\text{Risk}_{\text{exposed-sample}} = \frac{0.9 \times A}{(0.9 \times A + 0.9 \times c)} = \frac{0.9 \times A}{0.9 \times (A+C)} = \frac{A}{A+C}$$

Among the exposed, the same proportion of those with and without the outcome were lost to follow-up. For this reason, the risk among the exposed in the sample population is the same as in the source population.

## FIGURE 10.3 IMPACT OF SELECTION BIAS ON THE 2×2 TABLE IN THE HYPOTHETICAL COHORT STUDY OF MEDICAL CANNABIS USE AND OPIOID OVERDOSE

| Source Population No loss to follow-up | Medical Cannabis Users | Non-Cannabis Users |
|---|---|---|
| Opioid Overdose | A | B |
| No Opioid Overdose | C | D |
| Total | A+C | B+D |

| Sample Population With differential loss to follow-up | Medical Cannabis Users | Non-Cannabis Users |
|---|---|---|
| Opioid Overdose | 0.9×A | 0.7×B |
| No Opioid Overdose | 0.9×C | 0.9×D |
| Total | 0.9×A+0.9×C | 0.7×B+0.9×D |

Next, let's calculate the risk in the unexposed in both the source and sample populations:

$$\text{Risk}_{\text{unexposed-source}} = \frac{B}{(B+D)}$$

$$\text{Risk}_{\text{unexposed-sample}} = \frac{0.7 \times B}{(0.7 \times B + 0.9 \times D)} = \frac{0.7 \times B}{0.7 \times (B + \frac{9}{7}D)} = \frac{B}{B + \frac{9}{7}D}$$

Unlike in the exposed, the risk among the unexposed in the sample population does not simplify to the risk among the unexposed in the source population. The denominator of the risk calculation in the sample population ends up being too large (we divide by $B+\frac{9}{7}D$ instead of just B+D). The result is that the risk among the unexposed in the sample population is *too small*.

When we then compare the risks in the exposed and unexposed groups in the sample population by calculating the RR, the risk in the exposed is divided by a risk in the unexposed that is too small, thus making our RR larger than it should be.

This happened because the follow-up among the unexposed group (non-cannabis users) was *differential* by outcome status (those who were unexposed and experienced an opioid overdose were more likely to be lost to follow-up than those who were unexposed and did *not* experience an opioid overdose).

Though this is a hypothetical scenario, one could envision a situation in which this differential loss may occur if, for example, non-cannabis users (i.e., those who are not benefiting from potential pain relief from medical cannabis use) who are more likely to experience an opioid overdose are more likely to drop out of the study due to unmanageable pain and high-risk opioid use.

Now we must ask the question of whether this difference in measures is *meaningful*. The answer to this question is study-dependent and should be determined by the research team and subject matter experts who will consider factors such as how compelling the findings are in terms of impacting clinical decision-making and public health policy.

One question you may be asking yourself is how we can possibly know or even estimate the loss to follow-up in a longitudinal study. Sometimes, these values can be assumed based on what is known about the selection processes, participation, losses to follow-up, or nonresponses in previous studies of similar source populations. As we will describe in the text that follows, when this information isn't available, investigators may conduct **sensitivity analyses** using a range of hypothesized values. In sensitivity analyses, we use these different sets of plausible values and explore how these different sets of assumptions affect the results.

## Using Selection Probabilities to Find the Size of the Source and Sample Populations (LEARNING OBJECTIVE 10.6)

In the medical cannabis use and opioid overdose example, we were given information about the proportion of individuals who were lost to follow-up in each of the four cells of our study's 2×2 table. Epidemiologists will often use the inverse of these proportions, called **selection probabilities**, which are calculated in this example as: 100% – proportion lost to follow-up. Selection probabilities can be used to generate the R×C table for the sample population using data from the source population, or to generate the R×C table for the source population using data from the sample population. To distinguish between the cells for each of these populations, labels for the source population will appear in uppercase letters, and labels for the sample population will appear in lowercase letters. Note that although the following example uses selection probabilities to address loss to follow-up, this strategy can also be used when there are questions about selection into the study, participation, or response.

If you are given an R×C table with data from the source population along with the selection probabilities for each cell, you can generate the R×C table for the sample population by *multiplying* each of the cells of the source population's R×C table by the corresponding selection probabilities. For example, in **Figure 10.2**, we knew that there was 30% loss to follow-up among individuals in cell B (non-cannabis users who experienced an opioid overdose) of the source population. We'll begin by converting our information about loss to follow-up to a selection probability: 100% – 30% = 70%. Then, we multiply the number of individuals in cell B in the source population by this selection probability (150 × 70%) to find that our sample population should include a total of 105 non-cannabis users who experienced an opioid overdose.

More generally, the size of each cell in the sample population can be calculated as follows:

Sample population = Source population × Selection probability
= Source population × (100% lost to follow-up*)

Conversely, if you are given an R×C table with data from the sample population along with the selection probabilities for each cell, you can generate the R×C table for the source population by *dividing* each of the cells of the sample population's R×C table by the corresponding selection probabilities. Returning to **Figure 10.2**, there were 45 participants remaining in cell a of the sample population after a 10% loss, with a corresponding selection probability of 100% – 10% = 90%. By dividing the number of individuals in cell a (medical cannabis users who experienced an opioid overdose) in the sample population by this selection probability (45/90%), we find that our source population contained a total of 50 medical cannabis users who experienced an opioid overdose.

More generally, the size of each cell in the source population can be calculated as follows:

$$\text{Source polulation} = \frac{\text{Sample population}}{\text{Selection probability}}$$
$$= \frac{\text{Sample population}}{(100\% \text{ lost to follow-up*})}$$

At first, it may be confusing to think about going back and forth between the source and sample populations. One strategy to help keep you on track is to remember that the sample population is a *subset* of the source population; thus, the size of the source population should always be greater than or equal to that of the sample population. If you find that your sample population is larger than the source population, this is a good signal to go back and check your work!

*or other sources of selection bias

We just explored the situation where loss to follow-up was differential. Now let's see what happens if the loss to follow-up is **nondifferential**, meaning that it is not associated with both the exposure and outcome. Suppose that instead of 30% loss to follow-up in cell B of Figure 10.2, this group also had 10% loss to follow-up. This means that cell B in the sample population will contain 150×(100%) = 135 people. If 10% of the entire cohort is lost, then the relative sizes of each of your four cells will not change, and there will be no bias.

$$RR_{source} = \frac{\left[\frac{A}{(A+C)}\right]}{\left[\frac{B}{(B+D)}\right]} = \frac{\left[\frac{50}{(50+9,950)}\right]}{\left[\frac{150}{(150+9,850)}\right]} = 0.33$$

$$RR_{sample} = \frac{\left[\frac{0.9 \times A}{(0.9 \times A + 0.9 \times C)}\right]}{\left[\frac{0.9 \times B}{(0.9 \times B + 0.9 \times D)}\right]} = \frac{\left[\frac{45}{(45+8,955)}\right]}{\left[\frac{135}{(135+8,865)}\right]} = 0.33$$

Note that the formula for the risk ratio in the sample population reduces to the formula for the RR in the source population:

$$RR_{sample} = \frac{\left[\frac{0.9 \times A}{(0.9 \times A + 0.9 \times C)}\right]}{\left[\frac{0.9 \times B}{(0.9 \times B + 0.9 \times D)}\right]} = \frac{0.9 \times \left[\frac{A}{(A+C)}\right]}{0.9 \times \left[\frac{B}{(B+D)}\right]}$$

$$= \frac{\left[\frac{A}{(A+C)}\right]}{\left[\frac{B}{(B+D)}\right]} = RR_{source}$$

While this example illustrates what happens when loss to follow-up is nondifferential, the same thing is true for the three other factors that may cause selection bias. Selection bias will only occur if participant loss to follow-up, selection, participation, or nonresponse are *differential*.

We've explored one way that loss to follow-up may be nondifferential (i.e., all four exposure/outcome groups had 10% loss to follow-up). In **Pause to Practice 10.1** you will learn about a second way where loss to follow-up is nondifferential, and thus the results are not impacted by selection bias.

## Pause to Practice 10.1

### Exploring the Impact of Nondifferential Loss to Follow-Up

In this exercise, we will use the data from the source population in Figure 10.2 but will now consider the impact of non-differential follow-up that is only associated with the exposure. Consider a scenario where we observed 30% loss to follow-up among the exposed (i.e., in cells A and C) and 10% loss to follow-up among the unexposed (i.e., in cells B and D) during the follow-up period, which was 3 years.

1. Before calculating the measure of association from the sample population, do you think the resulting measure of association will be biased? Why or why not? If yes, in which direction?

2. Now construct the 2×2 table for the sample population and calculate the risk ratio.

3. Interpret this measure of association.

4. Is there any selection bias due to loss to follow-up? If so, what is the direction of the bias?

As you saw in **Pause to Practice 10.1**, if the proportion of people lost in cells A and C are equal, then the risk in the exposed remains the same as it was before the loss of participants. Similarly, if the proportion of people lost in cells B and D are equal, then the risk in the unexposed remains the same as it was before the loss of participants. Thus, when calculating a measure of association that compares the experience of the exposed and unexposed groups, there is no difference between what is calculated in the source and sample populations because within each exposure group, the loss to follow-up among those who get the outcome and those who don't are proportional to one another. **Pause to Practice 10.1** illustrates that selection bias will not occur if loss to follow-up is only associated with the exposure. As we've noted before, selection bias will only occur if the losses are *differential*, meaning related to both exposure and outcome statuses.

In summary, selection bias in longitudinal studies (e.g., controlled trials or cohorts) may arise when follow-up of the exposed and/or unexposed is differential by outcome status. This means selection bias can occur if (Learning Objective 10.6):

- A different proportion of exposed persons with the outcome are lost to follow-up compared to exposed persons without the outcome ($a/A \neq c/C$), and/or

- A different proportion of unexposed persons with the outcome are lost to follow-up compared to unexposed persons without the outcome ($b/B \neq d/D$)

Though we worked through examples using risk ratios, the same principles apply when calculating risk differences, rate ratios, or rate differences.

It can be difficult to track subjects over a longitudinal study, especially when follow-up is very long, the study procedures are onerous, or when studying populations that are relatively difficult to follow such as those that are highly mobile or unhoused. Generally, follow-up of greater than 80% of enrolled participants is viewed favorably. However, even a study with losses of 20% or less may have selection bias if the losses are related to both exposure and outcome statuses. Conversely, a study with 50% loss to follow-up may not have selection bias if the losses are not differential.

Loss to follow-up is not the only source of selection bias that can affect longitudinal designs. We will describe sources of selection bias that affect all study designs later in the chapter. We will also describe strategies to prevent and correct for selection bias, including strategies to maximize follow-up.

## Highlights

### Selection Bias in Longitudinal Designs

- A key underlying reason for selection bias in studies with longitudinal follow-up (e.g., controlled trials and cohorts) is differential loss to follow-up.

  - This occurs when outcome *and* exposure status influence the retention of participants in the sample population.

- Selection bias in longitudinal designs can occur if:

  - A different proportion of exposed persons with the outcome are lost to follow-up compared to exposed persons without the outcome ($a/A \neq c/C$), and/or

  - A different proportion of unexposed persons with the outcome are lost to follow-up compared to unexposed persons without the outcome ($b/B \neq d/D$)

## SELECTION BIAS IN CASE-CONTROL DEISGNS

Recall that in case-control studies, participants are selected on the basis of their outcome status and the appropriate measure of association is the exposure odds ratio (EOR), which compares the frequency of the exposure in cases to the frequency of exposure in the controls.

The exposure odds ratio calculated from the sample population may be affected by selection bias if selection of cases and/or controls is differential by exposure status. This means selection bias can occur in a case-control study when there is (Learning Objective 10.6):

- A different proportion of people in cells a versus b in the sample population relative to the source population (i.e., $a/A \neq b/B$) and/or

- A different proportion of people in cells c versus d in the sample population relative to the source population (i.e., $c/C \neq d/D$).

The main mechanisms leading to selection bias in case-control studies are related to **survival bias** and **differential participation**.

## Survival Bias in Case-Control Designs

As described in **Chapter 6, "Case-Control Designs,"** selection of prevalent cases in a case-control study may lead to survival bias if the exposure affects survival differentially by an individual's outcome status. The most common scenario is when exposed cases are more likely to die (and thus be unavailable for selection into a case-control study) than exposed controls. In this case, the frequency of exposure among the prevalent cases would be lower than that of all cases in the source population. More generally, survival bias in a case-control study could occur if:

- Exposed cases are more likely to survive longer than unexposed cases ($a/A > b/B$).
- Exposed controls are more likely to survive longer than unexposed controls ($c/C > d/D$).
- Unexposed cases are more likely to survive longer than exposed cases ($b/B > a/A$).
- Unexposed controls are more likely to survive longer than exposed controls ($d/D > c/C$).

### Pause to Practice 10.2

#### Assessing the Impact of Survival Bias in Case-Control Studies

Consider the following scenarios describing case-control studies and think about how the selection bias described would impact your 2×2 table. What is the direction of bias?

**Scenario 1**: A case-control study examined the association between prevalent overdoses (outcome) and prior use of propoxyphene, an analgesic (exposure). In the source population, patients who experienced an overdose and who had a history of propoxyphene use were more likely to die than patients who experienced an overdose and had no history of propoxyphene use.

**Scenario 2:** A case-control study assessed the association between access to harm reduction services (such as referral to treatment for substance use disorders and syringe service programs; exposure) and prevalent opioid overdoses (outcome). In the source population, patients who experienced an overdose and who had access to harm reduction services were more likely to survive than patients who experienced an overdose and did not have access to such services.

## Differential Participation in Case-Control Designs

In addition to survival bias when selecting prevalent cases, selection bias in case-control studies can occur because of differences in participation between cases and/or controls by exposure status. Thus, differential participation in a case-control study could occur if:

- Exposed cases are more likely to participate relative to unexposed cases ($a/A > b/B$).
- Exposed controls are more likely to participate relative to unexposed controls ($c/C > d/D$).
- Unexposed cases are more likely to participate relative to exposed cases ($b/B > a/A$).
- Unexposed controls are more likely to participate relative to exposed controls ($d/D > c/C$).

Consider a 2020 study describing an outbreak of HIV among people who inject drugs (PWID) in Massachusetts. The majority of cases in the study were unhoused. The investigators also reported that "[t]he investigation and publicity about the outbreak could have increased awareness among PWID of the outbreak and local services" (p. 43).[7] Now let's suppose that study investigators had conducted a case-control study to explore the association between being unhoused (exposure) and HIV (outcome) among PWID, and that it became known in the community that the investigators hypothesized that unhoused individuals were more affected by HIV than those who were housed. This could lead to unhoused cases being more willing to participate compared to housed cases due to increased risk perception (a self-selection bias) which motivated them to participate. To think through whether this could lead to bias in the measure of association, let's consider the potential impact on the study's 2×2 table, shown in **Figure 10.4**. Since exposed cases (cell A) are more likely to agree to participate relative to unexposed cases (cell B), the numerator of the odds ratio calculation will be too large, and the resulting exposure odds ratio will thus be biased away from the null. Similar concerns could arise for differential participation among controls if their likelihood of participating is differential by their exposure status.

## FIGURE 10.4 IMPACT OF DIFFERENTIAL PARTICIPATION ON THE 2×2 TABLE IN A CASE-CONTROL STUDY

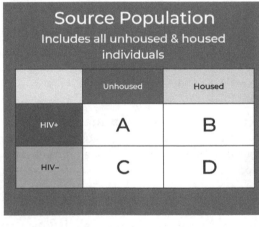

## Why Is Differential Participation *Not* a Main Concern in Cohorts and Trials?

Differential participation can introduce selection bias in case-control studies and cross-sectional studies. However, differential participation is not a main concern in controlled trials or cohorts because the outcome has not yet occurred when participants are eligible for the study. Therefore, while participation may be dependent on the exposure, it is unlikely to be related to whether someone develops the outcome during the study period, and therefore is less likely lead to selection bias.

### Selection Bias in Case-Control Designs

- The main mechanisms leading to selection bias in case-control studies are related to survival bias (a type of differential subject selection) and differential participation.

- Selection bias in case-control studies can occur if:

  - There is differential survival or participation for exposed and unexposed cases (i.e., $a/A \neq b/B$), and/or

  - There is differential survival or participation for exposed and unexposed controls (i.e., $c/C \neq d/D$).

## SELECTION BIAS IN CROSS-SECTIONAL DESIGNS

Recall that in cross-sectional studies, we often calculate a prevalence ratio (PR) or prevalence difference (PD) from a 2×2 table. Also recall that formulae for the calculation of prevalence ratios and prevalence differences from a 2×2 table are the same as for the risk ratios or risk differences, respectively, and thus the way selection bias may impact the calculation of the risk-based or prevalence-based measure of association follows the same rules. This means, as in cohort studies and controlled trials, selection bias in cross-sectional studies also occurs when the exposed and/or unexposed groups are selected differently by outcome status, meaning there is (Learning Objective 10.6):

- A different proportion of people in cells a versus c in the sample population relative to the source population (i.e., $a/A \neq c/C$) and/or

- A different proportion of people in cells b versus d in the sample population relative to the source population (i.e., $b/B \neq d/D$).

However, the main mechanisms leading to selection bias in cross-sectional studies, which do not have longitudinal follow-up (and thus no opportunities for participant loss to follow-up) are different. The main mechanisms leading to selection bias in cross-sectional studies are related to **survival bias** and **differential participation**.

### Survival Bias in Cross-Sectional Designs

One key form of selection bias in cross-sectional designs is **survival bias**. Recall that the prevalence of an outcome may be influenced both by exposure and the duration of the outcome. If the exposure influences survival time differently for those who get the outcome than for those who do not, then the measure of association calculated from a cross-sectional study may be biased. Thus, survival bias in a cross-sectional study could occur if:

- Exposed persons with the outcome are more likely to survive longer than exposed persons without the outcome ($a/A > c/C$).

- Exposed persons without the outcome are more likely to survive longer than exposed persons with the outcome ($c/C > a/A$).

- Unexposed persons with the outcome are more likely to survive longer than unexposed persons without the outcome ($b/B > d/D$).

- Unexposed persons without the outcome are more likely to survive longer than unexposed persons with the outcome ($d/D > b/B$).

For example, researchers have been interested in understanding the effect of polysubstance use (defined as consumption of more than one recreational substance simultaneously) and opioid overdose.[8-10] Let's consider a hypothetical cross-sectional study examining

## FIGURE 10.5 IMPACT OF SURVIVAL BIAS ON THE 2×2 TABLE IN THE HYPOTHETICAL CROSS-SECTIONAL STUDY OF POLYSUBSTANCE USE AND OPIOID OVERDOSE

| Source Population<br>Does not exclude those who died | Polysubstance Use | No Polysubstance Use |
|---|---|---|
| Opioid Overdose | A | B |
| No Opioid Overdose | C | D |
| Total | A+C | B+D |

| Sample Population<br>Impacted by survival bias | Polysubstance Use | No Polysubstance Use |
|---|---|---|
| Opioid Overdose | a ✳ | b |
| No Opioid Overdose | c | d |
| Total | a +c | b+d |

✳ Cell a is proportionally too small relative to cell c.

$$PR_{source} = \frac{A}{A+C} \Big/ \frac{B}{B+D}$$

$$PR_{sample} = \frac{a}{a+c} \Big/ \frac{b}{b+d}$$

this association and the possible effect of survival on the study findings (Figure 10.5). In this study, differential survivorship may impact who is recruited and may lead to a selection bias. Let's think through some ways in which this could occur. From a review of the literature, it might be reasonable to suspect that polysubstance users are more likely to experience a fatal opioid overdose.[9] How might that impact our 2×2 table? In this case, those exposed to polysubstance use who experience an opioid overdose are more likely to die compared to those exposed to polysubstance use who do not experience an opioid overdose (i.e., $a/A < c/C$). As shown in Figure 10.5, the size of cell $a$ in the sample population is smaller than it ought to be due to survival bias. The impact of this on the prevalence ratio is shown below the source and sample 2×2 tables: the size of the letter in cell $a$ is intentionally proportionally smaller relative to cell $c$. Having too few individuals in cell $a$ (i.e., those exposed to polysubstance use who experience an opioid overdose) relative to cell $c$ (i.e., those exposed to polysubstance use who do not experience an opioid overdose) will yield a prevalence in the exposed that is smaller than it should be. Thus, the prevalence ratio calculated from the sample population will also be smaller than it should be, resulting in bias toward the null. In this case, our study data would have underestimated the true association between polysubstance use and opioid overdose due to selective survival.

## Differential Participation in Cross-Sectional Designs

Differential participation in a cross-sectional study could occur if:

- Exposed persons with the outcome are more likely to participate relative to exposed persons without the outcome ($a/A > c/C$).

- Exposed persons without the outcome are more likely to participate relative to exposed persons with the outcome ($c/C > a/A$).

- Unexposed persons with the outcome are more likely to participate relative to unexposed persons without the outcome ($b/B > d/D$).

- Unexposed persons without the outcome are more likely to participate relative to unexposed persons with the outcome ($d/D > b/B$).

Differential participation is also sometimes called **self-selection bias**. One can imagine various factors that influence whether participants are motivated to join a study. For example, having a vested interest in the outcome under study (e.g., due to knowing a family member or friend affected by that outcome, or being in a demographic group disproportionately affected by that outcome) or having relatively more time to participate (e.g., due to being retired) may lead to increased participation. Conversely, a multitude of factors may decrease participation rates, for example, being uncomfortable answering study questions, uncomfortable with the procedures, or simply not having available time. As an example, it has been suggested that PWID may be significantly less likely to join studies because of fear of legal repercussions related to illicit drug use and stigma; persons who are unhoused may be less likely to agree to participate in studies for similar reasons.[4]

## Pause to Practice 10.3

### Assessing the Impact of Selection Bias in Cross-Sectional Studies

Consider the following scenarios describing cross-sectional studies and think about whether they are likely to lead to selection bias. If so, what is the likely direction of the bias? If not, explain why and what additional information would be helpful to have to determine whether selection bias is likely. As you think through these scenarios, it may be helpful to consider the impact of each scenario on the study's 2×2 table.

**Scenario 1:** In a cross-sectional study of mental illness (exposure) and illicit drug use (outcome), individuals diagnosed with mental illnesses in the source population who also used illicit drugs were less likely to agree to participate relative to those who didn't use illicit drugs due to concerns about stigma.

**Scenario 2:** In a cross-sectional study of previous versus current incarceration (exposure) and hepatitis C (outcome), individuals who were currently incarcerated were more likely to participate than those who had previously been incarcerated.

## Highlights

### Selection Bias in Cross-Sectional Designs

- The main mechanisms leading to selection bias in cross-sectional studies are related to survival bias (a type of differential subject selection) and differential participation.
- Selection bias in cross-sectional studies can occur if:
  - In the exposed group, there is differential survival or participation for those with and without the outcome of interest (i.e., $a/A \neq c/C$), and/or
  - In the unexposed group, there is differential survival or participation for those with and without the outcome of interest (i.e., $b/B \neq d/D$)

## SOURCES OF SELECTION BIAS THAT MAY AFFECT ANY DESIGN

While we have seen examples of how each of the study designs can be impacted by selection bias, it is notable that there are some selection-related issues that can affect any study design. The first of these is related to selection processes, which refers to the manner in which participants are selected from the source population into the sample population. For example, if some members of the source population are not considered for inclusion (e.g., because you didn't know they were in the source population or because of the sampling strategy used), or are unreachable (e.g., due to not having a phone or being highly mobile), this could lead to selection bias. Though differential selection processes can affect any study design, they are most problematic in case-control and cross-sectional designs since both outcome and exposure status are known and can therefore influence subject selection. As with the other selection-related concerns discussed previously, for selection processes to lead to selection bias, they must be associated with *both* exposure and outcome statuses.

## Berkson's Bias: An Example of a Selection Process That Can Cause Selection Bias

Berkson's bias is a form of selection bias that arises due to differential selection processes. Berkson's bias was first described by physician and statistician Joseph Berkson in 1964.[11] He described this bias within the context of case-control studies that recruited cases and controls from hospitals. Dr. Berkson noted how two diseases (let's consider one as an exposure and one as an outcome of interest) that are independent (i.e., not associated) in the source population may become noncausally associated in the sample population if persons with *both* diseases have a higher probability of being hospitalized than individuals with just one disease.

For example, assume that two diseases, sickle cell anemia (exposure) and asbestosis (outcome), are not associated in the source population—meaning that in the source population, those with sickle cell anemia are no more likely to have asbestosis and vice versa. However, individuals with *both* of these diseases are more likely to be hospitalized. Thus, if we select study participants for our sample population from a hospital, the proportion of individuals in cell *a* in the sample population are overrepresented relative to their frequency in cell *A* in the source population. Therefore, sickle cell anemia and asbestosis may become non-causally associated in the sample population.

Since its initial description, Berkson's bias has been known to arise in any type of study design, experimental or observational,[12] and can be generalized to occurring when the exposure and outcome of interest are both associated with attendance at a healthcare facility, and study selection takes place at these healthcare facilities.

A second way that any study type could be impacted by selection bias occurs once participants are enrolled. At any time, participants may refuse or be unable to provide outcome and/or exposure data, which is described as **participant nonresponse** and can lead to selection bias. As with all other sources of selection bias, participant nonresponse can only lead to selection bias if it is differential, meaning associated with both exposure and outcome statuses. For example, in a cross-sectional study exploring the association between two stigmatized behaviors, alcoholism (exposure) and illicit drug use (outcome), if all study participants were similarly likely to not respond to survey questions related to illicit drug use, and these nonresponses were not related to alcoholism, then there would be no selection bias. However, if persons struggling with alcoholism and illicit drug use (cell A) were more likely to not respond to survey questions assessing those behaviors relative to persons experiencing alcoholism only (cell C), this would result in a selection bias toward the null.

## WAYS TO ADDRESS SELECTION BIAS

Now that we have described some of the main ways selection bias can occur, we will turn our attention to strategies to address selection bias. There are two main opportunities to address selection bias: during the study design stage and during the data analysis stage.

## Addressing Selection Bias During the Study Design Stage
### (LEARNING OBJECTIVE 10.7)

**Maximizing follow-up in longitudinal studies.** In study designs with longitudinal follow-up, such as controlled trials and cohort studies, maximizing follow-up is key to reducing selection bias. Below is a non-exhaustive list of strategies that may be employed to maximize follow-up among study participants.

- Collect contact information at enrollment from all study participants that may facilitate future recontact of subjects (e.g., phone numbers, email addresses, physical addresses, and contact information for relatives/friends).

- Use an automatic study visit reminder system, with multiple reminders sent via different modes of contact (e.g., text, email, mail, phone calls) to nonresponders.

- Maintain regular contact with study participants, especially if scheduled visits are infrequent (e.g., if a participant is to be seen every 6 months, interim contact via phone or email may be useful).

- Share study progress and, when possible, interim study findings with participants.

- If possible, consider enrolling participants who are easier to follow (e.g., persons with homes, people with phones, people who do not plan on relocating). For example, high motivation to engage in long-term follow-up was one reason that the Nurses' Health Study enrolled nurses.[13]

- Provide incentives for attending follow-up visits to offset the opportunity cost of participant time. However, recalling the discussion of research ethics in **Chapter 1, "Introduction to Public Health and the Fundamentals of Epidemiology,"** the value of incentives must be balanced against possible coercion to participate.

- Consider how onerous the study procedures are (e.g., frequency of study visits, types of invasive procedures required) and strive to balance subject burden with answering the scientific question(s).

**Maximizing participation.** In case-control and cross-sectional studies in particular, maximizing initial study participation is key to preventing selection bias. Some of the previously described strategies may also be used to maximize participation.

- Consider how onerous the study procedures are and strive to balance subject burden with answering the scientific question(s).

- If possible, consider enrolling participants who are more likely to participate (e.g., highly motivated).

- Provide incentives for enrolling in the study to offset the opportunity cost of participant time.

**Minimizing participant nonresponse.** In all study designs, it is important to try to maximize response rates among participants, especially when collecting exposure and outcome data. Below is a non-exhaustive list of strategies that may be employed to maximize response rates among study participants, some of which have already been highlighted in the previous lists.

- Use reminders to follow-up with participants who have not completed exposure or outcome assessments.

- Provide incentives for providing complete exposure and outcome data.

- If collecting data electronically, make exposure and outcome measures required fields.

- When collecting self-reported data, assess measures using clear, simple questions to ensure comprehension.

- If asking survey questions on topics that may be stigmatized, consider use of audio-computer-assisted self-interviewing (ACASI) or other self-administered questionnaire methods.[14,15]

- When possible, consider use of measures that do not rely on self-report that may be relatively complete (e.g., from systematically collected medical records).

**Selecting incident cases in case-control studies.** To attempt to prevent survival bias in case-control studies, it is preferable to select *incident* rather than *prevalent* cases, which helps ensure that the frequency of exposure among cases selected for the study mirrors that of all individuals with the outcome of interest in the source population. However, there may be some impediments to identification and selection of incident cases:

- It may be difficult to identify and enroll incident (e.g., newly diagnosed) cases as they occur, for example, with diseases with ill-defined onset like obesity.

- Recruitment of incident cases may be resource intensive (e.g., deciding whether to use polymerase chain reaction (PCR) technology to identify incident cases of HIV or using less expensive antibody testing that will identify both prevalent and incident cases).

- For rare outcomes, prevalent cases may be more common and there may not be a sufficient number of incident cases available.

- Those who are newly diagnosed with an outcome might be less likely to join a study due to the mental and logistical burden of a new disease diagnosis than prevalent cases who have had the outcome for a longer amount of time.

**Using representative sampling strategies.** One way to prevent selection bias from arising due to selection processes is to begin with a **representative sampling strategy,** meaning a strategy that generates a sample population that mirrors the characteristics of the source population. From our discussion of identifying the source population in case-control studies in **Chapter 6, "Case-Control Designs,"** we know that the identification of the source population can be challenging, if not impossible. Further, even if the source population is well-identified, it is not always possible to enroll the entire source population (in fact, it is typically not necessary or logistically feasible to do so). Ideally, we would have a well-enumerated source population and are able to **randomly sample** from that group. Common sampling strategies are described in the text that follows and illustrated in **Figure 10.6**.

**Random sampling strategies (probability sampling).** Probability sampling involves random selection of study participants from a well-defined source population. Probability sampling means that every member of the source population has a predetermined chance of being selected into the sample population. This type of sampling allows investigators to make stronger inferences because the sample population is more likely to provide a good representation of the source population. A brief, non-exhaustive overview of some common types of probability sampling include:

- **Simple random sampling** is a sampling procedure in which individuals are selected from the source population for inclusion into the sample population at random, meaning they all have the same probability of being selected. Random sampling from a source population reduces the potential for selection bias and, as you'll learn in the text that follows, increases the **generalizability** of your study findings.

- **Stratified random sampling** involves dividing the source population into subgroups (strata) that differ by important characteristics (e.g., age, gender, etc.). Then participants are randomly sampled *within* those strata to ensure that every subgroup is represented in the sample population. This allows investigators to draw conclusions about these important characteristics.

- **Cluster sampling** involves dividing the source population into subgroups (clusters) where each subgroup has similar characteristics as the source population. Then entire subgroups are randomly selected. For example, in a study of an educational intervention for school aged children, investigators may decide to identify several schools (clusters) in a certain area which share characteristics (e.g., student demographics) of the source population and then randomly sample from this list of schools.

## FIGURE 10.6 COMMON SAMPLING METHODS USED IN EPIDEMIOLOGIC RESEARCH

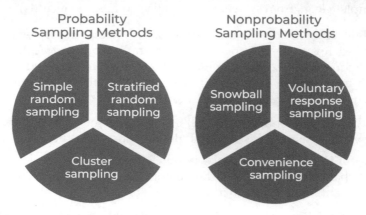

**Nonprobability sampling**. It may not be possible to employ a random sampling strategy. When random sampling strategies are not available, investigators may employ **nonrandom sampling strategies**, and must consider whether this type of sampling could introduce selection bias. Nonprobability sampling involves nonrandom participant selection, whereby not every individual has a pre-determined chance of being selected from the source population into the sample population. This type of sampling is easier and cheaper to implement but comes with a higher likelihood of bias, meaning that inferences from studies using nonprobability sampling are often weaker because it is unclear whether the sample population is a good representation of the source population. However, when conducting nonprobability sampling, investigators still strive to recruit study participants that represent the source population. A brief, non-exhaustive overview of some common types of nonprobability sampling include:

- **Convenience sampling.** Sample population includes individuals who are the most readily available to the researchers (e.g., students enrolled in a psychology class, or patients waiting to be seen in the emergency department).

- **Voluntary response sampling.** Sample population is comprised of participants who volunteered themselves (e.g., posting fliers in elevators and restrooms where individuals can learn about the study and learn how to contact the study team to enroll).

- **Snowball sampling**. Sample population is comprised of contacts of previously enrolled participants. Snowball sampling is a method whereby current study participants recruit additional participants (e.g., studies of hard-to-reach populations, like those with substance use disorders).

### Caution: Random Sampling Is Not the Same as Randomization!

Early students of epidemiology often confuse the terms *randomization* and *random sampling*. Although these contain the same root word (*random*) they are quite different!

Recall that **randomization** is a process by which every individual has an equal chance of being assigned to each exposure condition. Importantly, when the exposure is assigned randomly, that assignment is independent of patients' or study investigators' preferences. The benefit of randomization is that, on average, random assignment of the exposure should yield exposed and unexposed groups that are comparable on all factors except for the exposure status, thus isolating the effect of the exposure and preventing confounding of the measure of association.

Conversely, **random sampling** describes the process by which individuals are randomly *selected* from the source population into the sample population. Random sampling is attempting to address selection bias, not bias due to confounding.

Both randomization and random sampling can improve the validity of the study findings; however, one describes the allocation of the exposure while the other describes how the sample population was selected.

## Addressing Selection Bias During the Data Analysis Stage
### (LEARNING OBJECTIVE 10.8)

Once study data have been collected, adjustments can be made in the analysis stage in an attempt to quantitatively correct for selection bias. As you will see, this process requires several assumptions, and the information required to make those assumptions may not always be available. Although quantitative correction for selection bias during the data analysis stage is a handy tool to have in our toolbox, it is preferable to avoid or minimize selection bias before the data are even collected.

Since quantitative corrections for selection bias can be complicated for some case-control designs, we will focus solely on the use of **selection probabilities** to correct for selection bias in trials, cohort studies, or cross-sectional studies. Selection probabilities, which we will designate as $\alpha$, $\beta$, $\gamma$, and $\delta$, are defined as the probabilities of being selected from the source population into the sample population for each cell of the 2×2 table and are shown in Figure 10.7.

The 2×2 table on the left illustrates a sample population (denoted in green with lowercase letters) nestled within the source population (denoted in pink with uppercase letters). As we described previously, the selection probabilities are defined as the proportion of individuals from each cell of the R×C table that are selected from the source population into the sample population and are shown in the table on the right.

If the selection probabilities are known (or can be assumed), investigators can use these along with the information from the sample population to reweight the sample population data to reconstruct the source population.

## FIGURE 10.7 SELECTION PROBABILITIES FOR LONGITUDINAL AND CROSS-SECTIONAL DESIGNS

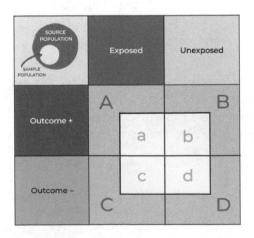

### Selection Probabilities

|  | Exposed | Unexposed |
|---|---|---|
| Outcome + | $\alpha = a/A$ | $\beta = b/B$ |
| Outcome – | $\gamma = c/C$ | $\delta = d/D$ |

Continuing with the convention of using uppercase and lowercase letters to represent the data from the source and sample populations, respectively, the source population data can be calculated as:

$$A = \frac{a}{\alpha} \quad B = \frac{b}{\beta} \quad C = \frac{c}{\gamma} \quad D = \frac{d}{\delta}$$

As you'll see in **Pause to Practice 10.4**, selection probabilities can be used not only to identify whether data from a sample population are subject to selection bias, but they can also be used to identify the direction of the bias.

## Pause to Practice 10.4

### Using Selection Probabilities to Correct for Selection Bias

Let's return to our previous example of a cohort study of polysubstance use and opioid overdose. It is likely that we could have trouble retaining people who experience an opioid overdose during the follow-up period. This could happen if those who experience an opioid overdose are more likely to die than those who do not experience an opioid overdose, and there may potentially be an even greater risk of death among the exposed (i.e., those with polysubstance use). Suppose that among those who experience an opioid overdose, we are only able to retain 60% of those with polysubstance use (i.e., O+E+) and 80% of those without polysubstance use (i.e., O+E−). Assume that all members of the cohort who do not experience an opioid overdose are retained. Thus, our selection probabilities are:

$$\alpha = 0.6 \quad \beta = 0.8 \quad \gamma = 1 \quad \delta = 1$$

Note that while these measures are called "selection" probabilities, they are used to correct for any sources of selection bias (e.g., participation, nonresponse, retention).

Data from the sample population, after loss to follow-up has occurred, are shown in **Table 10.2**.

TABLE 10.2 OBSERVED (SAMPLE POPULATION) DATA FOR THE ASSOCIATION BETWEEN POLYSUBSTANCE USE AND OPIOID OVERDOSE

|  | Polysubstance Use | No Polysubstance Use |
|---|---|---|
| Opioid Overdose | 120 | 24 |
| No Opioid Overdose | 1,000 | 1,000 |
| Total | 1,120 | 1,024 |

1. Calculate the risk ratio using data from the sample population (which is biased due to differential loss to follow-up).

2. Use the selection probabilities and the data from the sample population to create a 2×2 table for the source population.

3. Calculate the risk ratio that corrects for selection bias due to differential loss to follow-up.

4. What is the direction of the bias? In this example, is the corrected association between polysubstance use and opioid overdose weaker or stronger than what we observed in the sample population?

As we noted previously, one common question you may be asking is how we can possibly know or even estimate these selection probabilities. When selection probabilities are not known or cannot be assumed based on what is known about selection processes, participation, losses to follow-up, or nonresponses, investigators can conduct **sensitivity analyses** using a range of hypothesized selection probabilities. In sensitivity analyses, we would repeat the type of analysis shown in **Pause to Practice 10.4** multiple times to explore how different sets of plausible selection probabilities affect the results. For example, suppose that the investigators applied four different sets of selection probabilities, shown in **Table 10.3**, which were determined based on the investigators' educated guesses. Assume again that these experts expect to have trouble retaining people who experience an opioid overdose during the follow-up period (cells A and B), and that those with polysubstance use are at even greater risk of loss (cell A relative to cell B). Follow the same steps as in **Pause to Practice 10.4** to calculate the corrected risk ratios shown in **Table 10.3**. Note that while we use the term *corrected*, these results are based on educated guesses about the selection probabilities and generate results that are our best attempt at correcting the biased measures of association. Depending on how good our educated guesses are, the results that we refer to as *corrected* may not, in fact, fully correct for selection bias.

**TABLE 10.3 HYPOTHETICAL SENSITIVITY ANALYSIS TO CORRECT FOR SELECTION BIAS IN THE STUDY OF POLYSUBSTANCE USE AND OPIOID OVERDOSE**

| Selection Probabilities | | | | Risk Ratio Corrected for Selection Bias |
|---|---|---|---|---|
| $\alpha$ | $\beta$ | $\gamma$ | $\delta$ | |
| 0.6 | 0.8 | 1 | 1 | 5.72* |
| 0.5 | 0.8 | 1 | 1 | 6.65 |
| 0.6 | 0.7 | 1 | 1 | 5.03 |
| 0.5 | 0.7 | 1 | 1 | 5.84 |

*Calculated in Pause to Practice 10.4 question 3.

## Digging Deeper

## Inverse Probability Weighting and Imputation

Though beyond the scope of this textbook, we want to briefly mention two other strategies that are commonly used to quantitatively address selection bias: inverse probability weighting and imputation.

**Inverse probability weighting** is an extension of reweighting the sample population to approximate the source population using selection probabilities. Using this technique, investigators can weight the sample population data for additional factors, such as potential confounders. We've only considered weights for the four combinations of the exposure and outcome (E+O+, E+O−, E−O+, E−O−); however, we could add other covariates like employment status to create a total of eight categories:

E+O+ Employed, E+O− Employed, E−O+ Employed, E−O− Employed

E+O+ Unemployed, E+O− Unemployed, E−O+ Unemployed, E−O− Unemployed

For each of these combinations, investigators would explore the likelihood of participation. Groups with a lower likelihood of being in the sample population would carry more weight than those with a higher likelihood. For more on inverse probability weighting, see Mansournia and Altman's article "Inverse Probability Weighting."[16]

**Imputation** is the process of replacing missing data with substituted values that are assumed based on what is known about the sample population. The main assumption underlying this strategy is that the data are missing at random, meaning that there are no groups of individuals who are more likely to have missing data than others. For more on imputation of missing data see Sterne and colleagues' article, "Multiple Imputation for Missing Data in Epidemiological and Clinical Research: Potential and Pitfalls."[17]

A summary of the main ways that selection bias can occur within different study designs and opportunities to address these sources of selection bias is shown in **Table 10.4.**

**TABLE 10.4 SUMMARY OF PRIMARY SOURCES OF SELECTION BIAS AND OPPORTUNITIES TO ADDRESS, BY STUDY DESIGN**

| Study Design | Main Sources of Selection Bias | Addressing Selection Bias in the... | |
|---|---|---|---|
| | | Study Design Stage | Data Analysis Stage |
| Controlled trial and cohort (longitudinal studies) | Differential loss to follow-up | Use strategies to maximize follow-up | Weighting data from the sample population using:<br>• Selection probabilities<br>• Inverse probability weighting<br>• Imputation |
| Case-control | Survival bias | Select incident cases | |
| | Differential participation | Use strategies to maximize participation | |
| Cross-sectional | Survival bias | Best to avoid using a cross-sectional design when survival bias might be a concern | |
| | Differential participation | Use strategies to maximize participation | |
| Any design | Differential selection processes | Use representative sampling procedures if possible | |
| | Differential participant nonresponse | Use strategies to minimize participant nonresponse | |

# INTERNAL VALIDITY AND EXTERNAL VALIDITY

Now that we have discussed the concept of selection bias, we will revisit the distinction between internal validity and external validity introduced in **Chapter 9, "Error in Epidemiologic Research and Fundamentals of Confounding"** (Learning Objective 10.9).

**Internal validity** is related to whether the study results calculated from the sample population are valid (correct) with respect to the *source population.* All of the biases (systematic errors) discussed in this textbook (confounding, selection bias, and information bias) impact internal validity. Selection bias affects internal validity since selection bias occurs when the estimate in the sample population is different from what would have been obtained from the source population.

**External validity** (also called **generalizability**) is related to whether the results calculated from the sample population are valid (correct) with respect to some *target population.* The target population comprises the persons for whom the study results will be relevant (Learning Objective 10.10). See **Figure 10.8** for a schematic that differentiates these three populations: **source, sample,** and **target populations**. The target population is often an external population to which we want to generalize our findings. As shown in **Figure 10.8,** the target population could be the same as the source population (panel 1), slightly broader than the source population (panel 2), or completely external from the source population (panel 3).

# FIGURE 10.8 SOURCE, SAMPLE, AND TARGET POPULATIONS

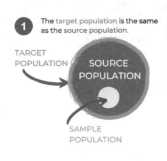

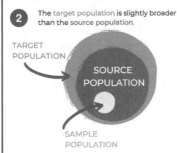

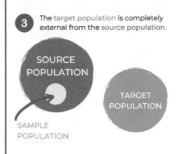

**SOURCE POPULATION**
- Population you are sampling from
- The population that gives rise to the outcome(s) of interest
- Defined by person, place, and/or time characteristics

**SAMPLE POPULATION**
- The people selected for inclusion in your study
- Usually a subset of the source population

**TARGET POPULATION**
- People you want to make inference to
- Can include the source population, but also may be an external group of individuals

**1** The target population is the same as the source population.

TARGET POPULATION — SOURCE POPULATION

SAMPLE POPULATION

**2** The target population is slightly broader than the source population.

TARGET POPULATION — SOURCE POPULATION

SAMPLE POPULATION

**3** The target population is completely external from the source population.

SOURCE POPULATION

SAMPLE POPULATION

TARGET POPULATION

## Caution: Selection Bias and Generalizability Are Not the Same Thing! (LEARNING OBJECTIVE 10.11)

It is common for new learners of epidemiology to confuse selection bias and generalizability. These concepts are illustrated in **Figure 10.9**. To help distinguish between these two, it is helpful to remember:

- **Selection bias** is related to a study's internal validity—if a study suffers from selection bias, this means that the results from the sample population do not reflect what would have been obtained from the source population due to selection processes.

- **Generalizability** (also called **external validity**)—if a study is not generalizable, the results obtained from a sample population will not be applicable to the target population.

## FIGURE 10.9 SELECTION BIAS VERSUS GENERALIZABILITY

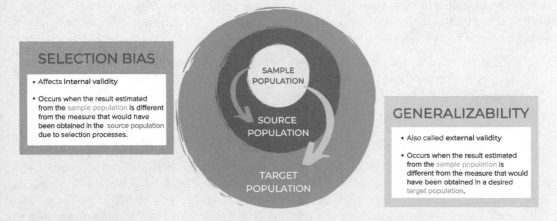

**SELECTION BIAS**
- Affects internal validity
- Occurs when the result estimated from the sample population is different from the measure that would have been obtained in the source population due to selection processes.

SAMPLE POPULATION

SOURCE POPULATION

TARGET POPULATION

**GENERALIZABILITY**
- Also called external validity
- Occurs when the result estimated from the sample population is different from the measure that would have been obtained in a desired target population.

A study that lacks internal validity cannot have external validity. This means that studies that suffer from selection bias are not generalizable—it wouldn't make sense to apply erroneous results to a target population!

### Defining Source, Sample, and Target Populations for the Framingham Heart Study

The Framingham Heart Study, introduced in **Chapter 5**, was one of the early cohort studies to explore the multi-factorial nature of heart disease. Let's explore the source, sample, and target populations for this landmark study.

- The **source population** of the original Framingham Heart Study included men and women aged 30 to 62 years who were residents of the town of Framingham, Massachusetts, in 1948.

- Not all men and women who were eligible to join the Framingham Heart Study were selected, and not all who were selected agreed to participate. The **sample population** was comprised of those who were invited and agreed to participate and were at-risk of developing cardiovascular disease at the start of the follow-up period.

- The **target population** comprised persons for whom the investigators wanted to apply the findings learned from the Framingham Health Study. The Framingham Heart Study has provided fundamental knowledge on cardiovascular disease epidemiology that is applied across industrialized countries.[18]

Internal validity is a prerequisite for external validity. Study results may be internally valid; however, the results may not apply to a target population of interest. For example, estimates from randomized controlled trials may have good internal validity if there is no loss to follow-up and the data are complete and correct; however, these trials may not be representative of every target population that could benefit from the trial findings. For example, this has historically been the case for clinical trials testing drugs and vaccines which have excluded pregnant people. While these study findings may have internal validity, they may not be generalizable to a target population that includes pregnant people who could potentially benefit from the drug or vaccine.

Consider a different example of studies of opioid use disorder treatment during pregnancy. Opioid use during pregnancy increased in the United States by 131% between 2010 and 2017,[19] and understanding the effect and safety of opioid use disorder treatments is of high clinical importance. Investigators undertook a **meta-analysis**, a special study design that combines data from many studies, to compare safety and pregnancy outcomes in those treated with either buprenorphine or methadone for opioid use disorder during pregnancy.[20] Pooled data from three randomized controlled trials (RCTs) and 15 cohort studies found that buprenorphine versus methadone use during pregnancy was associated with a lower risk of preterm birth, greater birth weight, and larger head circumference. The authors include the following statements in their publication:

> The RCTs included in this review were conducted rigorously, but suffered from relatively high levels of overall and differential attrition that increased the risk of selection bias and were not accounted for optimally in the published analyses.
>
> The addition of 1,923 participants in 15 cohort studies conducted in six additional countries and among a wider range of clinical settings increased the precision, statistical power and generalizability of our findings (pp. 2124–2125).[20]

The authors rightly differentiate between possible selection bias (in this case due to differential loss to follow-up) and generalizability (due to including studies from a variety of countries). This is an important reminder, however, that internal validity is a prerequisite for external validity. If the internal validity from some of the studies included in the meta-analysis are of concern, it is not appropriate to generalize the findings to other contexts.

## Efforts to Improve Internal Validity May Impact External Validity

Earlier we described ways that investigators might try to prevent selection bias when designing their studies, such as enrolling individuals who are easier to follow (and thus less likely to be lost to follow-up) or enrolling individuals who are more likely to agree to participate.

Such was the case in the Nurses' Health Study, which intentionally enrolled nurses because they were thought to be more invested in the research and thus more likely to agree to continued participation in the study compared to the general population.[13] If this assumption is true, this design choice will improve the internal validity of the study because it will reduce the likelihood for differential loss to follow-up during the study period. However, the decision to enroll nurses does come at a cost: nurses may be different in important ways from the general population, which could limit the generalizability of the findings.

While the decision to enroll nurses may raise questions about appropriate target populations for findings from the Nurses' Health Study, we must again remember that a study with poor internal validity cannot have external validity (i.e., cannot be generalizable). While there may be a tradeoff between some of the methods to prevent selection bias and generalizability, it's always best to err on the side of maximizing a study's internal validity to obtain meaningful results.

## Highlights

### Internal Validity, External Validity, Selection Bias, and Generalizability

- **Internal validity** is related to whether the study results calculated from the sample population are valid (correct) with respect to the source population.
  - **Selection bias** is related to **internal validity**. It occurs when the calculated measure of association estimated from your sample population is *meaningfully different* from the true measure of association that *would have* been estimated if you had data from all eligible subjects from the source population.
- **External validity** (also called **generalizability**) is related to whether the results from the sample population are valid (correct) with respect to a target population.
- Selection bias and generalizability are not the same thing.

## WHERE WE'VE BEEN AND WHAT'S UP NEXT

Selection bias occurs when the calculated measure of association estimated from your sample population is *meaningfully different* from the true measure of association that *would have* been estimated if you had data from all eligible subjects from the source population. Selection bias can arise due to differential (meaning associated with both the exposure and outcome) selection, participation, loss, or nonresponse of participants. The underlying reasons for selection bias usually differ by study design. Next, we will conclude our discussion of systematic error with information bias, which occurs when there is inaccurate measurement of the exposure and/or outcome (**Chapter 11, "Information Bias and Screening and Diagnostic Tests"**).

# END OF CHAPTER PROBLEM SET

Concern has arisen regarding the use of nonsteroidal anti-inflammatory drugs (NSAIDs), such as ibuprofen, and drug-induced liver toxicity.[21] Researchers undertook a case-control study to investigate this association. They enrolled 180 cases with drug-induced liver toxicity and 1,700 controls without drug-induced liver toxicity. Twenty percent of the cases reported NSAIDs use, and 10% of the controls reported NSAIDs use.

1. Use these data to fill in **Table 10.5** (round to the nearest whole number).

TABLE 10.5 **CASE-CONTROL STUDY OF NSAIDS USE AND DRUG INDUCED LIVER TOXICITY**

|  | NSAIDs Use (E+) | No NSAIDs Use (E−) |
|---|---|---|
| Cases | [A] | [B] |
| Controls | [C] | [D] |

NSAIDs, nonsteroidal anti-inflammatory drugs.

2. Given the study design, name and calculate the appropriate measure of association.

Let's assume that the previously noted data demonstrate the true (i.e., unbiased) association between NSAIDs use and drug-induced liver toxicity. Suppose that the researchers had no difficulties recruiting controls but were unable to recruit one-third of all eligible cases included in the table you completed in Question #1.

3. Fill in **Table 10.6** with the data that would result under this scenario (rounding to the nearest whole number).

TABLE 10.6 **CASE-CONTROL STUDY OF NSAIDS USE AND DRUG INDUCED LIVER TOXICITY (EXCLUDING ONE-THIRD OF ALL ELIGIBLE CASES)**

|  | NSAIDs Use (E+) | No NSAIDs Use (E−) |
|---|---|---|
| Cases | [a] | [b] |
| Controls | [c] | [d] |

NSAIDs, nonsteroidal anti-inflammatory drugs.

4. Calculate the measure of association reflecting this difficulty in recruiting cases.

5. Compared to the unbiased measure of association, is the measure of association reflecting the difficulty in recruiting cases biased? Explain how you determined whether this measure of association was biased.

Now suppose that people who experience drug-induced liver toxicity and *do* take NSAIDs are more likely to die than people who experience drug-induced liver toxicity and *do not* take NSAIDs.

6. What type of selection bias does this scenario describe?

7. What is the likely direction of bias for this scenario? Explain your answer.

Suppose that, due to concerns about survival bias affecting case-control studies, researchers instead conducted a cohort study to explore the association between NSAIDs use and drug-induced liver toxicity.

8. Given this study design, what is the main source of selection bias?

The tables that follow include the unbiased data from the source population as well as the data from the sample population of individuals who were recruited into a cohort study of NSAIDs and drug-induced liver toxicity (**Tables 10.7** and **10.8**, respectively).

**TABLE 10.7 COHORT STUDY OF NSAIDS USE AND DRUG INDUCED LIVER TOXICITY (SOURCE POPULATION)**

|  | NSAIDs Use (E+) | No NSAIDs Use (E−) |
|---|---|---|
| Drug-induced liver toxicity (O+) | 500 | 1,500 |
| No drug-induced liver toxicity (O−) | 2,000 | 15,000 |

NSAIDs, nonsteroidal anti-inflammatory drugs.

**TABLE 10.8 COHORT STUDY OF NSAIDS USE AND DRUG INDUCED LIVER TOXICITY (SAMPLE POPULATION)**

|  | NSAIDs Use (E+) | No NSAIDs Use (E-) |
|---|---|---|
| Drug-induced liver toxicity (O+) | 300 | 1,500 |
| No drug-induced liver toxicity (O−) | 1,800 | 15,000 |

NSAIDs, nonsteroidal anti-inflammatory drugs.

9. What are the selection probabilities?

10. Calculate the measures of association for the source and sample populations. Is there evidence of selection bias? If so, what is the direction?

11. Describe a hypothetical scenario relevant for a cohort study that may have led to the observed selection probabilities.

A type of selection bias called Berkson's bias can occur in studies if participants are selected from healthcare facilities, and people with *both* the exposure and outcome are more likely to attend those facilities than people with only the exposure or only the outcome. For example, researchers are exploring the association between diabetes and liver disease, and they recruit participants for a case-control study from hospitals. Assume that people with *both* diabetes and liver disease are more likely to be hospitalized (and thus selected into our study) relative to individuals who only have diabetes or only have liver disease.

12. How would this scenario affect the measure of association? Would the measure of association be biased?

Consider this quote: *"Women are more likely than men to respond to research inquiries, just as individuals with a higher socioeconomic status, a higher education, and a current employment. On the other hand, there is no such clear trend for age and ethnicity"* (p. 2).[22]

13. Does this quote describe the concept of selection bias or generalizability? How do you know?

## REFERENCES

1. Mattson CL, Tanz LJ, Quinn K, Kariisa M, Patel P, Davis NL. Trends and geographic patterns in drug and synthetic opioid overdose deaths—United States, 2013–2019. *MMWR Morb Mortal Wkly Rep*. 2021;70(6):202–207. https://doi.org/10.15585/mmwr.mm7006a4

2. Centers for Disease Control and Prevention. Understanding the opioid overdose epidemic. 2021. https://www.cdc.gov/opioids/basics/epidemic.html

3. Haffajee R, Mello MM. Drug Companies' liability for the opioid epidemic. *N Engl J Med*. 2017; 377(24):2301–2305. https://www.ncbi.nlm.nih.gov/pmc/articles/PMC7479783/

4. Zeng L, Li J, Crawford FW. Empirical evidence of recruitment bias in a network study of people who inject drugs. *Am J Drug Alcohol Abuse*. 2019;45(5):460–469. https://doi.org/10.1080/00952990 .2019.1584203

5. Campbell G, Hall W, Nielsen S. What does the ecological and epidemiological evidence indicate about the potential for cannabinoids to reduce opioid use and harms? A comprehensive review. *Int Rev Psychiatry*. 2018;30(5):91–106. https://doi.org/10.1080/09540261.2018.1509842

6. Shah A, Hayes CJ, Lakkad M, Martin BC. Impact of medical marijuana legalization on opioid use, chronic opioid use, and high-risk opioid use. *J Gen Intern Med*. 2019;34(8):1419–1426. https://doi .org/10.1007/s11606-018-4782-2

7. Alpren C, Dawson EL, John B, et al. Opioid use fueling HIV transmission in an urban setting: an outbreak of HIV infection among people who inject drugs-Massachusetts, 2015–2018. *Am J Public Health*. 2020;110(1):37–44. https://doi.org/10.2105/AJPH.2019.305366

8. Compton WM, Valentino RJ, DuPont RL. Polysubstance use in the U.S. opioid crisis. *Mol Psychiatry*. 2021;26(1):41–50. https://doi.org/10.1038/s41380-020-00949-3

9. Barocas JA, Wang J, Marshall BDL, et al. Sociodemographic factors and social determinants associated with toxicology confirmed polysubstance opioid-related deaths. *Drug Alcohol Depend*. 2019;200:59–63. https://doi.org/10.1016/j.drugalcdep.2019.03.014

10. Osborne V. Impact of survival bias on opioid-related outcomes when using death as an exclusion criterion. *Pharmacoepidemiol Drug Saf*. 2016;25(4):476. https://doi.org/10.1002/pds.3957

11. Berkson J. Limitations of the application of fourfold table analysis to hospital data. *Biometrics*. 1946;2(3):47–53. https://doi.org/10.2307/3002000

12. Westreich D. Berkson's bias, selection bias, and missing data. *Epidemiology*. 2012;23(1):159–164. https://doi.org/10.1097/EDE.0b013e31823b6296

13. Harvard T. H. Chan School of Public Health. The nutrition source: nurses' health studies. 2022. https://www.hsph.harvard.edu/nutritionsource/nurses-health-study

14. Napper LE, Fisher DG, Johnson ME, Wood MM. The reliability and validity of drug users' self reports of amphetamine use among primarily heroin and cocaine users. *Addict Behav*. 2010;35(4):350–354. https://doi.org/10.1016/j.addbeh.2009.12.006

15. Lind LH, Schober MF, Conrad FG, Reichert H. Why do survey respondents disclose more when computers ask the questions? *Public Opin Q*. 2013;77(4):888–935. https://doi.org/10.1093/poq/nft038

16. Mansournia MA, Altman DG. Inverse probability weighting. *BMJ*. 2016;352:i189. https://doi.org /10.1136/bmj.i189

17. Sterne JAC, White IR, Carlin JB, et al. Multiple imputation for missing data in epidemiological and clinical research: potential and pitfalls. *BMJ*. 2009;338:b2393. https://doi.org/10.1136/bmj.b2393

18. Mahmood SS, Levy D, Vasan RS, Wang TJ. The Framingham Heart Study and the epidemiology of cardiovascular disease: a historical perspective. *Lancet*. 2014;383(9921):999–1008. https://doi .org/10.1016/S0140-6736(13)61752-3

19. Centers for Disease Control and Prevention. About opioid use during pregnancy. 2021. https://www .cdc.gov/pregnancy/opioids/basics.html

20. Zedler BK, Mann AL, Kim MM, et al. Buprenorphine compared with methadone to treat pregnant women with opioid use disorder: a systematic review and meta-analysis of safety in the mother, fetus and child. *Addiction*. 2016;111(12):2115–2128. https://doi.org/10.1111/add.13462

21. Nonsteroidal Antiinflammatory Drugs. In: LiverTox: clinical and research information on drug-induced liver injury [Internet]. National Institute of Diabetes and Digestive and Kidney Diseases. Updated March 18, 2020. https://www.ncbi.nlm.nih.gov/books/NBK548614

22. Aigner A, Grittner U, Becher H. Bias due to differential participation in case-control studies and review of available approaches for adjustment. *PloS ONE*. 2018;13(1):e0191327. https://doi.org /10.1371/journal.pone.0191327

# CHAPTER 11

# INFORMATION BIAS AND SCREENING AND DIAGNOSTIC TESTS

## KEY TERMS

| | | |
|---|---|---|
| bias | measurement error | screening tests |
| diagnostic tests | misclassification | sensitivity |
| differential misclassification | negative predictive value | specificity |
| information bias | nondifferential | systematic error |
| interrater reliability | positive predictive value | |

## LEARNING OBJECTIVES

11.1 Define information bias.

11.2 Understand the common sources of information bias.

11.3 Distinguish between nondifferential and differential misclassification.

11.4 Calculate and interpret the sensitivity and specificity of the classification of exposures and outcomes.

11.5 Identify strategies for correcting information bias analytically.

11.6 Identify strategies for reducing information bias during the study design stage.

11.7 Differentiate between screening and diagnostic testing.

11.8 Calculate and interpret the sensitivity, specificity, positive predictive value, and negative predictive value of screening and diagnostic tests.

11.9 Understand considerations when deciding whether to implement a screening program.

11.10 Define and quantify the interrater reliability of screening and diagnostic tests.

# THE IMPACT OF MEDICAL ERRORS ON HEALTH IN THE UNITED STATES

Medical errors, generally defined as errors related to medical diagnoses, medication prescriptions, or other treatment decisions, are no minor issue. A review of 25 years of diagnosis-related malpractice claims in the United States found that diagnostic errors were the most common reason for claims, with the most common health outcomes after such errors being death and significant permanent injury.[1] Perhaps shockingly, a 2016 publication estimated that medical errors in the United States account for over a quarter of a million deaths annually, which would make medical errors the third leading cause of death (after heart disease and cancers) in the United States.[2] It has also been reported that medical errors in the United States are much higher than in other high-income countries (including Canada, Australia, New Zealand, Germany, and the United Kingdom).[3]

A recent example from 2022 came from the U.S. state of Nevada where state and local health officials contracted with a COVID-19 testing laboratory that failed to detect 96% of positive cases on a university campus using polymerase chain reaction (PCR) tests (PCR testing is considered the **gold standard**, meaning most definitive, COVID-19 testing method available). These errors resulted in people with COVID-19 going back to school and into their communities without knowing that they were infected.[4] As of this writing, there is an ongoing investigation into this public health failure.

Throughout this chapter, we will explore various sources and effects of **information bias**, which is bias that results from the incorrect measurement of exposure and/or outcome data. We will draw on studies that we have already discussed in this textbook as well as some new examples. As you read, we urge you to think not only about the impact of information bias on the internal validity of epidemiologic study results, but also the impact on people's lives due to, for example, misdiagnoses and subsequent incorrect patient management.

## INTRODUCTION TO INFORMATION BIAS (LEARNING OBJECTIVE 11.1)

As you've likely gathered, epidemiology relies heavily on measurement—measurement of exposures, outcomes, confounders, effect modifiers, and other variables. But what happens when we measure these variables incorrectly? This chapter explores why that might happen, and what we can do to either prevent or correct these errors.

### FIGURE 11.1 DEFINITION AND POTENTIAL SOURCES OF INFORMATION BIAS

Information bias occurs when...

there is error in the measurement of the exposure or outcome...

that leads to a measure of association that is meaningfully different from what would have been obtained if all variables had been measured correctly.

Potential sources of information bias

- Faulty measurement devices
- Poorly written questionnaires
- Incorrect self-report
- Data entry errors

**Information bias** occurs when there is error in the measurement of the exposure or outcome that leads to a measure of association that is meaningfully different from what would have been obtained if all variables had been measured correctly. **Figure 11.1** summarizes information bias and includes details that will be discussed in this chapter. Before we proceed, a quick note on terminology is helpful: information bias is often referred to as **measurement error**. When *categorical variables* are measured incorrectly, information bias is also referred to as **misclassification**, which leads us to place people into the incorrect cells of our R×C (row by column) tables.

In this chapter, you will learn about why information bias occurs, different types of information bias, and what can be done to address information bias. You will also learn about information bias as applied to medical screening and diagnostic testing, a topic that has large public health implications for almost everyone's lives.

# SOURCES OF INFORMATION BIAS
## (LEARNING OBJECTIVE 11.2)

Why might we measure our exposures and/or our outcomes of interest incorrectly? While not an exhaustive compendium, several common sources of information bias are detailed in the text that follows. A given study may be affected by one or multiple sources of information bias, and each source can affect measurement of the exposure, outcome, or both. It is additionally possible to misclassify other variables such as confounders or effect modifiers, which can also **bias** the measure(s) of association. Although a discussion of such misclassification is beyond the scope of this textbook, we will focus on how information bias affects the exposure and/or the outcome.

**Incorrect measurement devices or laboratory assays.** If your exposure and/or outcome of interest are measured using a device or laboratory assay, it is possible for those tools to yield incorrect results. For example, if study participants' weight was an exposure of interest, you would likely decide to weigh participants using a scale. If the scale were incorrectly calibrated, then your study team would incorrectly measure everyone's weight. Thus, weight would be subject to measurement error.

Another example that received attention during the COVID-19 pandemic is the finding that pulse oximetry measurements are systematically more likely to miss suboptimal levels of oxygen in the arteries in Black versus White patients. In one study, Black patients had roughly three times the incidence of occult hypoxemia (meaning undetected hypoxemia, defined as having a pulse oximetry reading greater than 92% despite an arterial blood oxygen saturation less than 88%) using pulse oximetry compared to their White counterparts.[5] Overestimation of blood oxygen levels by the most common pulse oximeters in use at the time were not tested on darker skin during development, and have subsequently been associated with overestimation of blood oxygen levels in persons with darker skin. The authors concluded: *"Given the widespread use of pulse oximetry for medical decision making, these findings have some major implications, especially during the current coronavirus disease 2019 (COVID-19) pandemic. Our results suggest that reliance on pulse oximetry to triage patients and adjust supplemental oxygen levels may place Black patients at increased risk for hypoxemia"* (p. 2478).[5]

Measurement devices or laboratory tests may also yield incorrect findings because the disease under study is subclinical. For example, certain laboratory tests may miss some subclinical disease. These **false negative** findings can contribute to worsening health outcomes if individuals who have a disease do not receive the care and treatment that they need. In the case of infectious diseases, false negative results can lead to uncontrolled transmission since those who are infected have not received information about treatment and self-isolation.

**Incorrect self-reported data.** Errors can arise when epidemiologists rely on study participants to provide information about their exposures and/or health outcomes. Broadly, these fall into two main categories: problems with the data collection instrument and participant barriers.

**Problems With the Data Collection Instrument.** Poorly constructed survey or interview questions (for example, those that use technical medical jargon, ambiguous language, or are not understood by participants) may prevent study participants from understanding the meaning of the questions posed. For example a UK survey on family planning[6] asked the question, *"Has it happened to you that over a long period of time, when you neither practiced abstinence, nor used birth control, you did not conceive?"* This question is complicated, and the time period is ambiguous. Both of these things could lead respondents to misinterpret the question and provide inconsistent answers.

**Participant Barriers.** Another source of information bias when using self-reported data can occur even with well-designed study or interview questions. **Recall bias** is a type of information bias that occurs when participants cannot remember certain behaviors or health information that occurred in the past. Additionally, participants with low health literacy, language barriers, or mental health concerns may struggle to accurately report the requested information. Finally, stigmatized behaviors or health outcomes may be intentionally misreported to investigators, especially when data are collected by human interviewers rather than computerized surveys; this is sometimes called **social desirability bias**. For example, heavy alcohol use and illicit drug use are often underreported in surveys due to the stigma associated with these behaviors.[7,8]

**Investigator error.** When investigators are collecting study data, they may draw incorrect conclusions about participant exposure and/or outcome status. This type of bias is also called **observer bias** and can occur due to fatigue, lack of time, limited knowledge, preconceptions, biases, beliefs, or preferences of the study investigators. For example, clinicians may have preconceived notions about a patient leading to inaccurate diagnoses, or investigators might influence participants' responses by their tone of voice or use of leading phrases. For example, in a study assessing sexual risk behaviors among both sex workers and married persons, information bias would likely occur if surveyors only asked sex workers about their number of sex partners while inputting "1" sexual partner for married persons rather than asking the question. In this example, the investigators' preconceived notions about the sexual behaviors of sex workers versus married persons would lead to collection of incorrect data. There are other examples of surveyors (and medical providers) assuming information about people based on characteristics such as race/ethnicity, sex, gender, weight, and occupation, which can lead to incorrect data collection or even decision-making.[9]

**Data management error.** Information bias can occur because of incorrect entry or coding of the exposure and/or outcome data. Data entry errors can occur because, for example, data entry personnel may not correctly interpret handwritten chart notes or simply due to incorrect keystrokes.

## Is Information Bias Affected by Sample Size?

It is good to remember that information bias, as with all **systematic error**, is *not* affected by sample size. Take the example of the miscalibrated scale used to measure study participant weight. If we are systematically incorrectly weighing our study participants, then enrolling more participants will not correct this error—in fact, we will just incorrectly weigh more people!

## Sources of Information Bias

As we learned in **Chapter 6, "Case-Control Designs,"** little is known about the causes of stillbirth.[2] To help address this gap, one study in the United States enrolled a group of individuals who experienced a stillbirth and a separate group whose babies were born alive. In this study, investigators interviewed women to determine whether there were any factors (including maternal age, maternal blood type, maternal education, previous pregnancy losses at less than 20 weeks' gestation, diabetes, obesity/overweight, smoking in the 3 months prior to pregnancy, alcohol consumption in the 3 months prior to pregnancy, history of drug addiction, history of infectious diseases, whether the pregnancy was unwanted) that were associated with stillbirth.[10]

1. Which of the listed questionnaire items might be subject to information bias and why?
2. Do you think investigator bias might influence the study results? Why or why not?
3. Do you think stillbirth is likely to be misclassified? Why or why not?

## Definition and Sources of Information Bias

- **Information bias** is occurs when there is error in the measurement of the exposure or outcome that leads to a measure of association that is meaningfully different from what would have been obtained if all variables had been measured correctly.
  - Information bias is also called **measurement error**.
  - Inaccurate measurement of categorical variables is called **misclassification**.
  - Confounders and effect measure modifiers may also be misclassified, which can lead to information bias.
- Common sources of information bias include:
  - Incorrect measurement devices or laboratory assays
  - Incorrect self-reported data:
    - problems with the data collection instrument
    - participant barriers
  - Investigator error
  - Data management error
- Information bias is not affected by sample size.

## THE IMPACT OF MISCLASSIFICATION ON R×C TABLES

Now that we have discussed how information bias may occur, let's explore its impact on study results. As previously noted, the exposure, outcome, or both may be misclassified in a given study. For simplicity, we will explore the impact of misclassification on the exposure and outcome separately.

**Misclassification of the exposure.** A schematic illustrating misclassification of the exposure of smoking is shown in **Figure 11.2A.** The first panel in this figure shows a 2×2 table comprised of the true data in which exposure status is correctly classified. The second panel illustrates individuals who will be misclassified with respect to smoking status, perhaps due to a data entry error. Finally, the third panel shows a 2×2 table comprised of the misclassified data. Individuals with misclassified smoking status are shown in magenta. When the exposure was accurately measured, both the risk ratio and the risk difference indicate that smoking is a risk factor for the outcome (true risk ratio = 2.67, true risk difference = 0.42). However, when the exposure was misclassified, we see evidence of switchover bias where smoking now appears to be protective for the outcome (biased risk ratio = 0.67, biased risk difference = -0.17; **Figure 11.2B**).

## FIGURE 11.2A MISCLASSIFICATION OF THE EXPOSURE OF SMOKING

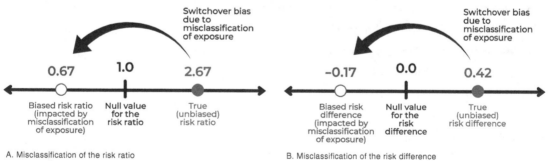

| Exposure Is Classified Correctly | Exposure Misclassification Occurs | Observed (Biased) Data With Exposure Misclassification |

True risk in exposed = 4/6 = 0.67
True risk in unexposed = 2/8 = 0.25

True (unbiased) risk ratio (RR)
= (4/6)/(2/8) = 2.67

True (unbiased) risk difference (RD)
= (4/6) – (2/8) = 0.42

Two smokers misclassified as nonsmokers.

Two nonsmokers misclassified as smokers.

Biased risk in exposed = 2/6 = 0.33
Biased risk in unexposed = 4/8 = 0.50

Biased risk ratio (RR)
= (2/6)/(4/8) = 0.67

Biased risk difference (RD)
= (2/6) – (4/8) = –0.17

## FIGURE 11.2B DIRECTION OF BIAS AFTER MISCLASSIFICATION OF THE EXPOSURE OF SMOKING ON THE RISK RATIO (A) AND RISK DIFFERENCE (B)

Switchover bias due to misclassification of exposure

0.67 — 1.0 — 2.67

Biased risk ratio (impacted by misclassification of exposure) | Null value for the risk ratio | True (unbiased) risk ratio

Switchover bias due to misclassification of exposure

–0.17 — 0.0 — 0.42

Biased risk difference (impacted by misclassification of exposure) | Null value for the risk difference | True (unbiased) risk difference

A. Misclassification of the risk ratio

B. Misclassification of the risk difference

*Note*: These figures are not drawn to scale.

**Misclassification of the outcome.** A schematic illustrating misclassification of the outcome of fever is shown in **Figure 11.3A**. The first panel in this figure shows a 2×2 table comprised of the true data in which outcome status is correctly classified. The second panel illustrates individuals who will be misclassified with respect to fever status perhaps due to a faulty measurement device. Finally, the third panel shows a 2×2 table comprised of the misclassified data. Individuals with misclassified fever status are shown in magenta. When the outcome was accurately measured, both the risk ratio and the risk difference indicate that the exposure is a risk factor for fever (true risk ratio = 2.00, true risk difference = 0.25). However, when the outcome was misclassified, we see that these associations are attenuated (i.e., there is evidence of bias toward the null). After misclassification of the outcome, the effect of the exposure on fever appears weaker than it really is (biased risk ratio = 1.33, biased risk difference = 0.17; **Figure 11.3B**).

## FIGURE 11.3A MISCLASSIFICATION OF THE OUTCOME OF FEVER

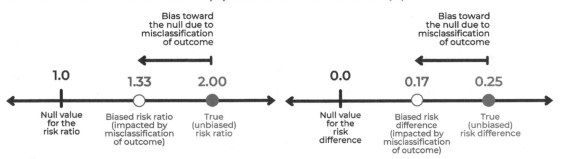

True risk in exposed = 3/6 = 0.50
True risk in unexposed = 2/8 = 0.25

True (unbiased) risk ratio (RR)
  = (3/6)/(2/8) = 2.00

True (unbiased) risk difference (RD)
  = (3/6) – (2/8) = 0.25

Everyone who has a fever is classified as having a fever.

However, three people without fever are misclassified as having a fever.

Biased risk in exposed = 4/6 = 0.67
Biased risk in unexposed = 4/8 = 0.50

Biased risk ratio (RR)
  = (4/6)/(4/8) = 1.33

Biased risk difference (RD)
  = (4/6) – (4/8) = 0.17

## FIGURE 11.3B DIRECTION OF BIAS AFTER MISCLASSIFICATION OF THE OUTCOME OF FEVER ON THE RISK RATIO (A) AND RISK DIFFERENCE (B)

Bias toward the null due to misclassification of outcome

1.0 — Null value for the risk ratio
1.33 — Biased risk ratio (impacted by misclassification of outcome)
2.00 — True (unbiased) risk ratio

Bias toward the null due to misclassification of outcome

0.0 — Null value for the risk difference
0.17 — Biased risk difference (impacted by misclassification of outcome)
0.25 — True (unbiased) risk difference

A. Misclassification of the risk ratio

B. Misclassification of the risk difference

*Note*: These figures are not drawn to scale.

**Misclassification of both the exposure and outcome.** Of course, it is possible to have misclassification of both the exposure and the outcome (and potentially other variables) at the same time. When there is only misclassification of the exposure, individuals are only moving between cells A and B and between cells C and D in a 2×2 table. Similarly, when there is only misclassification of the outcome, individuals are only moving between cells A and C and between cells B and D in a 2×2 table. When there is misclassification of both exposure and outcome, individuals can move from their true cell in an R×C table to any of the other cells.

## DIFFERENTIAL AND NONDIFFERENTIAL MISCLASSIFICATION
### (LEARNING OBJECTIVE 11.3)

Information bias can be broadly grouped into one of two categories: **nondifferential misclassification** and **differential misclassification**. These are defined in the text that follows and summarized in **Table 11.1**.

**TABLE 11.1 DIFFERENTIAL AND NONDIFFERENTIAL MISCLASSIFICATION OF THE EXPOSURE AND OUTCOME**

| | Exposure Misclassification | Outcome Misclassification |
|---|---|---|
| Nondifferential | Errors in exposure measurement are the same for O+ and O− | Errors in outcome measurement are the same for E+ and E− |
| Differential | Errors in exposure measurement are different for O+ and O− | Errors in outcome measurement are different for E+ and E− |

## Nondifferential Misclassification

**Nondifferential misclassification** occurs when the extent of misclassification of the exposure or outcome does *not* depend on the status of the other variable:

- **Nondifferential exposure misclassification** occurs when the exposure is misclassified, independent of outcome status. For example, in a case-control study of diabetes and dietary history, all study participants have similar difficulty accurately recalling their dietary history, regardless of their diabetes status. Thus, the extent of error in the reporting of dietary history is the same for those *with* diabetes as it is for those *without* diabetes.

- **Nondifferential outcome misclassification** occurs when the outcome is misclassified, independent of exposure status. For example, in a cohort study of COVID-19 vaccination and incident COVID-19 infection, a faulty COVID-19 diagnostic test was unknowingly used for all study participants, regardless of their COVID-19 vaccination status. Thus, the extent of error in identifying incident COVID-19 infections is the same for those who *received* a COVID-19 vaccine as it is for those who *did not receive* a COVID-19 vaccine.

## Differential Misclassification

**Differential misclassification** occurs when the extent of misclassification of the exposure or outcome *does* depend on the status of the other variable:

- **Differential exposure misclassification** occurs when the exposure is misclassified to a different degree for those who have the outcome than it is for those who do not have the outcome. For example, in a case-control study of diabetes and dietary history, we would expect differential exposure misclassification if only the cases (those with diabetes) had been taught to use food diaries to record dietary history. Thus, dietary history would likely be more accurately reported for the cases compared to the controls.

- **Differential outcome misclassification** occurs when the outcome is misclassified to a different degree for those who are exposed than it is for those who are not exposed. For example, in a cohort study of COVID-19 vaccination and incident COVID-19 infection, we would expect differential outcome misclassification if a faulty COVID-19 diagnostic test was only used among those who had received a COVID-19 vaccine. Thus, the identification of incident COVID-19 infections would be more likely to be inaccurate for those who had received a COVID-19 vaccine than it would be for those who had not.

If we can show quantitatively, as we will describe in the text that follows, or logically assume that any misclassification of binary exposure and outcome variables is **nondifferential**, then, in general, the resulting bias is *often* (though not always) toward the null.[11] If we can show quantitatively, as we will describe in the text that follows, or logically assume that any misclassification of the exposure or outcome is **differential**, then the direction of the resulting bias could be in any direction, even crossing the null.

## Highlights

### Differential and Nondifferential Misclassification of the Exposure and Outcome

- **Misclassification** of the exposure, outcome, or both, will affect the observed R×C table and thus the estimation of measures of frequency and association.
- **Nondifferential misclassification** occurs when the extent of misclassification of the exposure or outcome does *not* depend on the status of the other variable.
  - If misclassification of a binary exposure or outcome is **nondifferential**, then, in general, the resulting bias is *often* (though not always) toward the null.
- **Differential misclassification** occurs when the extent of misclassification of the exposure or outcome *does* depend on the status of the other variable.
  - If misclassification is **differential**, then the direction of the resulting bias could be in any direction, even crossing the null.

## QUANTIFYING INFORMATION BIAS (LEARNING OBJECTIVE 11.4)

The degree of misclassification, and whether misclassification is differential or nondifferential, can be explored using **misclassification tables**. Figure 11.4 shows two misclassification tables: an **exposure misclassification table** and an **outcome misclassification table**.

**FIGURE 11.4 EXPOSURE AND OUTCOME MISCLASSIFICATION TABLES**

**Exposure Misclassification Table**

| Classified | Truth*: E+ | Truth*: E− |
|---|---|---|
| E+ | True Positive | False ⚠ Positive |
| E− | False ⚠ Negative | True Negative |

**Outcome Misclassification Table**

| Classified | Truth*: O+ | Truth*: O− |
|---|---|---|
| O+ | True Positive | False ⚠ Positive |
| O− | False ⚠ Negative | True Negative |

⚠ The exposure (left) or outcome (right) status for individuals in these cells has been misclassified.

***Truth**: Reflects an individual's true exposure (left) or outcome (right) status.

Note that these misclassification tables are not oriented in the same way as the traditional 2×2 tables we have been using which show the allocation of *both* exposure and outcome within the same table. Misclassification tables orient the true data (meaning data that have not been misclassified and are not subject to any other sources of bias) in the columns and the data as classified (or misclassified!) in the rows. Using this orientation, the data that fall into cells A and D are correctly classified: these are **true positive** and **true negative** findings, respectively. Ideally, we would like all of our data to fall into these two cells. However, as we have seen, data may be misclassified. In these instances, individuals will fall into cells B or C: these are **false positive** and **false negative** findings, respectively.

Using the misclassification tables shown in Figure 11.4, we can quantify misclassification using measures of **sensitivity** and **specificity**. Sensitivity and specificity reflect the proportion of individuals who are correctly classified according to whether they truly have (sensitivity) or do not have (specificity) the attribute (exposure or outcome) under consideration.

**Sensitivity** is the proportion of those with the outcome or exposure who are correctly classified. Sensitivity can be reported as either a decimal or a percentage. The formula for sensitivity is shown in **Equation 11.1.**

$$\text{Sensitivity (Se)} = \frac{\text{True positives}}{\text{Total who truly have the attribute}}$$

$$= \frac{\text{True positives}}{\text{True positives + False negatives}} = \frac{A}{A+C} \tag{11.1}$$

**Specificity** is the proportion of those without the outcome or exposure who are correctly classified. Specificity can be reported as either a decimal or a percentage. The formula for specificity is shown in **Equation 11.2.**

$$\text{Specificity (Sp)} = \frac{\text{True negatives}}{\text{Total who truly do not have the attribute}}$$

$$= \frac{\text{True negatives}}{\text{False positives + True negatives}} = \frac{D}{B+D} \tag{11.2}$$

Let's practice quantifying exposure misclassification using the data shown in **Figure 11.5.** What are the sensitivity and specificity of the classification of the exposure in this example?

## FIGURE 11.5 QUANTIFYING EXPOSURE MISCLASSIFICATION

⚠ The exposure status for individuals in these cells has been misclassified.

*****Truth**: Reflects an individual's true exposure status

$$\text{Sensitivity} = \frac{200}{200+15} = 0.93 = 93\% \qquad \text{Specificity} = \frac{500}{25+500} = 0.95 = 95\%$$

A sensitivity of 93% means that 93% of individuals who are *truly* exposed were *correctly classified* as being exposed. A specificity of 95% means that 95% of individuals who were *truly* unexposed were *correctly classified* as being unexposed. Since sensitivity and specificity can range from 0 to 1 (or 0% to 100%), we would say that these are relatively high values for both sensitivity and specificity, a signal that our exposure classification methodology is performing well.

There is a trade-off between sensitivity and specificity, and thus it is important to identify classification methods which optimally balance the two. In general, tests with higher sensitivity have lower specificity. This means that while they are good at identifying true cases of the outcome, they also incorrectly identify people as having the outcome when they truly don't (i.e., there may be many false positives). For example, some screening tests for cancer such as mammograms have this profile where a proportion of women who do not truly have breast cancer have a positive mammogram and are referred for further testing. Conversely, in general, tests with high specificity generally have lower sensitivity. This means that while they have a lower probability of detecting false positive cases, they may miss many true positive cases. For example, use of pulse oximetry to detect hypoxemia in Black patients has this profile where a proportion of Black patients who truly do have hypoxia are not identified.

## Pause to Practice 11.2

### Quantifying Outcome Misclassification

In **Chapter 2, "Descriptive Epidemiology, Surveillance, and Measures of Frequency,"** we discussed how some gold standard (meaning the best available) laboratory diagnostics may not be available in certain settings due to limited resources or logistical constraints. For example, in much of sub-Saharan Africa, molecular testing (a highly sensitive and specific method) for diagnosis of sexually transmitted infections (STIs) is not currently available in many government-run health facilities. For this reason, STI cases are commonly classified syndromically (i.e., using clinical signs and symptoms, with no laboratory diagnostics), which is not as accurate as molecular testing.[12]

Between 2016 and 2019, the Rwanda Zambia Health Research Group conducted a study among symptomatic Rwandan women where they compared the classification of *Neisseria gonorrhoeae* and *Chlamydia trachomatis* using an evidence-based risk algorithm compared to the gold standard PCR molecular testing.[13] The study findings are shown in **Figure 11.6**. The evidence-based algorithm classified women as having *C. trachomatis* or *N. gonorrhoeae* if they had five or more risk factors such as being aged 25 years or younger, having no/primary education, not having full-time employment, and using condoms only sometimes.

### FIGURE 11.6 QUANTIFYING MISCLASSIFICATION OF CHLAMYDIA AND GONORRHOEAE

|  |  | Diagnosed with CT or NG by PCR (gold standard) | |
|  |  | CT/NG+ | CT/NG− |
| Classification using the algorithm | CT/NG+ | 132 | 142 ⚠ |
|  | CT/NG− | 30 ⚠ | 164 |

⚠ The outcome status for individuals in these cells has been misclassified.

CT, *Chlamydia trachomatis*; NG, *Neisseria gonorrhoeae*; PCR, polymerase chain reaction.
*Source*: Wall KM, Nyombayire J, Parker R, et al. Developing and validating a risk algorithm to diagnose *Neisseria gonorrhoeae* and *Chlamydia trachomatis* in symptomatic Rwandan women. *BMC Infect Dis.* 2021;21(1):392. https://doi.org/10.1186/s12879-021-06073-z

1. Calculate the sensitivity of the risk algorithm compared to PCR.

2. Calculate the specificity of the risk algorithm compared to PCR.

3. Calculate the proportion of false negatives among those who truly had chlamydia or gonorrhea.

4. Calculate the proportion of false positives among those who truly had chlamydia or gonorrhea.

5. The sensitivity of the risk algorithm was relatively high. What does the value for its sensitivity mean in words?

6. The specificity of the risk algorithm was relatively low. What does the value for its specificity mean in words?

## USING MISCLASSIFICATION TABLES TO DETERMINE WHETHER MISCLASSIFICATION IS DIFFERENTIAL OR NONDIFFERENTIAL

We have seen how to use misclassification tables to quantify the extent of exposure or outcome misclassification in a study. Now let's consider how to use misclassification tables to determine whether misclassification is differential or nondifferential. The following steps outline one strategy you can use to make this determination. **Pause to Practice 11.3** will show you an example in which you apply these steps.

**Steps to determine whether outcome misclassification is differential or nondifferential**

1. Create two separate outcome misclassification tables, one for those who are exposed and one for those who are unexposed.

2. Calculate and compare the sensitivity and specificity of the outcome misclassification in each table.

  – Outcome misclassification is *nondifferential* if the two sensitivities *and* the two specificities are the same for the exposed and the unexposed tables.

  – Outcome misclassification is *differential* if the two sensitivities *and/or* the two specificities are different for the exposed and the unexposed tables.

**Steps to determine whether exposure misclassification is differential or nondifferential**

1. Create two separate exposure misclassification tables, one for those who have the outcome and one for those who do not have the outcome.

2. Calculate and compare the sensitivity and specificity of the exposure misclassification in each table.

  – Exposure misclassification is *nondifferential* if the two sensitivities *and* the two specificities are the same for both *those who have the outcome* and *those who do not have the outcome*.

  – Exposure misclassification is *differential* if the two sensitivities *and/or* the two specificities are different for *those who have the outcome* and *those who do not have the outcome*.

**Table 11.2** is an extension of **Table 11.1**, which summarizes these rules for determining whether misclassification is nondifferential or differential using data from misclassification tables and measures of sensitivity and specificity.

**TABLE 11.2 DETERMINING WHETHER MISCLASSIFICATION IS NONDIFFERENTIAL OR DIFFERENTIAL**

|  | Exposure Misclassification | Outcome Misclassification |
|---|---|---|
| Nondifferential | **Se** among O+ = **Se** among O−<br>**AND**<br>**Sp** among O+ = **Sp** among O− | **Se** among E+ = **Se** among E−<br>**AND**<br>**Sp** among E+ = **Sp** among E− |
| Differential | **Se** among O+ ≠ **Se** among O−<br>**AND/OR**<br>**Sp** among O+ ≠ **Sp** among O− | **Se** among E+ ≠ **Se** among E−<br>**AND/OR**<br>**Sp** among E+ ≠ **Sp** among E− |

Se, sensitivity; Sp, specificity.

### Pause to Practice 11.3

### Determining Whether Exposure Misclassification Is Differential or Nondifferential

In **Chapter 5, "Cohort Designs,"** we explored a hypothesis tested by the Health Professionals Follow-Up Study to determine whether higher (vs. lower) red meat consumption was associated with coronary heart disease (CHD) among men in the United States. To test this hypothesis, analyses were conducted among a subset of men enrolled in the study who did not have CHD at enrollment.[14] CHD was defined as acute nonfatal myocardial infarction or fatal CHD. Red meat consumption was self-reported by participants. This study found that there was a positive association between red meat consumption and CHD diagnoses, which strengthened as the frequency of red meat consumption increased.

In a publication of the study findings, the authors stated that "*Inevitable measurement error in dietary assessment leading to inaccurate assessment or misclassification bias, even though reduced by using the average of repeated assessments, would have tended to underestimate the true associations with red meat. Because our study design was prospective, any measurement error would likely be independent of the outcome and therefore would attenuate the observed associations toward the null*" (p. 7).[14]

1. Do you think the exposure is likely to be misclassified in this study?
2. Do you think the outcome is likely to be misclassified in this study?
3. Do you think that the exposure misclassification is likely to be differential or nondifferential? Provide a brief explanation to support your answer.

These authors did not have a gold standard measure of red meat consumption to compare with participant self-report. However, let's hypothetically assume that a subsequent study was conducted among a random sample of the larger cohort which used a newly developed biomarker to quantitatively assess red meat intake, and that this biomarker was the gold standard (interestingly, though not yet available as of the writing of this book, such biomarkers are in development).[15,16] To determine whether there is evidence of differential exposure misclassification, we will follow the previously listed steps using data from this hypothetical study, which are shown in **Figure 11.7**. This figure provides two separate exposure misclassification tables: one for those who develop CHD and one for those who do not develop CHD.

**FIGURE 11.7 USING MISCLASSIFICATION TABLES TO DETERMINE WHETHER EXPOSURE MISCLASSIFICATION IS NONDIFFERENTIAL OR DIFFERENTIAL**

**CHD+**

| Classified based on self-report | Red meat consumption determined by biomarker*: High red meat consumption | Red meat consumption determined by biomarker*: Low red meat consumption |
|---|---|---|
| High red meat consumption | 500 | 25 ⚠ |
| Low red meat consumption | 100 ⚠ | 500 |

**CHD−**

| Classified based on self-report | Red meat consumption determined by biomarker*: High red meat consumption | Red meat consumption determined by biomarker*: Low red meat consumption |
|---|---|---|
| High red meat consumption | 250 | 50 ⚠ |
| Low red meat consumption | 50 ⚠ | 1000 |

⚠ The exposure status for individuals in these cells has been misclassified.

*Hypothetical gold standard
CHD, coronary heart disease

4. Calculate and compare the sensitivity and specificity of exposure misclassification for those with the outcome versus those without the outcome.
5. Is there evidence of misclassification of the exposure? If so, is this misclassification differential or nondifferential?
6. Given your answer to Question 5, what is the expected direction of the bias?
7. Use the information from the misclassification tables to construct a new 2×2 table for the association between self-reported red meat consumption and CHD. To do

this, sum the data across the rows such that you ignore the biomarker classification. This table reflects the biased data since it is not obtained using the gold standard exposure assessment method. Using this table, calculate the biased measure of association observed in the study.

8. Now sum the data across the columns such that you ignore the self-reported classification. What was the true measure of association (assuming no other sources of bias)?

9. What is the direction of the bias?

## Misclassification Tables, Sensitivity, Specificity, and Differential and Nondifferential Misclassification

- Using misclassification tables, we can quantify exposure or outcome misclassification using measures of **sensitivity** and **specificity**.

  - **Sensitivity** is the proportion of those with the outcome or exposure who are correctly classified.

  - **Specificity** is the proportion of those without the outcome or exposure who are correctly classified.

- Whether misclassification is differential or nondifferential can be explored using misclassification tables.

  - Create two separate **misclassification tables**, stratified by the nonmisclassified variable.

  - Calculate and compare the sensitivity and specificity of the classification in each table.

  - Misclassification is **nondifferential** if the two sensitivities *and* the two specificities are the same in each table.

  - Misclassification is **differential** if the two sensitivities *and/or* the two specificities are different in each table.

## OPPORTUNITIES TO CORRECT INFORMATION BIAS ANALYTICALLY (LEARNING OBJECTIVE 11.5)

In this section, we will discuss how to attempt to *correct* information bias during the data analysis stage using estimates of sensitivity and specificity. In the next section, we will discuss how to *minimize* information bias during the study design stage. While it is preferable to minimize information bias during the study design stage, you may find that you need to correct for it after a study has taken place.

To analytically address information bias, you will need a measure of the sensitivity and specificity of the classification of the variables of interest. If you know or can estimate the sensitivity and specificity of the classification, then any bias introduced by misclassification can be corrected. There are some options for accomplishing this.

**Validation studies.** Investigators may conduct validation studies to determine the sensitivity and specificity of different types of variable classification methods. For example, a self-reported instrument may undergo (or have already undergone) validation by either comparing self-reported data to other sources such as laboratory data. As another example, laboratory analysis of urine, blood, and/or hair samples are common validation approaches for self-reported substance use (both prescribed and illicit drugs). Think about the previous hypothetical example of applying biomarker validation to a random sample of participants in the cohort study to validate self-reported red meat intake. Though we used a hypothetical scenario and data, investigators are exploring biomarkers associated with consumption of animal protein from meats including various isotope ratios, anserine, carnosine, creatine, and creatinine, among others.[16] As another example, to validate self-reported sexual activity and condom usage, researchers have used detection of prostate-specific antigen which is transmitted through male ejaculate and can be detected in vaginal fluid with high sensitivity and specificity soon after unprotected sex.[17] When laboratory measures are not available, medical records, pharmacy prescription records, or reports from family or friends may be used to validate data. Importantly, when conducting validation studies, it is typically *not* necessary to perform validation on the entire sample, but rather just a random sample of the study population. This saves investigators both time and money and may also be preferred when the validation procedure is more costly or painful for participants.

## Digging Deeper

### Correcting for Information Bias Using Data From a Validation Study

Let's consider the scenario in the previous **Pause to Practice 11.3** where we explored the association between red meat consumption and CHD among men in the United States. Assume that we conducted a cohort study and generated the data shown in **Figure 11.8**, which are biased due to exposure misclassification.

### FIGURE 11.8 STUDY DATA BIASED DUE TO MISCLASSIFICATION OF RED MEAT CONSUMPTION

|  | High red meat consumption (E+) | Low red meat consumption (E−) |
|---|---|---|
| **CHD+ (Outcome +)** | 525 | 600 |
| **CHD− (Outcome−)** | 300 | 1,050 |

CHD, coronary heart disease.

We then conducted a (relatively expensive) validation study using biomarkers of red meat consumption on a random 30% of the study population and calculated that the exposure was misclassified with 83% sensitivity and 95% specificity. Misclassification of the exposure was not associated with outcome status, meaning there is nondifferential misclassification of the exposure.

Let's see how we can use the sensitivity and specificity estimates from the validation study to correct the observed 2×2 table data, which is biased due to exposure misclassification. While deriving these formulae is beyond what students need to know at this level, the text that follows shows the formulae relating observed data to corrected data using sensitivities and specificities, where capital letters denote *corrected* cell counts and lowercase letters denote *classified* cell counts. Note that different formulae are needed for misclassification of the exposure (**Equation 11.3**) versus misclassification of the outcome (**Equation 11.4**).

### Correcting Nondifferential Exposure Misclassification (11.3)

$$A = \frac{a \times \text{Specificity} - b \times (1 - \text{Specificity})}{\text{Sensitivity} + \text{Specificity} - 1}$$

$$B = \frac{b \times \text{Sensitivity} - a \times (1 - \text{Sensitivity})}{\text{Sensitivity} + \text{Specificity} - 1}$$

$$C = \frac{c \times \text{Specificity} - d \times (1 - \text{Specificity})}{\text{Sensitivity} + \text{Specificity} - 1}$$

$$D = \frac{d \times \text{Sensitivity} - c \times (1 - \text{Sensitivity})}{\text{Sensitivity} + \text{Specificity} - 1}$$

### Correcting Nondifferential Outcome Misclassification (11.4)

$$A = \frac{a \times \text{Specificity} - c \times (1 - \text{Specificity})}{\text{Sensitivity} + \text{Specificity} - 1}$$

$$B = \frac{b \times \text{Specificity} - d \times (1 - \text{Specificity})}{\text{Sensitivity} + \text{Specificity} - 1}$$

$$C = \frac{c \times \text{Sensitivity} - a \times (1 - \text{Sensitivity})}{\text{Sensitivity} + \text{Specificity} - 1}$$

$$D = \frac{d \times \text{Sensitivity} - b \times (1 - \text{Sensitivity})}{\text{Sensitivity} + \text{Specificity} - 1}$$

1. Use the appropriate set of formulae to correct for the exposure misclassification in this example.
2. Calculate the corrected measure of association.
3. What is the direction of the bias?

Note that there are also formulae for correcting differential exposure and outcome misclassification, as well as simultaneous misclassification of both the exposure and outcome.[18]

---

**Sensitivity analyses.** In general, sensitivity analyses are defined as analyses in which investigators seek to understand how study findings may change under different sets of plausible assumptions. When we do not know the exact sensitivity and specificity nor do we have one "best guess," we can perform multiple corrections using a range of plausible sensitivity and specificity estimates using educated guesses for these values. We would repeat the type of analysis shown in **Digging Deeper, Correcting for Information Bias Using Data From a Validation Study,** multiple times using different sets of plausible sensitivities and specifies to learn how different sets of assumptions affect the results.

Recall from **Chapter 10, "Selection Bias,"** that we explored various research questions related to opioid use. One cross-sectional study evaluated the association between experiences of past year major depressive episodes and self-reported opioid use disorder.[19] In this study, investigators found an unadjusted prevalence odds ratio for the association between experiences of past year major depressive episodes and opioid use disorder of 5.4 (**Figure 11.9**). Information bias may be of concern in this study participants may underreport illicit drug use to study investigators due to concerns about legal repercussions as well as stigma, or they may misreport their drug use history due to recall bias.[20] Thus, in the observed data shown in **Figure 11.9**, the outcome is likely misclassified.

## FIGURE 11.9 OBSERVED DATA FROM A CROSS-SECTIONAL STUDY OF DEPRESSION AND OPIOID USE DISORDER

|  | Major depressive episode in the last year (E+) | No major depressive episode in the last year (E−) |
|---|---|---|
| **Opioid use disorder (O+)** | 1,416 | 3,679 |
| **No opioid use disorder (O−)** | 25,995 | 367,872 |

Prevalence odds ratio (POR)

$$= \frac{1{,}416 \times 367{,}872}{3{,}679 \times 25{,}995} = 5.4$$

*Source*: Ashrafioun L, Allan NP, Stecker TA. Opioid use disorder and its association with self-reported difficulties participating in social activities. *Am J Addict*. 2022;31(1):46–52. https://doi.org/10.1111/ajad.13220

While the investigators did not undertake a sensitivity analysis, they did note that "*Data were based on self-report, which are subject to memory and social desirability biases among other limitations*" (p. 51).[19] Other investigators who conducted validation studies comparing self-reported drug use with urine analyses found that the specificity of self-report was generally higher (often greater than 80%–90%) while the sensitivity was generally lower, as low as 40%.[21,22] This supports the notion that non-drug users are more likely to report their true behaviors, while some proportion of drug users are likely to underreport their drug use. **Figure 11.10** shows a hypothetical sensitivity analysis that could have been conducted to correct for possible nondifferential outcome misclassification in this study. We apply four different scenarios (i.e., assumed sensitivities and specificities based on findings from previous validation studies) to see how our observed data (shown in **Figure 11.9**) would change using the formulae for correcting for nondifferential outcome misclassification presented in **Digging Deeper, Correcting for Information Bias Using Data From a Validation Study**. Note the impact of the sensitivity analysis assumptions on the prevalence odds ratio, shown in the leftmost table of **Figure 11.10**. The observed prevalence odds ratio of 5.4 is closer to the null than the corrected prevalence odds ratios. Given these sensitivity analyses, we might conclude that the true association between experiences of past year major depressive episodes and self-reported opioid use disorder is stronger than what was observed in the cross-sectional study (i.e., the true prevalence odds ratio is likely to be greater than 5.4).

**FIGURE 11.10 HYPOTHETICAL SENSITIVITY ANALYSIS TO CORRECT FOR NONDIFFERENTIAL MISCLASSIFICATION OF THE OUTCOME OF OPIOID USE FROM A CROSS-SECTIONAL STUDY**

| Estimates of Outcome Misclassification | | Prevalence odds ratio (POR) corrected for misclassification of the outcome |
|---|---|---|
| Sensitivity | Specificity | |
| 0.40 | 1.00 | 5.84 |
| 0.55 | 1.00 | 5.65 |
| 0.65 | 1.00 | 5.58 |
| 0.75 | 1.00 | 5.53 |

**CORRECTED DATA**

*Sensitivity = 0.40, Specificity = 1.0*

| | Major depressive episode in the last year (E+) | No major depressive episode in the last year (E−) |
|---|---|---|
| Opioid use disorder (O+) | 3,540 $$= \frac{1{,}416 \times 1.0 - 25{,}995 \times (1 - 1.0)}{0.4 + 1.0 - 1}$$ | 9,197 $$= \frac{3{,}679 \times 1.0 - 367{,}872 \times (1 - 1.0)}{0.4 + 1.0 - 1}$$ |
| No opioid use disorder (O−) | 23,871 $$= \frac{25{,}995 \times 0.4 - 1{,}416 \times (1 - 0.4)}{0.4 + 1.0 - 1}$$ | 362,354 $$= \frac{367{,}872 \times 0.4 - 3{,}679 \times (1 - 0.4)}{0.4 + 1.0 - 1}$$ |

$$\text{Corrected POR}_{Se=0.40,\ Sp=1.0} = \frac{3{,}540 \times 362{,}354}{9{,}197 \times 23{,}871} = 5.84$$

# OPPORTUNITIES TO REDUCE INFORMATION BIAS IN THE STUDY DESIGN STAGE (LEARNING OBJECTIVE 11.6)

When designing an epidemiologic study, decisions can be made at the outset to attempt to reduce the likelihood for information bias. A brief overview of such strategies is described in the text that follows.

**Masking**. Preventing investigators from knowing participants' exposure or outcome status may reduce bias since it may be less likely for investigators' preconceived beliefs to influence their interactions with study participants or their assessment of study participant data. Masking participants from knowing their exposure status, which can potentially be achieved in an experimental study, may reduce bias since participants may be less likely to differentially report outcomes or adhere to study procedures.

**Use validated, ideally gold standard, exposure and outcome classification methods.** Whenever possible, use the most objective and accurate method for measurement of exposure and outcome that are feasible in your study.

**Support accurate self-report**. It is often the case that data must be self-reported. If collecting self-reported data, it is often preferred to use self-administered surveys like audio computer-assisted self-interviewing (ACASI), especially for sensitive or stigmatized questions,[20,23] as opposed to interviewer-administered surveys. Use of short, simple, unambiguous, nonleading survey questions without technical jargon is preferred.[24]

**Support accurate recall.** It is sometimes the case that self-reported data collection must rely on study participant recall. Use of memory aids or diaries and framing questions to use short recall periods (for example, asking participants about behaviors occurring during the past week instead of during the past year, which may be more difficult to remember) may support accurate recall.

**Use multiple, independent assessors.** Depending on the type of assessment tool, it may be possible to have multiple independent assessors review findings from data collection tools to adjudicate discrepant results. For example, if collecting data from MRI scans, two different radiologists could be trained to read the scans and discuss where their assessments disagreed.

**Plan and budget for validation studies.** In the study design stage, it may be prudent to plan and budget for validation studies using gold standard measurement tools among a random subset of study participants, if feasible.

## Highlights

### Correcting and Preventing Information Bias

- Investigators may attempt to correct information bias **during the data analysis stage** using estimates of sensitivity and specificity.
  - **Validation studies** may be used to determine the sensitivity and specificity of different measurement tools.
  - **Sensitivity analyses** may be used in which investigators make multiple corrections using a range of plausible estimates of sensitivity and specificity.
- Investigators may attempt to minimize information bias **during the study design stage** using:
  - Masking
  - Validated, ideally gold standard exposure and outcome assessment techniques

- Strategies to support accurate self-report
- Strategies to support accurate recall
- Multiple, independent assessors
- Validation studies

• While it is preferable to minimize information bias during the study design stage, you may find that you need to correct for it after a study has taken place.

## SCREENING AND DIAGNOSTIC TESTING (LEARNING OBJECTIVE 11.7)

One source of information bias that is relevant to almost everyone's lives is related to screening and diagnostic testing. The purpose of a medical test is to provide information that will alter subsequent diagnostic, treatment, or management plans and improve health outcomes. In a perfect world, tests would always be correct and have no negative effects. However, test results may be incorrect, which can lead to misdiagnosis and a potential cascade of other unintended consequences. As described at the beginning of this chapter medical errors can have major repercussions for patient health and healthcare costs. Let's begin by defining and differentiating screening tests from diagnostic tests.

**Screening tests** are often used in individuals who appear to be healthy but may be at-risk for a disease of interest, with the goal of classifying them with respect to their likelihood of having that disease. Screening tests are useful because they may detect the presence of a disease at an early stage (before symptoms begin), which can lead to earlier treatment and thereby reduce subsequent morbidity and mortality. Often, people with a positive screening test will undergo diagnostic testing.

**Diagnostic tests** are used in individuals with abnormal signs or symptoms (or individuals with a positive screening test) to either establish or rule out a disease which would then go on to be treated or managed.

The process by which individuals receive screening and/or diagnostic tests is shown in **Figure 11.11**. To quantify how well screening and diagnostic tests classify individuals on the basis of their outcome status, we calculate the sensitivity and specificity of the tests compared to a gold standard measure as we have done previously. In addition, there are two new measures used to describe the performance of screening and diagnostic tests in given populations: **positive predictive value** and **negative predictive value**. These metrics estimate the likelihood that someone actually has or does not have the outcome of interest given their test result.

## FIGURE 11.11 SCREENING AND DIAGNOSTIC TESTING PROCESS

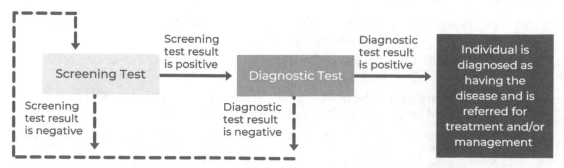

*Those with a negative screening or diagnostic test result may undergo screening testing again at a later time.*

**Positive predictive value (PPV)** is the proportion of those who test positive who truly *do* have the disease. PPV can be reported as either a decimal or a percentage. The formula for PPV is shown in **Equation 11.5**.

$$PPV = \frac{A}{A+B} = \frac{\text{True positives}}{\text{Total who test positive}} = \frac{\text{True positives}}{\text{True positives + False positives}} \tag{11.5}$$

**Negative predictive value (NPV)** is the proportion of those who test negative who truly *do not* have the disease. NPV can be reported as either a decimal or a percentage. The formula for NPV is shown in **Equation 11.6**.

$$NPV = \frac{D}{D+C} = \frac{\text{True negatives}}{\text{Total who test negative}} = \frac{\text{True negatives}}{\text{True negatives + False negatives}} \tag{11.6}$$

From a patient's point of view, the PPV and NPV may answer the first questions that come to mind after receiving the results of a test from their medical provider: *If the test is positive, how concerned should I be? What is the likelihood that I actually have this disease? Conversely, if the test is negative, how relieved should I be? What is the likelihood that I don't actually have this disease?*

## What Is the Gold Standard When Evaluating Screening Tests?

We need a measure of the "truth" to quantify the performance of a measurement tool. We previously defined the **gold standard** as the best classification method available. When assessing the performance of screening tests, the gold standard may be a more accurate (and sometimes more expensive or invasive) diagnostic test, or it might be the final consensus diagnosis based on the results from multiple diagnostic tests.

## Pause to Practice 11.4

### Quantifying the Performance of Screening and Diagnostic Testing for Breast Cancer
(LEARNING OBJECTIVE 11.8)

Breast cancer is the second most common type of cancer among American women,[25] and screening is recommended in the United States.[26] Screening asymptomatic women, typically with mammography, increases the likelihood of earlier detection and treatment to improve survival.[27] As of 2023, the United States Preventive Services Task Force (USPSTF) recommends that women aged 40 to 74 years receive a mammogram every 2 years.[26] Suppose investigators undertook a cross-sectional study whereby 1,000 women were screened for breast cancer using mammography. The mammography results are compared below to true cancer status. Results of the screening test are shown in the leftmost 2×2 table in **Figure 11.12** (phase 1).

1. Calculate and interpret the sensitivity of screening mammography.
2. Calculate and interpret the specificity of screening mammography.
3. Calculate and interpret the PPV of screening mammography.
4. Calculate and interpret the NPV of screening mammography.

Though these are hypothetical 2×2 table data, a systematic review that generated evidence for the USPSTF found that, over a 1-year screening interval among U.S. women aged 40 to 74 years, first screening mammography has sensitivity, specificity, PPV, and NPV estimates that generally correspond to the estimates found here.[28]

## FIGURE 11.12 QUANTIFYING THE PERFORMANCE OF SCREENING AND DIAGNOSTIC TESTING FOR BREAST CANCER

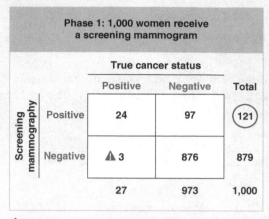

▲ Breast cancer cases missed by mammography (n = 3) and core needle biopsy (n = 2).

▲ Erroneously identified breast cancer after undergoing both screening and diagnostic testing (n = 3).

In this example, 121 women (24 + 97) had a positive screening mammogram result. These women were then referred for core needle biopsy followed by histopathology, which is a common diagnostic test if breast cancer is suspected.[29] Hypothetical results comparing core needle biopsy to true cancer status are shown in the rightmost 2×2 table in Figure 11.12 (phase 2). The following questions pertain to the assessment of the performance of core needle biopsy relative to true cancer status.

5. Calculate and interpret the sensitivity of core needle biopsy.
6. Calculate and interpret the specificity of core needle biopsy.
7. Calculate and interpret the PPV of core needle biopsy.
8. Calculate and interpret the NPV of core needle biopsy.

Though these are hypothetical data, these values for the performance of core needle biopsy compared to true cancer status are also reasonable based on prior studies.[30-32]

## The Trade-Off Between Sensitivity and Specificity

We previously noted that there is a trade-off between sensitivity and specificity. Deciding which is more important depends on the specific situation. For example, when measuring a disease that is fatal and for which treatment of individuals who truly do not have the outcome is not harmful, we may prioritize having high sensitivity to avoid missing many cases (i.e., we prefer to have a low proportion of false negative findings). In contrast, when measuring a disease that is not fatal nor associated with severe morbidity, but for which treatment of individuals who truly don't have the outcome is harmful, we may prioritize having high specificity to avoid misdiagnosing many people without disease (i.e., we prefer to have a low proportion of false positive findings).

Let's now consider what happened as this population of 1,000 women progressed through the process of both screening (mammography) and diagnostic (core needle biopsy) testing (Figure 11.13). The initial probability of breast cancer in the population of 1,000 women who underwent screening was just 3% ([24 + 3]/1,000). In addition, 121 of the 1,000 women who had a positive mammography screening test were then sent for core needle biopsy. The

## FIGURE 11.13 THE SCREENING (MAMMOGRAPHY) AND DIAGNOSTIC (CORE NEEDLE BIOPSY) TESTING PROCESS FOR A POPULATION OF 1,000 WOMEN

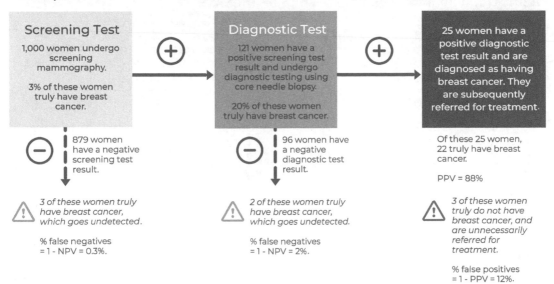

NPV, negative predictive value; PPV, positive predictive value.

probability of breast cancer among these 121 women was much higher, at 20% ([22 + 2]/121). Of the 121 women who had a positive core needle biopsy, 88% (PPV) truly had breast cancer. Of the 121 women who had a negative core needle biopsy, 98% (NPV) truly did not have breast cancer. This means that only 2% (1 – NPV) of those who received a negative core needle biopsy test actually had breast cancer. **Figure 11.13** illustrates how the purpose of screening and diagnostic testing is to provide information to inform subsequent diagnostic, treatment, or management plans and improve health outcomes.

While sensitivity and specificity are descriptions of the accuracy of a test, PPV and NPV provide information about the probability of disease given either a positive or negative test result. Sensitivity and specificity are attributes of the tests themselves and are not impacted by the prevalence of the disease in the population. PPV and NPV, on the other hand, are dependent not only upon test sensitivity and specificity, but they also change depending on the prevalence of the disease in a population. As the prevalence of disease increases, positive test results are more likely to be predictive of having the outcome (i.e., PPV increases); however, as the prevalence of disease increases, negative test results are not as informative for ruling out disease (i.e., NPV decreases).

## The Dependence of Positive Predictive Value and Negative Predictive Value on the Prevalence of Disease

The performance of a test as measured by its PPV and NPV is determined by its sensitivity and specificity, as well as the prevalence of the disease in the population under study. Specifically, the PPV increases as the prevalence of disease in the population *increases*. In contrast, the NPV increases as the prevalence of disease in the population *decreases*.

Let's consider the example of screening for breast cancer in women of different ages. We know that the prevalence of breast cancer increases with increasing age,[33] and we can show how this impacts both PPV and NPV. Consider **Figure 11.14**, which shows two 2×2 tables comparing the performance of mammography (a screening tool) versus true cancer status. The table on the left is data we have already seen and is comprised of women of eligible screening ages 40 to 74 (Group 1). The table on the right is a subset of those women who are aged 64 to 74 years (Group 2).

## FIGURE 11.14 THE DEPENDENCE OF POSITIVE PREDICTIVE VALUE AND NEGATIVE PREDICTIVE VALUE ON THE PREVALENCE OF DISEASE

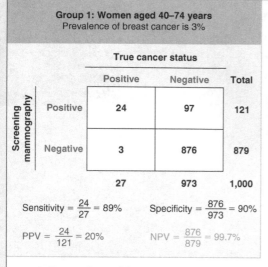

As the prevalence of the outcome in the population increases, **positive predictive value (PPV) increases** and negative predictive value (NPV) decreases. However, both **sensitivity and specificity remain the same**.

NPV, negative predictive value; PPV, positive predictive value.

The prevalence of breast cancer is lower in the 2×2 table on the left ([24 + 3]/1,000 = 3%), which is comprised of women aged 40 to 74 years, compared to the 2×2 table on the right ([16 + 2]/58 = 31%), which is comprised of women aged 64 to 74 years.

Notice that the sensitivity and specificity, which are fixed characteristics of the testing method, do not change as the prevalence of the disease changes. However, the PPV increases from 20% to 80% and the NPV decreases from 99.7% to 95% as the prevalence of breast cancer increases from 3% to 31%.

Given that positive test results are more likely to be true when the prevalence of disease is higher, public health officials may decide to allocate tests to populations known to be at greater risk for the disease. This may be an important strategy when affordability or feasibility of the test is limited, for example, as may occur in some low resource settings or when the tests themselves are very expensive or in short supply.

## Highlights

### Screening and Diagnostic Testing

- **Screening tests** are often used in individuals who appear to be healthy but may be at-risk of disease to identify or rule out the possibility of disease.

- **Diagnostic tests** are used in individuals with abnormal signs or symptoms (or individuals with a positive screening test) to either establish or rule out a disease which would then go on to be treated or managed.

- Test performance is quantified using measures of sensitivity, specificity, PPV, and NPV.
  - **Sensitivity** and **specificity** describe how well a test correctly classifies those who truly have or truly do not have the disease, respectively, and are not impacted by the prevalence of the disease in the population.

- **Predictive values** are dependent upon test sensitivity and specificity, as well as the prevalence of the disease in the population, and provide information about how likely it is that an individual has the disease given that they have a positive or negative test result.

  - **Positive Predictive Value (PPV)** is the proportion of those who test positive who truly *do* have disease.

  - **Negative Predictive Value (NPV)** is the proportion of those who test negative who truly *do not* have disease.

  - As the prevalence of disease increases in a population, PPV increases and NPV decreases. Similarly, as the prevalence of disease decreases in a population, PPV decreases and NPV increases.

## CONSIDERATIONS FOR SCREENING PROGRAMS (LEARNING OBJECTIVE 11.9)

The purpose of a screening test is to identify and address disease earlier, before symptoms even occur, therefore leading to better health outcomes. However, screening is not always appropriate, nor is it always beneficial. When should we screen for diseases? Some considerations that support screening include:

- The disease is serious (i.e., is associated with severe morbidity and/or mortality).

- The proportion of disease that is detectable by screening (before symptoms begin) is relatively high.

- Screening enables early identification of disease AND early treatment/management leads to better outcomes.

- Screening tests exist which are accurate (i.e., high sensitivity and specificity), reliable, affordable, straightforward to administer, and have few or acceptable side effects.

Breast cancer screening provides a good example for an instance where screening is recommended. Breast cancer is associated with severe morbidity and mortality, mammography screening can detect a considerable proportion of asymptomatic disease, earlier treatment leads to better health outcomes, and mammography has an acceptable profile relative to its side effects.[27,28]

The benefits of screening must be weighed against potential harms and limitations. When should we not screen for diseases? Some considerations that *do not* support screening include:

- Overdiagnosis and overtreatment may occur if a screening test leads to the identification of many asymptomatic cases that would have not required any intervention. For example, many gallstones remain asymptomatic and never require surgery.

- Undertreatment may occur if the screening test results in a high proportion of false negative findings. The seriousness of the consequences of false negative results should be considered.

- A screening test may cause physical and psychologic side effects. For example, it may be preferable to avoid radiation from x-rays or psychologic distress from false positive findings.

- Some screening tests may have high costs or be unaffordable.

- Ethical concerns include: Are screening tests widely available to everyone in the target population? Are adequate and timely diagnostic tests widely available for those to screen positive?

## Biases That Influence Screening Programs

**Self-selection bias.** The so-called "worried well" are individuals who may be more likely to participate in screening programs because they are health conscious and want as much information about their health status as possible. These may be people who are asymptomatic but are at higher risk for certain diseases (e.g., due to a family history of cancer). Such self-selection into a screening program may make the screening tool look better (especially in terms of PPV) than the program would in the general population because these people may be more likely to actually have the disease given their family history.

**Lead time bias (Figure 11.15).** We often define disease-specific survival as the time between diagnosis and death. If screening results in earlier diagnosis but not in decreased mortality (e.g., no gains in survival) relative to obtaining a diagnosis only after symptoms arise, there may be the false appearance of increased survival due to screening. In Figure 11.15, we consider what could happen to an individual with a disease of interest under two scenarios: the disease is detected using a screening test, and the disease is diagnosed only after symptoms have occurred. Regardless of whether the disease was detected with screening or after symptoms develop, the individual has the same time of death. What differs, though, is that the time from diagnosis to death is greater under the scenario where they have been diagnosed through screening because the disease was recognized earlier, thus giving the appearance that survival is longer. In reality, there was no difference in the individual's life span, it is just that their disease was identified earlier through screening.

## FIGURE 11.15 LEAD TIME BIAS

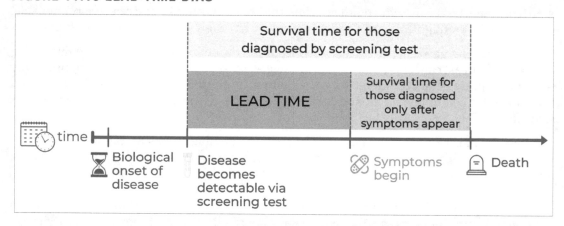

**Length time bias (Figure 11.16).** The length of time when disease is asymptomatic but detectable by screening can vary widely for different people with the same disease. Some people may have more aggressive diseases with a shorter asymptomatic and detectable phase and therefore have less of an opportunity to be detected via screening. These people are more likely to be detected after symptoms develop. Meanwhile, some people may have a very long asymptomatic but detectable phase and therefore have an increased opportunity for detection of more benign disease by screening. Thus, diseases detected by screening tend to be less aggressive and associated with better outcomes than more aggressive diseases detected after symptoms develop. This difference is due to the additional period during which screening programs are able to catch less aggressive diseases.

## FIGURE 11.16 LENGTH TIME BIAS

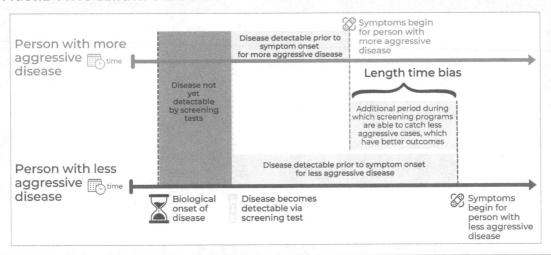

## Weighing Risks and Benefits: Screening for Breast Cancer

### Benefits

- Early identification of breast cancer can result in earlier treatment and improved survival.

### Risks

- False positive screening tests can lead to unnecessary diagnostic tests and treatments which may be costly, invasive, and cause psychologic stress.
- False negative test results may delay cancer identification and treatment.

### Benefit or Risk?

Some true positive screening tests will occur among individuals who will be told they have breast cancer earlier than they would have been told if diagnosed after symptoms develop, but with no subsequent prolonged survival (i.e., the lead time will not result in increased survival). This may cause unnecessary stress among some individuals. However, while someone's true survival might not be changed, by detecting their cancer earlier they have more opportunity to do things that they hope to do before they potentially become ill and die. A delayed diagnosis would shorten this period. Whether this is perceived as a benefit or risk would depend on the individual. It is worth noting, however, that an individual would only experience one of these scenarios, and it would be impossible to know how they would have felt about a counterfactual timing of diagnosis (i.e., earlier or later).

## INTERRATER RELIABILITY OF SCREENING AND DIAGNOSTIC TESTS (LEARNING OBJECTIVE 11.10)

To conclude this overview of screening and diagnostic testing, we will describe one common measure of **interrater reliability**, also called interobserver reliability, which considers the reproducibility of test results by two or more raters. For example, findings from two raters can be oriented as shown in **Figure 11.17** where findings from one rater are presented in the rows and those from the other rater are presented in the columns. In some instances, the raters will agree on the test results (cells A and D), while in other instances the raters will not agree on the test results (cells B and C).

## FIGURE 11.17 QUANTIFYING THE INTERRATER RELIABILITY OF SCREENING OR DIAGNOSTIC TESTS

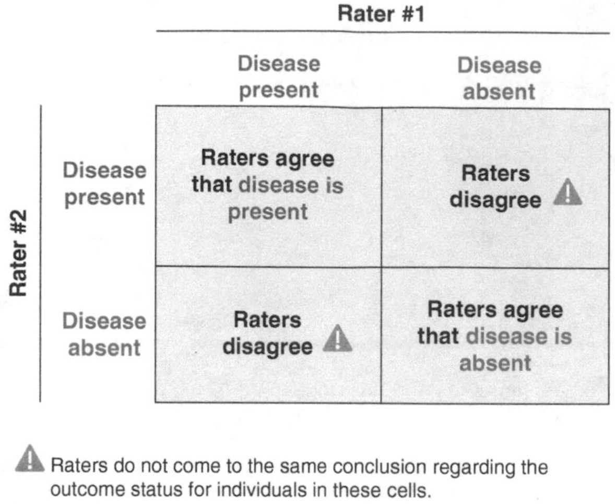

▲ Raters do not come to the same conclusion regarding the outcome status for individuals in these cells.

For example, one study examined the interrater reliability when different specialists were grading diabetic retinopathy severity from photographic images of the eye (**Figure 11.18**).[34] In some instances, both specialists agreed on the diagnosis of disease severity (cells A and D), whereas in other instances they disagreed (cells B and C). One simple measure, the **percent agreement**, can quntify the interrater reliability of testing using this retinal photography method.

## FIGURE 11.18 QUANTIFYING INTERRATER RELIABILITY

▲ Raters do not come to the same conclusion regarding the outcome status for individuals in these cells.

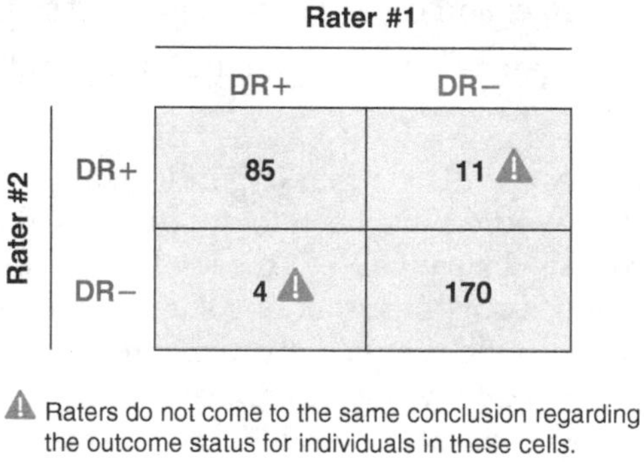

DR, diabetic retinopathy.

**Percent agreement.** The percent agreement is a simple measure of interrater agreement. Percent agreement is calculated as the proportion of the reviews in which the raters reach the same conclusion (**Equation 11.7**):

$$\text{Percent agreement} = \frac{(A+D)}{(A+B+C+D)} \times 100\% \tag{11.7}$$

Data adapted from the study of the interrater reliability of specialists grading diabetic retinopathy severity from photographic images are shown in **Figure 11.18**.[34] The percent agreement is calculated as:

$$\text{Percent agreement} = \frac{(85+170)}{(85+11+4+170)} \times 100\% = 94.4\%$$

The percent agreement is interpreted as the percent of reviews that the raters agree on. The percent agreement ranges from 0% (the raters agree on none of their conclusions) to 100% (the raters agree on all of their conclusions). In this case, the raters agreed on the classification of 94.4% of the reviews. One limitation to the use of percent agreement is that it does not account for agreement that arises due to chance alone. Also, percent agreement only estimates absolute agreement (yes vs. no) and does not consider the degree of agreement when agreement is measured using a numerical scale or more than 2 categories. There are other statistical measures of interrater reliability that take into account agreement due to chance or the degree of agreement (e.g., Kappa statistics and correlation coefficients, respectively), which are described elsewhere.[35]

## Highlights

### Considerations for Screening Programs and Interrater Test Reliability

- Screening is not always appropriate, nor is it always beneficial.
- The strengths and limitations of specific screening programs must be weighed.
- Some biases influence screening programs:
  - Self-selection bias
  - Lead time bias
  - Length time bias
- **Interrater reliability** (also called interobserver reliability) refers to the reproducibility of test results by two or more raters.
- **Percent agreement** is one measure of the interrater reliability of testing.

## WHERE WE'VE BEEN AND WHAT'S UP NEXT

Information bias is an error in the estimation of a measure of frequency or association which occurs when measurement of the exposure and/or outcome is inaccurate. In this chapter, you have learned about why information bias occurs, different types of information bias, and what can be done to address information bias. You have also learned about information bias as applied to screening and diagnostic testing which is an area that affects almost everyone's lives. This concludes our section on bias (i.e., systematic error). Up next is a discussion of random error and precision in epidemiologic studies (**Chapter 12, "Random Error in Epidemiologic Research"**).

## END OF CHAPTER PROBLEM SET

Decide whether the following scenarios describe concerns about misclassification of the exposure or outcome, and whether the potential misclassification is differential or nondifferential.

1. Due to concern that people who have given birth may report alcohol and cigarette consumption differently by pregnancy outcome status (stillbirth, small for gestational age, congenital malformations, preterm birth, and low birthweight), investigators assessed alcohol and cigarette use both retrospectively and prospectively.[36]

2. In a study that used electronic health records (EHR) to collect exposure and outcome data, the investigators noted that many outcomes are recorded inconsistently in terms of quality and availability by potential exposures of interest.[37]

3. A case-control study on radiofrequency exposure from mobile phones and acoustic neuroma risk used network operator data to validate participants' recall of the start of their mobile phone use.[38] No differences were found in the accuracy of the self-reported cell phone use initiation between those with and without acoustic neuroma.

## Questions 4 to 9 refer to the following description and the data shown in Table 11.3.

Numerous studies have found racial bias in healthcare providers' assessment of patients' pain levels[39-41] largely due to implicit biases and providers' false beliefs about biologic differences in pain experienced in Black versus White people. These biased perceptions of patient pain are associated with negative outcomes such as suboptimal access to care and treatment. Questions 4 to 9 use hypothetical cross-sectional study data to illustrate radifferences in physicians' perceptions of patient pain after surgery, by patient race (**Table 11.3**).

**TABLE 11.3 HYPOTHETICAL STUDY DATA TO ILLUSTRATE DIFFERENCES IN PHYSICIANS' PERCEPTIONS OF PATIENT PAIN AFTER SURGERY, BY PATIENT RACE**

| Black Patients | | Actual Patient Pain | |
|---|---|---|---|
| | | + | − |
| Patient pain classified by physicians | + | 100 | 5 |
| | − | 50 | 95 |
| | Total | 150 | 100 |

| White Patients | | Actual Patient Pain | |
|---|---|---|---|
| | | + | − |
| Patient pain classified by physicians | + | 125 | 5 |
| | − | 25 | 95 |
| | Total | 150 | 100 |

4. Calculate the prevalence of actual patient pain among Black and White patients.

5. Calculate the sensitivity of pain classification among Black patients.

6. Calculate the sensitivity of pain classification among White patients.

7. Calculate the specificity of pain classification among Black patients.

8. Calculate the specificity of pain classification among White patients.

9. Is this an example of differential or nondifferential classification of patient pain after surgery? How do you know?

## Questions 10 to 13 refer to the study description that follows.

In 2020, investigators in China developed a serologic test to identify antibody response to SARS-CoV-2 infection.[42] IgM antibody detection was compared to the gold standard of PCR (i.e., nucleic acid testing for SARS-CoV-2) to evaluate its ability to identify individuals with COVID-19. A total of 126 individuals underwent antibody testing; 51 of them were correctly classified as being COVID-19 positive and 60 were correctly classified as being COVID-19 negative. The sensitivity of the antibody test was 77.3% and the specificity was 100%.

10. Use the information given to construct a 2×2 misclassification table.

11. Calculate and interpret the PPV and NPV of the antibody test.

12. What would happen to the sensitivity and specificity of this antibody test if it were applied in a population that had a higher prevalence of COVID-19 infection?

13. What would happen to the PPV and NPV of this antibody test if it were applied in a population that had a higher prevalence of COVID-19 infection?

**Questions 14 and 15 refer to the study description that follows and the data shown in Table 11.4.**

The following data are from the case-control study on radiofrequency exposure from mobile phones and acoustic neuroma risk described earlier in this problem set (**Table 11.4**). Recall that these investigators used network operator data to validate participants' recall of the start of their mobile phone use.[38]

**TABLE 11.4 DATA FROM THE CASE-CONTROL STUDY ON RADIOFREQUENCY EXPOSURE FROM MOBILE PHONES AND ACOUSTIC NEUROMA RISK**

| Observed Data | | Initiation of Cell Phone Use From Operator Data | | | |
|---|---|---|---|---|---|
| | | <5 years ago | 5–9 years ago | >=10 years ago | Total |
| Initiation of cell phone use from self-report | <5 years ago | 33 | 23 | 2 | 58 |
| | 5–9 years ago | 11 | 70 | 10 | 91 |
| | >=10 years ago | 9 | 21 | 28 | 58 |
| | Total | 35 | 114 | 40 | 207 |

14. Calculate the percent agreement comparing self-report and operator data.

15. Interpret the value that you calculated for the percent agreement.

## REFERENCES

1. Saber Tehrani AS, Lee H, Mathews SC, et al. 25-Year summary of US malpractice claims for diagnostic errors 1986–2010: an analysis from the National Practitioner Data Bank. *BMJ Qual Saf.* 2013;22(8):672–680. https://doi.org/10.1136/bmjqs-2012-001550

2. Macdorman MF, Kirmeyer S. The challenge of fetal mortality. *NCHS Data Brief.* 2009;(16):1–8. https://www.cdc.gov/nchs/products/databriefs/db16.htm

3. Schoen C, Osborn R, Huynh PT, et al. Taking the pulse of health care systems: experiences of patients with health problems in six countries. *Health Aff.* 2005;(Suppl Web Exclusives):W5–509. https://doi.org/10.1377/hlthaff.w5.509

4. Damon A. The COVID testing company that missed 96% of cases. ProPublica. May 16, 2022. https://www.propublica.org/article/covid-testing-nevada-false-negatives-northshore

5. Sjoding MW, Dickson RP, Iwashyna TJ, Gay SE, Valley TS. Racial bias in pulse oximetry measurement. *N Engl J Med.* 2020;383(25):2477–2478. https://doi.org/10.1056/NEJMc2029240

6. Lewis-Faning E. *Report on an Enquiry Into Family Limitation and Its Influence on Human Fertility During the Past Fifty Years.* Vol. 1. His Majesty's Stationery Office; 1949.

7. McGregor K, Makkai T. Self-reported drug use: how prevalent is under-reporting? *Trends Issues Crime Crim. Justice.* 2003(260):1–6. https://www.aic.gov.au/publications/tandi/tandi260

8. Kilian C, Manthey J, Probst C, et al. Why is per capita consumption underestimated in alcohol surveys? Results from 39 surveys in 23 European countries. *Alcohol Alcohol.* 2020;55(5):554–563. https://doi.org/10.1093/alcalc/agaa048

9. FitzGerald C, Hurst S. Implicit bias in healthcare professionals: a systematic review. *BMC Med Ethics.* 2017;18(1):19. https://doi.org/10.1186/s12910-017-0179-8

10. Stillbirth Collaborative Research Network Writing Group. Association between stillbirth and risk factors known at pregnancy confirmation. *JAMA.* 2011;306(22):2469–2479. https://doi.org/10.1001/jama.2011.1798

11. Jurek AM, Greenland S, Maldonado G, Church TR. Proper interpretation of non-differential misclassification effects: expectations vs observations. *Int J Epidemiol.* 2005;34(3):680–687. https://doi.org/10.1093/ije/dyi060

12. Ghebremichael M. The syndromic versus laboratory diagnosis of sexually transmitted infections in resource-limited settings. *ISRN AIDS.* 2014;2014:103452. https://doi.org/10.1155/2014/103452

13. Wall KM, Nyombayire J, Parker R, et al. Developing and validating a risk algorithm to diagnose *Neisseria gonorrhoeae* and *Chlamydia trachomatis* in symptomatic Rwandan women. *BMC Infect Dis.* 2021;21(1):392. https://doi.org/10.1186/s12879-021-06073-z

14. Al-Shaar L, Satija A, Wang DD, et al. Red meat intake and risk of coronary heart disease among US men: prospective cohort study. *BMJ.* 2020;371:m4141. https://doi.org/10.1136/bmj.m4141

15. Cuparencu C, Rinnan Å, Dragsted LO. Combined markers to assess meat intake-human metabolomic studies of discovery and validation. *Mol Nutr Food Res.* 2019;63(17):e1900106. https://doi.org/10.1002/mnfr.201900106

16. Cuparencu C, Praticó G, Hemeryck LY, et al. Biomarkers of meat and seafood intake: an extensive literature review. *Genes Nutr.* 2019;14(1):35. https://doi.org/10.1186/s12263-019-0656-4

17. Macaluso M, Lawson L, Akers R, et al. Prostate-specific antigen in vaginal fluid as a biologic marker of condom failure. *Contraception.* 1999;59(3):195–201. https://doi.org/10.1016/s0010-7824(99)00013-x

18. Brenner H, Savitz DA, Gefeller O. The effects of joint misclassification of exposure and disease on epidemiologic measures of association. *J Clin Epidemiol.* 1993;46(10):1195–1202. https://doi.org/10.1016/0895-4356(93)90119-l

19. Ashrafioun L, Allan NP, Stecker TA. Opioid use disorder and its association with self-reported difficulties participating in social activities. *Am J Addict.* 2022;31(1):46–52. https://doi.org/10.1111/ajad.13220

20. Napper LE, Fisher DG, Johnson ME, Wood MM. The reliability and validity of drug users self reports of amphetamine use among primarily heroin and cocaine users. *Addict Behav.* 2010;35(4):350–354. https://doi.org/10.1016/j.addbeh.2009.12.006

21. Substance Abuse and Mental Health Services Administration. Comparing and evaluating youth substance use estimates from the National Survey on Drug Use and Health and other surveys [Internet]. 2012. https://www.ncbi.nlm.nih.gov/books/NBK533885

22. Patnode CD, Perdue LA, Rushkin M, O'Connor EA. *Screening for Unhealthy Drug Use in Primary Care in Adolescents and Adults, Including Pregnant Persons: Updated Systematic Review for the U.S. Preventive Services Task Force.* Evidence Synthesis No. 186. AHRQ Publication No. 19-05255-EF-1. Agency for Healthcare Research and Quality (US); 2020. https://www.ncbi.nlm.nih.gov/books/NBK558174/

23. Lind LH, Schober MF, Conrad FG, Reichert H. Why do survey respondents disclose more when computers ask the questions? *Public Opin Q.* 2013;77(4):888–935. https://doi.org/10.1093/poq/nft038

24. Choi BCK, Pak AWP. A catalog of biases in questionnaires. *Prev Chronic Dis.* 2005;2(1):A13. https://www.ncbi.nlm.nih.gov/pmc/articles/PMC1323316

25. Centers for Disease Control and Prevention. Breast cancer statistics. 2021. https://www.cdc.gov/cancer/breast/statistics/index.htm

26. U.S. Preventive Services Task Force. Breast cancer: screening. 2023. https://www.uspreventiveservicestaskforce.org/uspstf/draft-recommendation/breast-cancer-screening-adults#fullrecommendationstart

27. Centers for Disease Control and Prevention. What is breast cancer screening? 2021. https://www.cdc.gov/cancer/breast/basic_info/screening.htm

28. Humphrey LL, Helfand M, Chan BK, Woolf SH. Breast cancer screening: a summary of the evidence for the U.S. Preventive Services Task Force. *Ann Intern Med.* 2002;137(5_Part_1):347–360. https://doi.org/10.7326/0003-4819-137-5_part_1-200209030-00012

29. American Cancer Society. Core needle biopsy of the breast. Updated January 14, 2022. https://www.cancer.org/cancer/breast-cancer/screening-tests-and-early-detection/breast-biopsy/core-needle-biopsy-of-the-breast.html

30. Bukhari MH, Akhtar ZM. Comparison of accuracy of diagnostic modalities for evaluation of breast cancer with review of literature. *Am Can Soc.* 2009;37(6):416–424. https://doi.org/10.1002/dc.21000

31. Lacambra MD, Lam CC, Mendoza P, et al. Biopsy sampling of breast lesions: comparison of core needle- and vacuum-assisted breast biopsies. *Breast Cancer Res Treat.* 2012;132(3):917–923. https://doi.org/10.1007/s10549-011-1639-3

32. Wang M, He X, Chang Y, Sun G, Thabane L. A sensitivity and specificity comparison of fine needle aspiration cytology and core needle biopsy in evaluation of suspicious breast lesions: a systematic review and meta-analysis. *Breast.* 2017;31:157–166. https://doi.org/10.1016/j.breast.2016.11.009

33. American Cancer Society. Cancer facts and figures. 2003. https://www.cancer.org/research/cancer-facts-statistics/all-cancer-factsfigures/2023-cancer-facts-figures.html

34. Srinivasan S, Suresh S, Chendilnathan C, et al. Inter-observer agreement in grading severity of diabetic retinopathy in wide-field fundus photographs. *Eye*. 2023;37(6):1231–1235. https://doi.org/10.1038/s41433-022-02107-1

35. Hallgren KA. Computing inter-rater reliability for observational data: an overview and tutorial. *Tutor Quant Methods Psychol*. 2012;8(1):23–34. https://doi.org/10.20982/tqmp.08.1.p023

36. Verkerk PH, Buitendijk SE, Verloove-VanHorick SP. Differential misclassification of alcohol and cigarette consumption by pregnancy outcome. *Int J Epidemiol*. 1994;23(6):1218–1225. https://doi.org/10.1093/ije/23.6.1218

37. Chen Y, Wang J, Chubak J, Hubbard RA. Inflation of type I error rates due to differential misclassification in EHR-derived outcomes: empirical illustration using breast cancer recurrence. *Pharmacoepidemiol Drug Saf*. 2019;28(2):264–268. https://doi.org/10.1002/pds.4680

38. Pettersson D, Bottai M, Mathiesen T, Prochazka M, Feychting M. Validation of self-reported start year of mobile phone use in a Swedish case-control study on radiofrequency fields and acoustic neuroma risk. *J Expo Sci Environ Epidemiol*. 2015;25(1):72–79. https://doi.org/10.1038/jes.2014.76

39. Hoffman KM, Trawalter S, Axt JR, Oliver M. Racial bias in pain assessment and treatment recommendations, and false beliefs about biological differences between Blacks and Whites. *Proc Natl Acad Sci U S A*. 2016;113(16):4296–4301. https://doi.org/10.1073/pnas.1516047113

40. Staton LJ, Panda M, Chen I, et al. When race matters: disagreement in pain perception between patients and their physicians in primary care. *J Natl Med Assoc*. 2007;99(5):532–538. https://pubmed.ncbi.nlm.nih.gov/17534011

41. Tait RC, Chibnall JT. Racial/ethnic disparities in the assessment and treatment of pain: psychosocial perspectives. *Am Psychol*. 2014;69(2):131–141. https://doi.org/10.1037/a0035204

42. Xiang F, Wang X, He X, et al. Antibody detection and dynamic characteristics in patients with coronavirus disease 2019. *Clin Infect Dis*. 2020;71(8):1930–1934. https://doi.org/10.1093/cid/ciaa461

# CHAPTER 12

# RANDOM ERROR IN EPIDEMIOLOGIC RESEARCH

## KEY TERMS

confidence interval

meaningful significance

null hypothesis significance testing

*p*-value

precision

point estimate

population parameter

random error

statistical significance

## LEARNING OBJECTIVES

12.1 Define random error and understand why it occurs.

12.2 Describe the relationship between random error and precision and their relationship with sample size.

12.3 Construct a null hypothesis and its associated one- and two-sided alternative hypotheses in words and using measures of association.

12.4 Define null hypothesis significance testing, and explain the uses and limitations of this practice.

12.5 Define and distinguish between the two types of random error.

12.6 Describe the relationship between random error, study power, and sample size.

12.7 Define *p*-values, including the two key assumptions.

12.8 Describe how *p*-values are used for null hypothesis significance testing, and explain the uses and limitations of this practice.

12.9 Distinguish between one- and two-tailed *p*-values.

12.10 Interpret a *p*-value associated with a given research question.

12.11 Describe the difference between statistical and meaningful significance.

12.12 Explain how *p*-values are expected to change with sample size and/or outcome prevalence.

12.13 Define confidence intervals (CIs) using the concept of hypothetical study replications.

12.14 Describe how confidence intervals are used for null hypothesis significance testing.

12.15 Explain the relationship between confidence intervals, precision, and sample size.

12.16 Describe the relationship between *p*-values and confidence intervals.

# SMALL NUMBERS, GREAT IMPORTANCE

An essential component of public health is working toward the elimination of health inequities, which requires that investigators consider the health of diverse sets of populations. Sometimes, individuals who are at increased risk of some poor health outcomes also belong to groups that are relatively small in number. Without careful planning, it can be difficult (if not impossible!) to enroll enough of these individuals in a sample population to draw meaningful conclusions about factors that impact their health.

Prior to 2020, there was little research about the health of transgender individuals (i.e., those whose gender identity does not align with the sex that they were assigned at birth), who are estimated to compose 0.3% to 0.5% of the U.S. adult population.[1] Transgender individuals are more likely to report being in poor health than their cisgender counterparts (i.e., those whose gender identity aligns with the sex that they were assigned at birth). However, findings have been mixed or limited about specific health disparities due to limited enrollment of transgender individuals in epidemiologic studies.[2]

In this chapter's **Pause to Practice** series, you will be introduced to a groundbreaking study that leveraged electronic medical records to better understand the health of transgender individuals enrolled in an integrated healthcare system.[3] This study overcame many of the barriers of previous research to identify a sizable number of transgender individuals through medical records to learn about factors that particularly impact this group.

## INTRODUCTION TO RANDOM ERROR (LEARNING OBJECTIVE 12.1)

As discussed in **Chapter 9, "Error in Epidemiologic Research and Fundamentals of Confounding,"** there are two types of error in epidemiologic research: **systematic error** and **random error** (see **Figure 9.1**). In the previous three chapters, we discussed the ways in which the systematic errors of confounding, selection bias, and information bias can influence epidemiologic research. We now turn our attention to random error, which occurs because our studies are conducted among a sample of individuals, rather than the entire source population. In epidemiologic research, we often do not have the time or other resources, nor is it necessary, to enroll the entire **source population** (the group of people from which study participants are selected) into a study. Instead, we enroll a subset of these individuals in our sample population. **Random error** (also called **sampling error**) can be thought of as the error introduced because we conduct a study among a sample rather than the entire source population. The act of sampling leads to random error because, just by chance, our **sample population** (those enrolled in our study) may not be representative of the source population.

In **Chapter 4, "Randomized Controlled Trial Designs"**; **Chapter 5, "Cohort Designs"**; **Chapter 6, "Case-Control Designs"**; and **Chapter 7, "Cross-Sectional Designs,"** we learned about the four major epidemiologic study designs and the related measures of association. In those chapters, we focused on using each design to test hypotheses about the relationship between an exposure and an outcome of interest. We did this by calculating difference or ratio measures of association and compared these measures to their null values (0 or 1 for difference and ratio measures, respectively). As we move into a discussion of random error, we will take this one step further to determine whether our measures of association are different from the null value from a *statistical* perspective. This determination is made using **statistical inference**, which allows us to quantify the impact of random error on our study results. In this chapter, we will return to the example of factors associated with stillbirth to illustrate how the quantification of random error can enhance the interpretation of our study findings. However, as you will learn, we caution against relying on statistical inference alone when considering the implications of study findings.

# Conceptualizing Random Error

In **Chapter 9, "Error in Epidemiologic Research and Fundamentals of Confounding,"** we introduced the concepts of **population parameters** and **point estimates**. Recall that the population parameter is the unobserved true value in the source population, and that the point estimate is the measure that is calculated using data from the sample population to make inference (i.e., evidence-based conclusions) about the population parameter. For example, in **Chapter 6, "Case-Control Designs,"** we took a close look at a case-control study that sought to identify risk factors for stillbirth in the United States (in the United States, stillbirths are defined as pregnancy losses occurring anytime from the 20th week of pregnancy onward[4]). In **Pause to Practice 6.2**, we explored the age of the birthing parent as a potential risk factor for stillbirth and found that 2.1% (28/1,354) of the control group (i.e., those who had a live birth) was aged 40 years or older. Recall that the purpose of the control group in a case-control study is to provide an estimate of the frequency of the exposure in the source population (here, the source population was comprised of five distinct geographic areas associated with each of the study's participating universities). In this study, the controls provided an estimate of the proportion of birthing parents in the source population who were aged 40 years or older (a measure of prevalence). Using these data, we can infer that 2.1% of pregnant people living in the source population were aged 40 years or older.

Let's consider, though, what might have happened if the investigators had hypothetically ended up with a different group of 1,354 individuals who had a live birth (this could have happened, for example, if control sampling had taken place a few months earlier or later). In this situation, it is very unlikely that investigators would have enrolled exactly 28 individuals aged 40 years or older, and thus this hypothetical alternate control group would yield a different estimate of the proportion of birthing parents in this age group—even if the investigators used the exact same recruitment methods. Barring any systematic error, any differences that might be observed between these two different control groups would be due to random error (i.e., sampling error).

It may seem strange to consider these two different hypothetical samples, since, in practice, studies are conducted only among a single sample population. However, the concept of drawing **hypothetical independent samples** from the same source population, and the related concept of **hypothetical study replications** (i.e., a hypothetical scenario in which the study is repeated an infinite number of times), are foundational to understanding random error. Independent sampling means that whether a person is selected for one sample has no bearing on whether they are selected for another; an individual could be selected for one, some, all, or neither of the hypothetical samples.

An illustration of independent sampling is shown in **Figure 12.1**, where three different sample populations have been selected from the same source population. For illustrative purposes, we are considering a source population of 48 pregnant individuals, one of whom was aged 40 years or older. Thus, the true proportion of pregnant people aged 40 years or older (i.e., the population parameter) in the source population is 2.1%. Both the first and the second sample populations shown in **Figure 12.1** include 10 individuals, yet they yield different point estimates of the proportion of pregnant people aged 40 years or older. In the first sample, none of the 10 sampled individuals were aged 40 years or older, yielding a point estimate of 0%. In the second sample, one of the 10 sampled individuals was aged 40 years or older, yielding a point estimate of 10%. In the third sample, we see what might happen if we were to increase our sample size to 25 individuals. This time, we obtain a point estimate of 4%. While our estimate from the third sample population still differs from the population parameter (i.e., the true prevalence of 2.1%), it is closer than estimates from the first two samples, which contained only 10 individuals each.

It is important to note that just by chance, a random sample of 25 individuals could happen to exclude the one person who was aged 40 years or older, again yielding a point estimate of 0%. Since those who are aged 40 years or older compose such a small proportion of our source

## FIGURE 12.1 ESTIMATING THE PREVALENCE OF BIRTHING PARENTS AGED 40 YEARS AND OLDER: SELECTING DIFFERENT SAMPLE POPULATIONS FROM THE SAME SOURCE POPULATION

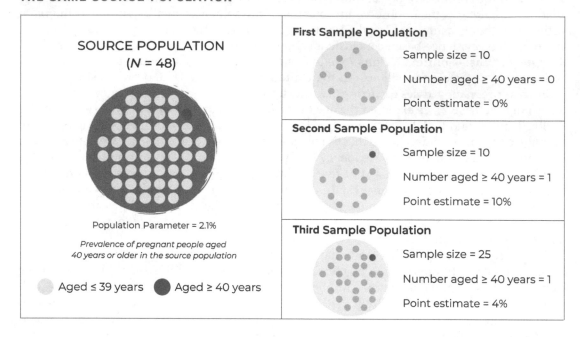

population, our point estimates are likely to be very different from the population parameter when our sample populations are small (such as in the first two scenarios). Considering the other extreme, if we were to enroll all 48 people from the source population in our sample population, there would be no random error because there was no sampling, and our point estimate would equal the population parameter (2.1%).

## Random Error, Precision, and Sample Size (LEARNING OBJECTIVE 12.2)

There is a balance between random error and a concept called **precision**. Measures that are subject to less random error are said to be more precise, while those that are subject to more random error are said to be less precise. The balance between random error and precision is illustrated in **Figure 12.2**. The study with a smaller sample population (**Figure 12.2–Panel A**) is subject to more random error, and thus the point estimate is less precise. The study with a larger sample population (**Figure 12.2–Panel B**) is subject to less random error, and thus the point estimate is more precise. On average, as the sample population gets larger (and thus closer to the size of the source population), there is *less* random error affecting the results, and thus our estimates are *more* precise. As previously noted, if a study includes everyone in the source population, the results are not subject to random error since there was no sampling. We will discuss how to quantify the precision of a point estimate using **confidence intervals** later in this chapter.

When reading reports of epidemiologic studies in the popular press, you will notice that authors often call attention to the number of participants included in a study, particularly when it is in the thousands. The emphasis on large sample populations as a study strength is related to the notion that these studies are less subject to random error. While it can be reassuring that a larger study may be less prone to *random* error, we must remember that even large studies are not immune to *systematic* error.

## FIGURE 12.2 RANDOM ERROR, PRECISION, AND SAMPLE SIZE

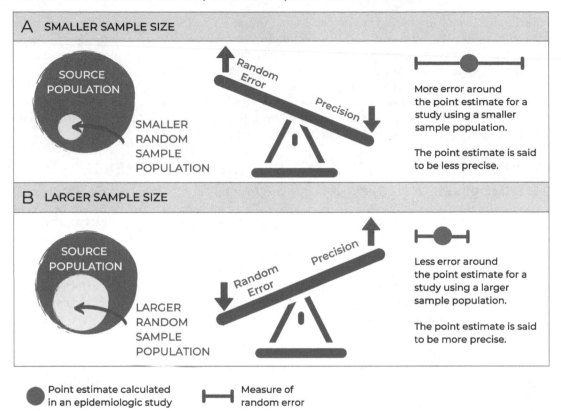

A SMALLER SAMPLE SIZE

SOURCE POPULATION

SMALLER RANDOM SAMPLE POPULATION

Random Error

Precision

More error around the point estimate for a study using a smaller sample population.

The point estimate is said to be less precise.

B LARGER SAMPLE SIZE

SOURCE POPULATION

LARGER RANDOM SAMPLE POPULATION

Random Error

Precision

Less error around the point estimate for a study using a larger sample population.

The point estimate is said to be more precise.

● Point estimate calculated in an epidemiologic study

⊢●⊣ Measure of random error

---

## Highlights

### Overview of Error in Epidemiologic Research

- Epidemiologic studies are designed to estimate a **population parameter**, which is the unobserved true value in the source population.
- The measures calculated using data from a sample population are called **point estimates** and are used to make inferences about the population parameter.
- Two categories of error occur in epidemiologic research:
  - **Random Error** (i.e., **sampling error**)
    - a difference between the population parameter and our point estimate that occurs solely because we study a sample rather than an entire source population.
  - **Systematic Error** (i.e., **bias**)
    - a difference between the population parameter and our point estimate that occurs because of a flaw in the study that leads to incorrect conclusions.
- Impact of sample size:
  - Random error can be reduced by increasing a study's sample size.
  - Systematic error is not influenced by a change in the study's sample size.
- There is an inverse relationship between random error and **precision**.

# INTRODUCTION TO STATISTICAL INFERENCE

Thus far, we have learned that study results are influenced by random error because we study a sample, rather than the entire source population. As we previously noted, the process by which we quantify random error is called statistical inference. Statistical inference can be useful for understanding the degree of uncertainty in our data due to sampling. This chapter focuses on two forms of statistical inference that are foundational to conducting and interpreting epidemiologic research: **null hypothesis significance testing** and **interval estimation**. Before we dive into the details of these two inferential tools, we must first understand how to construct hypotheses for statistical inference.

## STRUCTURING HYPOTHESES FOR STATISTICAL INFERENCE
### (LEARNING OBJECTIVE 12.3)

As noted in **Chapter 3, "Introduction to Analytic Epidemiologic Study Designs and Measures of Association,"** etiologic hypotheses—statements that describe the research questions at hand—are foundational to analytic epidemiology. When considering hypotheses for statistical inference, we distinguish between two types of hypotheses: the **null hypothesis ($H_0$)** and the **alternative hypothesis ($H_A$)**, which we introduced in **Chapter 8, "Effect Measure Modification and Statistical Interaction."** As a reminder, the null hypothesis posits that the population parameter is *not different* from the null value from a statistical perspective. On the other hand, the alternative hypothesis posits that the population parameter *is different* from the null value from a statistical perspective.

We distinguish between two types of alternative hypotheses. A **two-sided alternative hypothesis ($H_{A2}$)** posits that there is an association between the exposure and the outcome of interest; however, it does not specify whether the direction of this association is positive or negative (meaning above or below the null, respectively; revisit **Figure 3.14**). A **one-sided alternative hypothesis ($H_{A1}$)** not only posits that there is an association between the exposure and the outcome of interest, but also specifies the hypothesized direction of the association.

Returning to the case-control study to identify factors associated with stillbirth,[5] the null and alternative hypotheses for the relationship between the age of the birthing parent and stillbirth could be structured as follows:

- $H_0$: The odds of being aged 40 years or older among those who experienced a stillbirth *are not statistically significantly different* from the odds of being aged 40 years or older among those who had a live birth.

- $H_{A2}$: The odds of being aged 40 years or older among those who experienced a stillbirth *are statistically significantly different* from the odds of being aged 40 years or older among those who had a live birth.

- $H_{A1}$: The odds of being aged 40 years or older among those who experienced a stillbirth *are statistically significantly higher* than the odds of being aged 40 years or older among those who had a live birth.

  - Note that this is how investigators would structure the one-sided alternative hypothesis under the assumption that stillbirth is more likely to occur among older birthing parents. This is a reasonable hypothesis given that older age is known to be a risk factor for many adverse pregnancy and health outcomes.[6]

The term *statistically significant* simply refers to whether the association is different from the null from a *statistical* perspective—it implies neither that the difference is meaningful from a public health perspective, nor that the exposure *causes* the outcome. We will continue to revisit this matter throughout the chapter.

While the previous null and alternative hypotheses have been structured in words, we can also structure them in terms of the relevant measure of association. Returning to the case-control study to identify factors associated with stillbirth, researchers compared the distribution of various exposures among a group of cases (those who experienced a stillbirth) and a group of controls (those who had a live birth). Given the study design, the appropriate measure of association is the exposure odds ratio (EOR). For example, the exposure odds ratio for the association between older age (≥40 years) of the birthing parent and stillbirth is:

$$EOR = \frac{\text{Odds of being aged 40 years or older among cases}}{\text{Odds of being aged 40 years or older among controls}}$$

We can equivalently structure the previous null and alternative hypotheses in terms of the exposure odds ratio as follows:

- $H_0$: EOR = 1 (the null value for a ratio measure of association)
- $H_{A2}$: EOR ≠ 1
- $H_{A1}$: EOR > 1

## Pause to Practice 12.1

### Formulating Statistical Hypotheses

Gender-affirming hormone therapy (GAHT, sometimes referred to as cross-sex hormone therapy), is a treatment given to some transgender individuals to help their bodies better align with their gender identity.[7] While GAHT is associated with increased quality of life and decreased depression and anxiety, there are concerns about the potential for GAHT to have a negative impact on cardiovascular health.[8] For this reason, researchers conducted a cohort study using electronic medical records to evaluate the association between GAHT and cardiovascular health.[3]

For the following questions, we will consider just one of several exposure-outcome relationships that the investigators considered in their cohort study: cross-sex estrogen use and ischemic stroke. The exposed group is comprised of transfeminine individuals (i.e., those whose gender identity does not align with their male sex designation at birth) who received gender-affirming estrogen therapy. The unexposed group is comprised of cisgender men (i.e., individuals who identify as men and who were assigned male sex at birth).[3]

Construct the null and alternative hypotheses (both one- and two-sided) that correspond to the association between cross-sex estrogen use and ischemic stroke using words *and* in terms of the rate ratio.

When evaluating a given association, researchers will develop and test either a one- or two-sided alternative hypothesis, but not both. A two-sided alternative hypothesis is useful when exploring an association where it is unknown whether the exposure is likely to increase or decrease the occurrence of the outcome. On the other hand, a one-sided alternative hypothesis may be chosen when there is existing evidence supporting a direction of the association, such as the example in **Pause to Practice 12.1,** where researchers suspected that cross-sex estrogen use was associated with an increase in ischemic stroke.[3] While it might be intuitive to construct one-sided alternative hypothesis (e.g., smoking is generally bad for health, and so we would hypothesize that smoking *increases* the likelihood of some negative health outcome), we will see that there are some reasons to avoid one-sided alternative hypotheses, and researchers often use two-sided alternative hypotheses even when there is prior evidence supporting the likely direction of the association.

# NULL HYPOTHESIS SIGNIFICANCE TESTING (LEARNING OBJECTIVE 12.4)

Null hypothesis significance testing is a common practice used to test whether our study results differ from the null hypothesis from a *statistical* perspective (i.e., whether the results are **statistically significant**). Another way to think about this is that we use null hypothesis significance testing to determine whether our data are more consistent with the null hypothesis or with the alternative hypothesis. Let's consider the two possible scenarios:

**The data are more consistent with the null than the alternative hypothesis.** Under this scenario, our data do not provide sufficient evidence that the population parameter (i.e., the truth we're trying to estimate) is different from its null value, and thus we *do not reject the null hypothesis*. When the data are more consistent with the null hypothesis, we say that the measure *is not statistically significant*, which means that from a statistical perspective, the measure *is not* significantly different from its null value.

**The data are more consistent with the alternative hypothesis than the null hypothesis.** Under this scenario, our data provide evidence that the population parameter is different from its null value, and thus we *reject the null hypothesis*. When the data are not consistent with the null hypothesis, we say that the measure *is statistically significant*, which means that from a statistical perspective, the measure *is* significantly different from its null value.

## Words Matter

The phrases "reject the null" and "do not reject the null" can feel very technical, and sometimes learners are tempted to restructure these phrases. Unfortunately, doing so can lead you astray. Some examples of *incorrect* interpretations of these phrases are shown in the text that follows.

We do not reject the null when the data suggest that there *is not* a statistically significant association between the exposure and outcome. This should *not* be interpreted as:

- ✘ The null hypothesis is true.
- ✘ The data prove that the null hypothesis is true.
- ✘ We accept the null hypothesis.

We reject the null when the data suggest that there *is* a statistically significant association between the exposure and outcome. This should *not* be interpreted as:

- ✘ The alternative hypothesis is true.
- ✘ The data prove that the alternative hypothesis is true.
- ✘ We accept the alternative hypothesis.

While these incorrect interpretations may be grammatically correct, they are not appropriate interpretations of null hypothesis significance testing. When conducting research, we can never *prove* whether a hypothesis is correct, and we certainly do not know whether we have been able to identify the truth. Finally, although the use of the word *accept* seems more natural than *reject* or *do not reject*, this phrasing is also inappropriate.

When describing your conclusions related to null hypothesis significance testing, it is best to say that you either "reject the null hypothesis" or "do not reject the null hypothesis" and avoid creative interpretations.

We now know that we will either reject, or not reject, the null hypothesis. At this point, we need to think about the four different ways in which our study results (i.e., the point estimates) could align with the population parameters that we aim to estimate, which are shown in **Table 12.1**. Whether there is truly an association between the exposure and the outcome is presented in the columns, while the rows include information about the conclusions we reach using our study data. The four possible ways that our study results could compare to the population parameter are as follows:

TABLE 12.1 **HOW THE POINT ESTIMATE CAN ALIGN WITH THE POPULATION PARAMETER: TYPE I AND TYPE II ERRORS**

| | | Population Parameter (i.e., the unobserved true value in the source population) | |
| --- | --- | --- | --- |
| | | $H_0$ Is True<br>There truly is NO association between the exposure and outcome. | $H_0$ Is NOT True<br>There truly IS an association between the exposure and outcome. |
| **Point Estimate** (i.e., what we calculate using data from our sample population) | **Do not reject $H_0$**<br>Study data do NOT provide evidence of a statistically significant association between the exposure and outcome. | Quadrant 1<br>Correct Inference<br>Probability = $1 - \alpha$ | Quadrant 2<br>Type II Error<br>*False negative*<br>Probability = $\beta$ |
| | **Reject $H_0$**<br>Study data do provide evidence of a statistically significant association between the exposure and outcome. | Quadrant 3<br>Type I Error<br>*False positive*<br>Probability = $\alpha$ | Quadrant 4<br>Correct Inference<br>Probability = $1 - \beta$<br>*Also called study power* |

$H_0$, null hypothesis.

- **Quadrant 1:** We do not reject $H_0$ and $H_0$ is true.
  - ✓ A correct inference
- **Quadrant 2:** We do not reject $H_0$ and $H_A$ is true.
  - ✗ An incorrect inference, called **type II error** (i.e., a **false negative** conclusion)
- **Quadrant 3:** We reject $H_0$ and $H_0$ is true.
  - ✗ An incorrect inference, called **type I error** (i.e., a **false positive** conclusion)
- **Quadrant 4:** We reject $H_0$ and $H_A$ is true.
  - ✓ A correct inference

## A Note About Null Study Findings

As discussed previously, the goal of an analytic epidemiologic study is to obtain an estimate of the association between the exposure and the outcome that is both valid *and* precise. Our goal is not to achieve results that support our hypotheses; rather, our findings should be a good estimate of the true population parameters, whatever they may be. This means that we want our conclusions to fall in either the first or the fourth quadrants of **Table 12.1**.

Some researchers become disappointed when they do not observe an association between their exposure and outcome of interest. However, null results that are valid can be quite helpful! Generating evidence that there is not an association can be just as important as generating evidence that there is one, and publishing null findings may prevent other researchers from investing resources to study the same relationships or making inappropriate public health recommendations.

In fact, the scientific literature has been influenced by **publication bias**, which occurs when studies with statistically significant findings are more likely to be published while those that have null findings are less likely. To emphasize the importance of publishing null findings, some investigators have asked journals to give equal consideration to studies with null findings, and some specialty journals have even been created solely for the publication of null results.

## Type I and Type II Errors (LEARNING OBJECTIVE 12.5)

In all studies, there is a possibility that our point estimates will not align with the population parameters simply due to random error. As previously noted, this occurs when our results fall within the second or third quadrants of **Table 12.1**.

We can quantify the likelihood of making an incorrect inference using **probabilities**. A probability quantifies how likely it is that something will occur and ranges from 0 (certain that the event will not occur) to 1 (certain that the event will occur). Probabilities are sometimes expressed as a percentage, and thus range from 0% to 100%.

We must determine the probability of making erroneous inferences that we are willing to accept because we have enrolled only a sample of the source population. Since there are two types of erroneous inference (**type I error** and **type II error**), we set two thresholds for acceptable probabilities:

- How often are we willing to say there *is* an association when there truly *is not*? This is the acceptable threshold for type I error.

- How often are we willing to say there *is not* an association when there truly *is*? This is the acceptable threshold for type II error.

A **type I error** occurs when we reject the null hypothesis, and infer a non-null association between our exposure and outcome, when the null hypothesis is actually true (also called a **false positive finding**). The acceptable probability of a type I error is denoted using the Greek letter **alpha** ($\alpha$) and is sometimes referred to as the **significance level**. The value for $\alpha$ (i.e., the probability of a type I error that we are willing to accept in our study) should be decided on before conducting a study because it informs how many people should be enrolled and how long they should be followed (for clinical trial and cohort designs). Additionally, setting the alpha level prior to conducting the study avoids making decisions about what is considered statistically significant after seeing the results. The alpha is typically set at 0.05 (or 5%), which means that there is a 5% probability that we will reject the null hypothesis when, in fact, it is true.

A **type II error** occurs when we do not reject the null hypothesis when the null hypothesis is actually false (also called a **false negative finding**). The acceptable probability of a type II error is denoted using the Greek letter **beta** ($\beta$). As with type I error, the probability of type II error that we are willing to accept in our study should be decided in advance. The $\beta$ is typically set at 0.20 (or 20%), which means that there is a 20% chance that we fail to reject the null hypothesis when, in fact, the null hypothesis is false. On the other hand, if there truly is an association between our exposure and outcome, there is an 80% ($1 - \beta$) probability that our study findings will provide sufficient evidence to reject the null hypothesis. This probability ($1 - \beta$) is referred to as **study power**.

Returning to the association between the age of the birthing parent and stillbirth, $\alpha$, $\beta$, and study power would be interpreted as follows:

- **Alpha ($\alpha$):** This refers to the acceptable probability that we would reject the null hypothesis when it is true, possibly leading us to incorrectly conclude that there *is* an association between being aged 40 years or older and stillbirth when there truly *is no* association.

- **Beta ($\beta$):** This refers to the acceptable probability that we would not reject the null hypothesis when it is false, possibly leading us to incorrectly conclude that there *is not* an association between being aged 40 years or older and stillbirth when there truly *is* an association.

- **Study power ($1 - \beta$):** This refers to the probability that we would reject the null hypothesis when it is false, possibly leading us to accurately conclude that there *is* an association between being aged 40 years or older and stillbirth when there truly *is* an association.

## Pause to Practice 12.2

### Type I and Type II Errors in the Study of Gender-Affirming Estrogen Therapy and Ischemic Stroke

In the study of the association between cross-sex estrogen use and ischemic stroke, researchers set the acceptable probability of a type I error to 0.05.[3] Their publication does not provide information about the threshold for type II error, but let's suppose that it was set to 0.1.
    Use this information to interpret alpha, beta, and study power.

# The Relationship Between Sample Size and Type I Error, Type II Error, and Power (LEARNING OBJECTIVE 12.6)

The conventional thresholds for α and β—set to 0.05 and 0.2, respectively—mean that researchers are generally more willing to accept false negative rather than false positive findings. While this is the typical convention, investigators should think critically about their choice of acceptable type I and type II error levels. Whether a false negative or a false positive finding is more acceptable depends on the research question at hand, and may be different for different stakeholders interested in the study's results.

For example, the consequences of failing to identify an association between elevated blood lead levels and poor child development could be quite severe; thus, researchers might decide to decrease the threshold for β from 0.2 to 0.1 (thus increasing power [1 – β] from 0.8 to 0.9).

On the other hand, a study designed to evaluate whether there are any unintended negative consequences of using certain types of sunscreen might prefer the conventional thresholds for α and β. Given the known benefits of sunscreen, there may be concern about falsely identifying negative consequences, which could then impact sunscreen use and inadvertently increase rates of skin cancer. However, manufacturers of sunscreen, users of sunscreen, and regulators of sunscreen may all have different views about what should be the acceptable probability of type I and type II errors.

As reflected in **Figure 12.2**, when we are willing to accept less random error, either type I or type II, we must enroll more people into our study (or follow the enrolled group for a longer time to accrue more cases, for clinical trials and cohort designs). If we decide that we are willing to accept more random error, either type I or type II, we can enroll fewer people into our study (or follow individuals in a clinical trial or cohort design for a shorter duration).

## Digging Deeper

### Calculating Sample Size

There are several considerations in addition to acceptable levels of type I and type II errors that must be considered to determine how many people should be enrolled in an epidemiologic study. These factors can include the size of the population from which you are sampling, how common the exposure and/or outcome are, and how strong of an association you aim to observe.[9] The formulae used to conduct a **sample size calculation** vary depending on study design.

There are ample sample size calculators available online (including OpenEpi,[10] which we introduced in **Chapter 8, "Effect Measure Modification and Statistical Interaction"**) that readers can use to modify different inputs to see how they affect the required sample size. In general, you must increase your sample size if you want to:

- Decrease acceptable type I error.

- Decrease acceptable type II error (and thus increase study power).

- Be able to find evidence of statistically significant differences for weaker measures of association.

Let's expand on the final bullet point. The further a measure of association is from the null, the easier it is to conclude that it is statistically significantly different from the null. For this reason, larger sample sizes are needed when investigators hypothesize that the exposure may have a meaningful, but small, effect on the outcome. For example, a larger sample size will be needed to conclude that a risk ratio of 1.2 is statistically different from 1 than to conclude that a risk ratio of 5.0 is statistically different from 1, all other considerations being held constant.

To determine the size of the measure of association you wish to detect, you can ask yourself questions such as:

- Given background knowledge, what is the magnitude of the association that I should reasonably expect?

- What magnitude of the measure of association would justify the use of a more expensive treatment?

- What magnitude of the measure of association would be important for making recommendations about treatment strategies or prevention interventions?

- What magnitude of the measure of association would be meaningful to the patient to improve their quality of life?

## What if We Make a Type I or Type II Error?

While we do our best to obtain a valid and precise estimate of the population parameter, we must recognize that we will make mistakes along the way (bias) and our results will be subject to error due to sampling (random error). While this can be unsettling, it is important to note that it is rare for public health practice or policy to change due to the results of a single study. Rather, public health professionals and policy makers consider the body of scientific evidence. This means that changes to public health practice often occur only after several studies have produced similar findings.

### Highlights

### Type I and Type II Errors

- Type I error ($\alpha$)
  - This is the acceptable probability of false positive findings.
- Type II error ($\beta$)
  - This is the acceptable probability of false negative findings.
  - Type II error is related to study power ($1 - \beta$), which is the probability that a study will reject the null hypothesis when it is false, leading to an inference that correctly identifies a non-null association between the exposure and the outcome.
- There is an inverse relationship between random error and sample size. Thus, more study participants are needed if...
  - Type I error ($\alpha$) is lowered (e.g., from 0.05 to 0.01).
  - Type II error ($\beta$) is lowered (e.g., from 0.2 to 0.1).
  - Study power is increased (e.g., from 0.8 to 0.9).

### *p*-Values (LEARNING OBJECTIVE 12.7)

Once we have formulated our null and alternative hypotheses, set values for alpha and beta, and have our data in hand, we are finally ready to assess the degree to which our data are consistent with the null hypothesis. This assessment can be made using a ***p*-value**, which is defined as:

> The **probability** of obtaining a result **as or more extreme** than the result observed in your study, **if the null hypothesis is true** and **there is no bias**.

The conceptualization of *p*-values relies on the idea of hypothetical study replications that we discussed earlier. We must imagine a hypothetical scenario where we have replicated our study an infinite number of times, with two key assumptions:

1.  There is truly no association between the exposure and the outcome of interest.

2.  Each of those hypothetical study replications has happened without the influence of systematic error (i.e., bias).

The different components of the definition of the *p*-value are shown in **Figure 12.3** and described further in the text that follows.

## FIGURE 12.3 SUMMARY OF THE DEFINITION OF A *P*-VALUE

| *p*-value | |
|---|---|
| The **probability** of obtaining a result **as or more extreme** than the result observed in your study, if the **null hypothesis is true** *and* there is **no bias** | |
| **probability** | P-values are probabilities and range from 0 to 1. P-values < alpha (α) indicate that the data are *not* consistent with the null hypothesis (i.e. there *is* a statistically significant association) and values ≥ alpha (α) indicate that the data *are* consistent with the null hypothesis (i.e. there *is not* a statistically significant association). |
| **as or more extreme** | This can also be thought of as "as strong or stronger." Results that are stronger than what was observed in your study are all of the possible values that are further away from the null than the one that you observed. |
| **null hypothesis is true** | Null hypothesis significance testing is an evaluation of whether our data support the null hypothesis. One of the underlying assumptions is that the null hypothesis is true (i.e. there is truly no association between the exposure and outcome). |
| **no bias** | A second, and critically important, assumption of null hypothesis significance testing is that the results have not been influenced by bias (i.e., systematic error). |

*p* **is for probability.** A *p*-value is a probability and thus it ranges from 0 to 1. We will revisit exactly what this probability tells us (and what it doesn't!) after reviewing the other components of the definition.

**As or more extreme.** A *p*-value reflects the probability that infinite hypothetical study replications would yield results that are as strong or stronger, relative to the null, than the one that we actually observed in our study under the previously described assumptions. **Figure 12.4** illustrates what results are considered "as or more extreme" than the result that was observed in a given study. Each plot represents the range of possible values that a measure of association could take on ([-1, 1] for difference measures; [0, ∞) for ratio measures). The measure of association observed in a given study is indicated in blue, and the red arrows represent the values of the hypothetical measures of association that are as strong or stronger, relative to the null, than what was actually observed. In all cases, the arrows point *away* from the null value (0 for difference measures; 1 for ratio measures).

Notice that there is a difference in which values are considered "as or more extreme" depending on whether an one- or two-sided alternative hypothesis is considered. Recall that a one-sided alternative hypothesis is directional; that is, the researcher states whether they believe that the association is positive (above the null) or negative (below the null). For a one-sided alternative hypothesis, the values that are considered as or more extreme than the observed association will fall to the right of positive associations (**Figure 12.4–Panel A1**) and to the left of negative associations (**Figure 12.4–Panel A2**).

## FIGURE 12.4 ILLUSTRATING MEASURES OF ASSOCIATION THAT ARE "AS OR MORE EXTREME" THAN THE OBSERVED RESULT

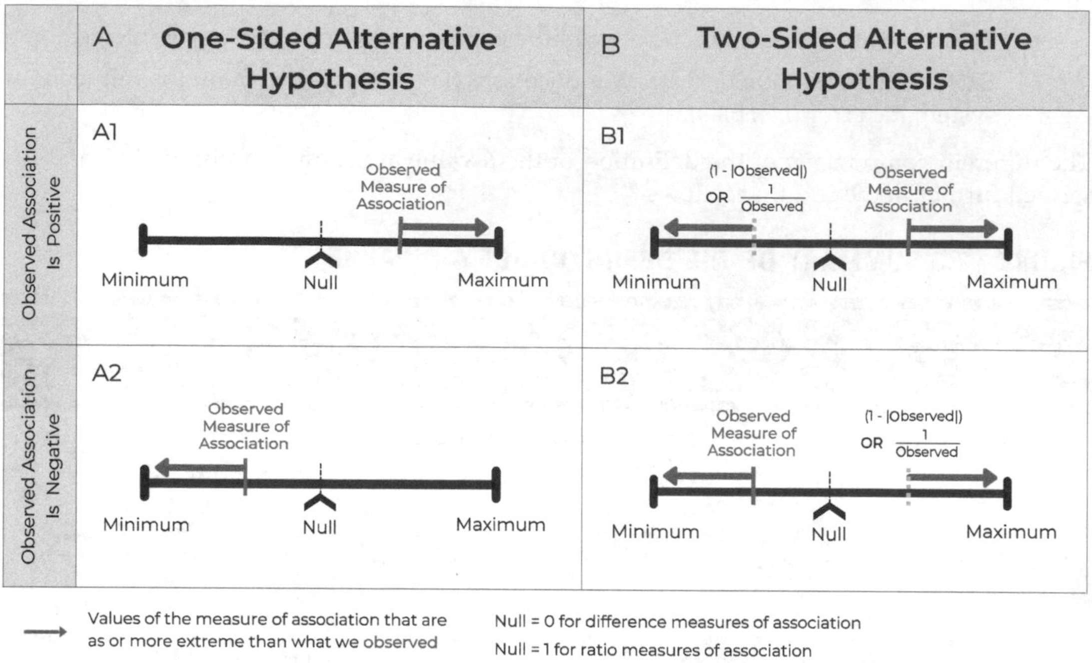

| A | One-Sided Alternative Hypothesis | B | Two-Sided Alternative Hypothesis |
|---|---|---|---|

→ Values of the measure of association that are as or more extreme than what we observed

Null = 0 for difference measures of association

Null = 1 for ratio measures of association

Since two-sided alternative hypotheses do not posit whether the association is positive or negative, the values that are considered "as or more extreme" must fall on *both* sides of the null (Figure 12.4–Panel B). Regardless of whether we observe a positive association (Figure 12.4–Panel B1) or a negative association (Figure 12.4–Panel B2), we must consider the values that are as strong or stronger than the one we observed, as well as the equivalent association on the other side of the null value. These values are denoted in Figure 12.4–Panel B, using a gray dotted line. For difference measures, we find this by subtracting the absolute value of the observed value from 1 (i.e., $1 - |\text{observed}|$), and for ratio measures, we take the inverse of the observed association $\left( \text{i.e., Observed}^{-1} \text{ or } \dfrac{1}{\text{Observed}} \right)$. For example, if we observed a risk ratio of 2, the values that would be considered as or more extreme for a two-sided alternative hypothesis would be $[0, \frac{1}{2}]$ and $[2, \infty)$; if we observed a risk difference of -0.3, the corresponding range of values would be $[-1, -0.3]$ and $[0.7, 1]$.

Tests of one- and two-sided alternative hypotheses will yield **one-tailed $p$-values** and **two-tailed $p$-values**, respectively. This is because one-sided alternative hypotheses consider only values that are "as or more extreme" on one side of the null, while two-sided alternative hypotheses consider values that are as or more extreme on both sides of the null. For a given measure of association, the two-tailed $p$-value will always be larger than the one-tailed $p$-value. We will discuss this further when interpreting $p$-values.

**If the null hypothesis is true.** In null hypothesis significance testing, we are evaluating the degree to which our data are consistent with the null hypothesis. The $p$-value gives us an idea of how likely it would be to get the result that we did observe (or something even stronger) *if there truly were no association* between the exposure and outcome.

**There is no bias.** A key, but often forgotten, assumption of the $p$-value is that the study results are not biased. $p$-values only quantify the influence of random, not systematic, error. Thus, any deviation of the point estimate from the population parameter is assumed to be due to random error (i.e., sampling error) alone.

## Calculating *p*-Values

The formulae for calculating *p*-values vary depending on the measure of interest as well as the sample size, and a discussion of these details is beyond the scope of this text. However, readers can use online calculators, such as OpenEpi,[10] to obtain *p*-values for their measures of interest.

Let's revisit the study of the association between the age of the birthing parent and stillbirth, where the investigators considered four different exposure categories: aged younger than 20 years, aged 20 to 34 years, aged 35 to 39 years, and aged 40 years or older.[5] The group of individuals who were aged 20 to 34 years was used as the reference group. Data adapted from this study comparing just those aged 40 years or older to those who were aged 20 to 34 years are shown in Figure 12.5, along with corresponding output related to the *p*-value from OpenEpi.[10] The exposure odds ratio for the association between the age of the birthing parent (aged 40 years or older vs. aged 20–34 years) and stillbirth is 2.4, with a corresponding two-tailed (mid-*p* exact) *p*-value of 0.002. Although OpenEpi provides many more decimal places than what we have included here, recall from **Chapter 2, "Descriptive Epidemiology, Surveillance, and Measures of Frequency,"** that we want to be mindful of the number of significant figures that we use when reporting our study findings.

## FIGURE 12.5 DATA AND *P*-VALUE FOR THE CRUDE ASSOCIATION BETWEEN THE AGE OF THE BIRTHING PARENT AND STILLBIRTH

|  | Aged 40 years or older (E+) | Aged 20–34 years (E−) |
|---|---|---|
| Stillbirth (Cases) | 28 | 427 |
| Live Birth (Controls) | 28 | 1,024 |

**2×2 Table Statistics**

Single Table Analysis

Exposure

|  | (+) | (−) | |
|---|---|---|---|
| Disease (+) | 28 | 427 | 455 |
| (−) | 28 | 1,024 | 1,052 |
|  | 56 | 1,451 | 1,507 |

Chi Square and Exact Measures of Association

| Test | Value | *p*-value(1-tail) | *p*-value(2-tail) |
|---|---|---|---|
| Uncorrected chi square | 10.83 | 0.0005002 | 0.001000 |
| Yates corrected chi square | 9.873 | 0.0008388 | 0.001678 |
| Mantel-Haenszel chi square | 10.82 | 0.0005022 | 0.001004 |
| Fisher exact |  | 0.001217 | 0.002435 |
| Mid-P exact |  | 0.0008435 | 0.001687 |

*Source*: Data from Stillbirth Collaborative Research Network Writing Group. Association between stillbirth and risk factors known at pregnancy confirmation. *JAMA*. 2011;306(22):2469-2479. https://doi.org/10.1001/jama.2011.1798

To interpret the two-tailed *p*-value of 0.002, we would say that there is a 0.2% (0.002 × 100%) chance that the researchers would have observed an exposure odds ratio of 2.4 or greater *or* an exposure odds ratio between 0 and 0.42 $\left(\dfrac{1}{2.4}\right)$ if there were truly was no association between being aged 40 years or older (vs. being aged 20 to 34 years) and stillbirth (and there was no bias!). Thus, if sampling were the only source of error in this study, it is very unlikely that there is truly no association between the age of the birthing parent and stillbirth.

# Using *p*-Values for Null Hypothesis Significance Testing
## (LEARNING OBJECTIVE 12.8)

*P*-values are used to make decisions about whether to reject the null hypothesis. If we reject the null hypothesis, we are saying that there *is* a statistically significant association between the exposure and the outcome. We already know that there is a chance that we could say that there is an association when there truly isn't (a type I error). In order to reject the null hypothesis, our *p*-value must be *less* than the threshold that we've set for type I error. Thus, we compare our *p*-value against alpha, which is used as the cutoff for **statistical significance**.

*p*-value $\geq \alpha$: Do not reject $H_0$.

- The measure of association *is not* statistically significantly different from the null.
- The data *do not* provide sufficient evidence to infer that the population parameter is different from the null.

*p*-value $< \alpha$: Reject $H_0$.

- The measure of association *is* statistically significantly different from the null.
- The data provide sufficient evidence to infer that the population parameter *is* different from the null.

Considering the association between the age of the birthing parent and stillbirth, we can compare our *p*-value of 0.002 to an alpha of 0.05. Since 0.002 is less than 0.05, we reject the null hypothesis that there is truly no association between the age of the birthing parent and stillbirth. Put another way, we conclude that there is a statistically significant association between the age of the birthing parent and stillbirth.

**One- and two-tailed *p*-values (Learning Objective 12.9).** As you might guess, one- and two-tailed *p*-values correspond to the one- and two-sided alternative hypotheses, respectively. As previously described, two-sided alternative hypotheses consider values that are "as or more extreme" on *both* sides of the null, and thus will always yield a greater *p*-value than that calculated for a one-sided alternate hypothesis. This means that it will be harder to reject the null for two-sided versus a one-sided alternative hypothesis because the two-tailed *p*-value will be larger. To be cautious and avoid overstating findings, researchers will often test a two-sided alternative hypothesis, and thus use a two-tailed *p*-value for null hypothesis significance testing—even when they have an idea of whether the association between their exposure and outcome of interest is likely to be positive or negative.

# Interpreting *p*-Values (LEARNING OBJECTIVE 12.10)

Recall that a *p*-value is defined as the probability of obtaining a result as or more extreme than the result observed in your study if the null hypothesis is true and there is no bias. This can be a cumbersome definition, and students and epidemiologists alike often have trouble interpreting *p*-values. Consider again the association between the age of the birthing parent and stillbirth.

What the *p*-value of 0.002 tells us:

- ✓ If our data have not been influenced by bias, it is unlikely that there is no true association between the age of the birthing parent and stillbirth.
- ✓ The study data are *not* consistent with the null hypothesis.
- ✓ At an α level of 0.05, there is a statistically significant association between the age of the birthing parent (those aged 40 years and older compared to those aged 20 to 34 years) and stillbirth.

What the $p$-value of 0.002 does *not* tell us:

✗ Whether we have identified the true association between the age of the birthing parent and stillbirth.

✗ There is a 0.2% chance that the null hypothesis is true.

✗ There is a 0.2% chance that the observed result is due to chance alone.

✗ The magnitude of the association between the age of the birthing parent and stillbirth in our study. Without additional information, there's no way to know if the EOR was 1.2 or 8.7!

✗ Whether or not the observed association is meaningfully significant from a public health perspective.

## Common Misinterpretations of the $p$-Value

The $p$-value is a measure that is often misinterpreted as the probability that the measure of association observed in a study occurred due to chance, or even the probability that a type I error has occurred. These incorrect interpretations are made by new and experienced epidemiologists alike. In fact, a top-tier journal prepared a guide to assist journalists in interpreting epidemiologic research that included an erroneous interpretation,[11] which was then denounced by a substantial number of epidemiologists who raised concerns about the misinterpretation and misuse of $p$-values.[12]

Another common pitfall is forgetting that the $p$-value encompasses not just the probability of the observed result, but also the probabilities associated with results that are stronger than what was observed.

Finally, we must remember that $p$-values only provide information about the influence of random error on the study findings; $p$-values cannot tell us anything about the influence of systematic error. Thus, all $p$-values must be interpreted under the (often unrealistic) assumption that the results are unbiased.

## Pause to Practice 12.3

### $p$-Values in the Study of Cross-Estrogen Use and Ischemic Stroke

The data in **Table 12.2** are adapted from the previously described cohort study that evaluated the association between cross-sex estrogen use and ischemic stroke.[3] Use these data to answer the questions that follow.

**TABLE 12.2 DATA ADAPTED FROM THE COHORT STUDY THAT EVALUATED THE ASSOCIATION BETWEEN CROSS-SEX ESTROGEN USE AND ISCHEMIC STROKE**

| | Transfeminine Persons Who Used Hormone Treatment (E+) | Cisgender Men (E−) |
|---|---|---|
| Cases of Ischemic Stroke | 17 | 356 |
| Person-Years | 2,576 | 122,786 |

*Source:* Getahun D, Nash R, Flanders WD, et al. Cross-sex hormones and acute cardiovascular events in transgender persons: a cohort study. *Ann Intern Med.* 2018;169(4):205–213. https://doi.org/10.7326/M17-2785

1. Calculate and interpret the rate ratio that describes the association between cross-sex estrogen use and ischemic stroke, comparing transfeminine persons who used hormone treatment (the exposed group) to cisgender men (the unexposed group).

*Recall that the formula for the rate (incidence density) ratio (IDR) is given by:*

$$IDR = \frac{\text{Rate exposed}}{\text{Rate unexposed}} = \frac{\left(\dfrac{\text{Cases among exposed}}{\text{person-time among exposed}}\right)}{\left(\dfrac{\text{Cases among unexposed}}{\text{person-time among unexposed}}\right)}$$

2. Enter these data in OpenEpi using the "Compare 2 Rates" feature. You can find the one-tailed $p$-value for the rate ratio calculated in Question 1 listed next to the z-score and should find that this value is 0.00033. Using the definition of a $p$-value, how do you interpret this result? If $\alpha$ were set at 0.05, and there is no bias, would the findings lead you to reject the null hypothesis?

3. In the OpenEpi output, you should find that the two-tailed $p$-value for the rate ratio is 0.00066. Using the definition of a $p$-value, how do you interpret this result? If $\alpha$ were set at 0.05, and there is no bias, would the findings lead you to reject the null hypothesis?

4. Compare your answers to Questions 2 and 3. Do you reach the same conclusion for each test?

5. Suppose that the one- and two-tailed $p$-values had been 0.04 and 0.08, respectively. How would you interpret these results? If $\alpha$ were set at 0.05, and there is no bias, would the findings lead you to reject the null hypothesis?

## Digging Deeper

### Where Do $p$-Values Come From?

While we have described $p$-values as telling us how likely it is that we would observe results as strong as or stronger than the ones that we observed (if the null hypothesis were true *and* there were no bias!), we have not described how $p$-values are calculated.

Although the specifics are beyond the scope of this text, readers should know that $p$-values are generated using **probability density functions (PDFs)**, which are functions that describe the probability of observing different outcomes. **Figure 12.6** graphs one such PDF where the outcome of interest is a measure of association, with one-tailed $p$-values illustrated in **Figure 12.6–Panel A**, and two-tailed $p$-values illustrated in **Figure 12.6–Panel B**.

The range of possible values for a given measure of association is plotted on the $x$-axis. The $y$-axis (not depicted on the graphs) plots the probabilities indicating how likely it would be to observe a given measure of association *if the null hypothesis were true* (i.e., their probability of occurrence). Since the PDF describes probability densities, the area under the curve is equal to one.

Let's think through why the PDFs peak around the null value. If the null hypothesis is true (i.e., if there is truly no association between the exposure and the outcome), then it is most likely that our study would yield a result that is close to the null. Similarly, measures of association that are further from the null would be increasingly less likely to occur, which is why the probability densities in the tails of the distribution are much smaller. To calculate a $p$-value associated with a particular measure of association, we begin by finding where our observed result falls on the $x$-axis. We then sum the probability densities under the curve corresponding to all of the measures of association that are stronger than the result that we observed.

Returning to **Figure 12.6**, the solid blue line in each panel represents the value of the measure of association that was observed in a given study, and the red arrows represent all of the values for the measure of association that are "as or more extreme" than our observed result.

## FIGURE 12.6 ILLUSTRATING ONE- AND TWO-TAILED *p*-VALUES USING PROBABILITY DENSITY FUNCTIONS

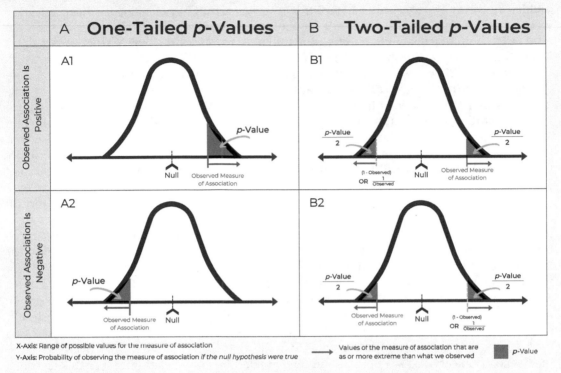

X-Axis: Range of possible values for the measure of association
Y-Axis: Probability of observing the measure of association *if the null hypothesis were true*

Values of the measure of association that are as or more extreme than what we observed

*p*-Value

To calculate a one-tailed *p*-value (**Figure 12.6–Panel A**), we sum the probability densities that are associated with our observed measure of association, and all possible values that are *further* from the null than what we observed. In all cases, we sum *away* from the null value: if we observe a positive association, we sum to the right of the observed result (**Figure 12.6–Panel A1**); if we observe a negative association, we sum to the left (**Figure 12.6–Panel A2**). The *p*-value is given by the area of the blue shaded region under the curve associated with these values.

The calculation of a two-tailed *p*-value (**Figure 12.6–Panel B**) is slightly more complicated because we must consider results that are as or more extreme than what we observed on *both* sides of the null value. We identify both our observed measure of association *and* the corresponding measure of association on the other side of the null value. As its name suggests, a two-tailed *p*-value is given by summing the probability densities from both tails of this distribution.

## Statistical Significance Does Not Imply Meaningful Significance
### (LEARNING OBJECTIVE 12.11)

As we noted previously, we caution against relying on null hypothesis significance testing to make conclusions about whether there is a true association between an exposure and an outcome.

Suppose there was a second team of researchers who also used a case-control design to study the association between the age of the birthing parent and stillbirth, and who also used an acceptable type I error rate of 5% ($\alpha = 0.05$) but enrolled fewer participants. Further, this study estimated an odds ratio for this association of 2.3 and an associated two-tailed *p*-value of 0.07. Recall that data from the Stillbirth Collaborative Research Network (SCRN)[5] generated an estimated odds ratio for the association between the age of the birthing parent and stillbirth of 2.4, with an associated *p*-value of 0.002. The major difference between this second team's study and that of the SCRN was that the second team did not have as much research funding and thus enrolled fewer participants (making it *more* subject to random error than the original study).

If we compare the point estimates alone (2.3 and 2.4), it is clear that these two studies yielded findings of very similar magnitude. However, null hypothesis significance testing would result in not rejecting the null for the smaller study (since 0.07 is greater than the alpha threshold of 0.05) while rejecting the null hypothesis for the SCRN study (since 0.002 is less than the alpha threshold of 0.05). If we based our public health conclusions solely on these statistical inferences, we might mistakenly conclude that these results are contradictory since one found a statistically significant association between the age of the birthing parent and stillbirth, while the other did not. Relying solely on statistical significance ignores that both studies found that the odds of being aged 40 years or older among those who had a stillbirth are roughly 2.4 times the odds of being aged 40 years or older among those who had a live birth. This information suggests that older birthing parents may be more likely to experience a stillbirth and that additional education and monitoring may be warranted for these patients.

Although this is a hypothetical example, misguided interpretations of the public health significance of studies relying solely on null hypothesis significance testing are abundant in the epidemiologic literature. For example, consider a randomized controlled trial to determine whether vitamin D and calcium supplementation decrease the incidence of cancer among women aged 55 years and older compared to a placebo.[13] Investigators estimated a hazard ratio (a measure of association that is interpreted similarly to a rate ratio) of 0.70 with an associated two-tailed $p$-value of 0.06. In their abstract, the authors conclude that "supplementation with vitamin $D_3$ and calcium compared with placebo did not result in a significantly lower risk of all-type cancer at 4 years." While it is true that this result does not reach *statistical* significance (since 0.06 is greater than the alpha threshold of 0.05), a decrease in the incidence of cancer of 30% is notable and likely to be clinically meaningful. For this reason, a focus on the magnitude of the association should have also been highlighted as part of their conclusions. This interpretation has also been critiqued for a lack of consideration of potential biases that may violate one of the assumptions of the $p$-value.[14]

This example leads us to consider the difference between *statistical* and *meaningful* differences in epidemiologic research. Two results may be statistically significantly different from one another, or a study result may be statistically significantly different from the null; however, this does not imply that these differences have **meaningful significance**. An association that is meaningfully significant is one that would have an impact on public health, such as leading to a change in clinical care, policy, or public health resource allocation. As we discussed previously, random error is influenced by sample size; thus, a very large sample could yield a measure of association that is *just* above the null but has an associated $p$-value less than alpha. It is typically unlikely that a very small, but statistically significant, increase in the likelihood of the outcome would have any public health impact. The converse is also true: a study that yields an estimate showing a strong association between the exposure and outcome may have important implications for public health but may not have been statistically significant due to a small sample size.

When interpreting study results, a focus on null hypothesis significance testing can lead readers—including public health decision-makers—to reach erroneous, and potentially harmful, conclusions if they incorrectly assume that statistical significance equates to meaningful significance. It is for this reason that the American Statistical Association issued a statement on statistical significance and $p$-values that outlines many of the concerns included here.[15]

## Factors That Influence *p*-Values (LEARNING OBJECTIVE 12.12)

To enhance our ability to think critically about the utility of $p$-values for interpreting findings from epidemiologic studies, let's take a closer look at the data from the randomized

## FIGURE 12.7 IMPACT OF SAMPLE SIZE AND FREQUENCY OF OUTCOME ON $p$-VALUES

| | Observed Study Data | | | Alternative scenario #1 | | | | Alternative scenario #2 | | |
|---|---|---|---|---|---|---|---|---|---|---|
| | Vitamin D and Calcium Supplement-ation (E+) | Placebo (E−) | | Increase All Cell Sizes by 50% | Vitamin D and Calcium Supplement-ation (E+) | Placebo (E−) | | Increase Incidence of the Outcome | Vitamin D and Calcium Supplement-ation (E+) | Placebo (E−) |
| Incident Cancer During Follow-Up Period (O+) | 45 | 64 | | Incident Cancer During Follow-Up Period (O+) | 45 × 1.5 = 67.5 | 64 × 1.5 = 96 | | Incident Cancer During Follow-Up Period (O+) | 578 | 1,147 × 0.71 = 814.4 |
| No Incident Cancer During Follow-Up Period (O−) | 1,111 | 1,083 | | No Incident Cancer During Follow-Up Period (O−) | 1,111 × 1.5 = 1,666.5 | 1,083 × 1.5 = 1,624.5 | | No Incident Cancer During Follow-Up Period (O−) | 578 | 1,147−814.4 = 332.6 |
| TOTAL | 1,156 | 1,147 | | TOTAL | 1,156 × 1.5 = 1,734 | 1,147 × 1.5 = 1,720.5 | | TOTAL | 1,156 | 1,147 |

| Measure of Interest | Observed Study Data ($N = 2,303$) | Alternative Scenario #1 ($N = 3,454.5$) | Alternative Scenario #2 ($N = 2,303$) |
|---|---|---|---|
| Risk$_{exposed}$ | 3.89% | 3.89% | 50% |
| Risk$_{unexposed}$ | 5.58% | 5.58% | 71.0% |
| Risk Ratio | 0.70 | 0.70 | 0.70 |
| $p$-value | 0.06 | 0.02 | <0.0001 |

controlled trial of vitamin D and calcium supplementation to better understand some of the factors that can influence $p$-values. Figure 12.7 contains the data that were observed in the randomized controlled trial,[13] along with two alternative scenarios for consideration.

In the first alternative scenario, we consider a study population that is 50% larger than the original (i.e., all of the cell sizes have been multiplied by 1.5). Since all four cells have been changed in the same way, we notice that the risk in the exposed and unexposed are identical to the original study, and thus the risk ratio also remains the same. The only difference is that the $p$-value for the study that is 50% larger is 0.02, compared to 0.06 from the original study. Simply by increasing the sample size, the study results have gone from not being statistically significant to being statistically significant at an alpha of 0.05.

In the second alternative scenario, we consider a study population where the incidence of cancer is much higher than in the original study. We have set the incidence of cancer in the exposed group to be 50%. To keep the risk ratio at 0.70, we have set the risk in the unexposed group to 71%. Although the risk ratio hasn't changed, increasing the incidence of cancer in this alternative scenario also yields a much smaller $p$-value compared with the original study.

In all three cases, vitamin D and calcium supplementation are associated with a 30% decrease in the incidence of cancer compared to the placebo. However, we see that increasing either the sample size or the incidence of the outcome both yielded smaller $p$-values than the original study. It is for this reason that we must consider the influence that the sample size and frequency of the outcome may have had on the results of studies that we aim to interpret.

Not shown in these figures is the influence of systematic error on $p$-values. As we discussed, null hypothesis significance testing is influenced by the magnitude of the measure of association. For this reason, a measure of association that is biased away from the null may have a $p$-value less than alpha, even if the null hypothesis is true. This underscores the importance of the assumption of no bias when interpreting a $p$-value.

## *p*-Values

- *p*-values are one tool used to quantify the influence of random error (specifically type I error) on study results.
- A *p*-value is the probability of observing a result as or more extreme than the one that you observed in your study if...
  - the null hypothesis were true, *and*
  - there were no bias.
- Null hypothesis significance testing using *p*-values:
  - Is a practice that is widespread but should not be used to interpret whether study findings are meaningfully significant.
  - Involves comparing *p*-values against a selected acceptable type I error rate ($\alpha$):
    - $p \geq \alpha \rightarrow$ do not reject the null hypothesis
    - $p < \alpha \rightarrow$ reject the null hypothesis
- Limitations of *p*-values and null hypothesis significance testing:
  - They provide no indication of how results may have been influenced by systematic error.
  - They provide no information about the strength, direction, or precision of the related measure of association.
  - They are influenced by sample size—thus, large samples will typically yield small *p*-values and vice versa.
  - Results that are statistically significant might not be meaningfully significant and vice versa.

## CONFIDENCE INTERVALS (LEARNING OBJECTIVE 12.13)

Like *p*-values, **confidence intervals (CIs)** can be used for statistical inference to quantify the impact that random (but not systematic!) error may have had on our study results. They may also be used for null hypothesis significance testing. Unlike *p*-values, confidence intervals provide additional information about the strength, direction, and precision of our measure of association. The most general conceptualization of a confidence interval is:

Measure of association ± Measure of random error

The **lower limit of the confidence interval** is calculated as: measure of association - measure of random error. Similarly, the **upper limit of the confidence interval** is calculate as: measure of association + measure of random error. Since the confidence interval is constructed around the measure of association, the measure of association calculated for a given study will always fall somewhere between the lower and upper confidence limits.

Most often, investigators calculate **95% confidence intervals**. We will describe the reason for this as we move along but will use this convention as we formally define confidence intervals, once again using the conceptualization of hypothetical study replications:

**95% of the confidence intervals generated from infinite unbiased study replications** would include the **population parameter**.

**Infinite unbiased study replications**. We first imagine that we have replicated our study an infinite number of times, again under the assumption that each of these replications have happened without the influence of systematic error. Each of these study replications would generate a point estimate, and each point estimate would have its own confidence interval.

**Population parameter**. Each of those infinite unbiased study replications would attempt to estimate the population parameter in the source population. The goal is that the population parameter will be contained within the confidence interval constructed around the point estimate.

**95%.** We quantify the proportion of the hypothetical study replications that would contain the population parameter. This proportion corresponds to $(1-\alpha)$, and since $\alpha$ is typically set to 0.05 (or 5%), investigators typically calculate 95% confidence intervals.

A schematic of the conceptualization of the confidence interval is shown in **Figure 12.8**. Of course, we cannot illustrate an infinite number of hypothetical study replications; however, the results of these 10 study replications help us to understand the overarching concept. The vertical black line represents the population parameter that we aim to estimate; the circles reflect the point estimate obtained from each study replication; and the bars represent the confidence intervals around each point estimate. The measures noted in blue are the ones where the confidence interval contains (i.e., overlaps) the population parameter, while the red confidence interval does not contain the population parameter.

**FIGURE 12.8 CONCEPTUALIZING THE CONFIDENCE INTERVALS AND ITS RELATIONSHIP TO THE POPULATION PARAMETER**

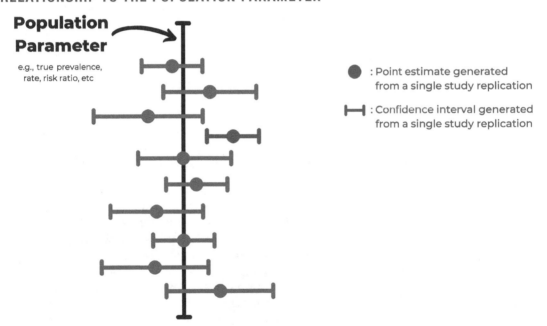

While we conceptualize these study replications, in reality, we only conduct one study that yields one confidence interval for our measure of association. To apply the principle of hypothetical study replications to our single study, we can interpret our confidence interval as a range of more plausible values for the population parameter than those outside the range, given what we observed in our study.[16]

## Calculating Confidence Intervals

The formulae for calculating confidence intervals around point estimates vary depending on the measure of interest as well as the sample size, and a discussion of these details is beyond the scope of this text. However, readers can use online calculators, such as OpenEpi,[10] to obtain confidence intervals for measures of interest.

Data adapted from the study of the association between the age of the birthing parent and stillbirth[5] are shown in **Figure 12.9**, along with corresponding output from OpenEpi.[10] Using this information, we see that the odds ratio for this association is 2.4 with a 95% confidence interval of (1.4, 4.1). This means that, based on our data and assuming that there is no bias,

## FIGURE 12.9 DATA AND OpenEpi OUTPUT FOR THE ASSOCIATION BETWEEN THE AGE OF THE BIRTHING PARENT AND STILLBIRTH

| | Aged 40 years or older (E+) | Aged 20–34 years (E−) |
|---|---|---|
| Stillbirth (Cases) | 28 | 427 |
| Live Birth (Controls) | 28 | 1,024 |

**2×2 Table Statistics**

**Single Table Analysis**
Exposure

| | | (+) | (−) | |
|---|---|---|---|---|
| | (+) | 28 | 427 | 455 |
| Disease | (−) | 28 | 1,024 | 1,052 |
| | | 56 | 1,451 | 1,507 |

**Odds-Based Estimates and Confidence Limits**

| Point Estimates | | Confidence Limits |
|---|---|---|
| | Value | Lower, Upper |
| CMLE Odds ratio | 2.397 | 1.395, 4.117 |
| | | 1.35,  4.255 |
| Odds ratio | 2.398 | 1.403, 4.098 |

CMLE, conditional maximum-likelihood estimate.
*Source*: Data from Stillbirth Collaborative Research Network Writing Group. Association between stillbirth and risk factors known at pregnancy confirmation. *JAMA*. 2011;306(22):2469-2479. https://doi.org/10.1001/jama.2011.1798

the population parameter (i.e., the true odds ratio for the association between the age of the birthing parent and stillbirth) is more likely to lie between 1.4 and 4.1 than outside this range.

## Confidence Intervals and Null Hypothesis Significance Testing
### (LEARNING OBJECTIVE 12.14)

Confidence intervals are related to type I error ($\alpha$) and can thus be used for null hypothesis significance testing. It is important for readers to understand the correct use of confidence intervals for null hypothesis significance testing by putting this information into context alongside other information (e.g., strength of the association, public health importance of the finding, and possible sources of bias).

To draw inference about the statistical significance of the point estimate using a confidence interval, we evaluate whether the confidence interval contains the null value. Recall that we can interpret a confidence interval as a more plausible range of values for the population parameter than those outside the range, given what we have observed in our study and assuming no bias.

An illustration of how confidence intervals are used for null hypothesis significance testing is shown in **Figure 12.10**. If a confidence interval contains the null value, the null value is thus a plausible value for the population parameter. This means that the measure of association is not statistically significantly different from the null, the associated *p*-value will be greater than or equal to $\alpha$, and we would not reject the null hypothesis. In **Figure 12.10–Panel A**, we see three different examples of confidence intervals that contain the null value: in the first and second examples, the point estimate falls either below or above the null value, respectively. However, in the third example, the point estimate is the same as the null value.

If a confidence interval does *not* contain the null value, the null value is a *less* plausible value for the population parameter given what we observed in our study. This means that the measure of association *is* statistically significantly different from the null, the associated *p*-value will be less than alpha, and we would reject the null hypothesis. In **Figure 12.10–Panel B**, we see two possible ways that this can happen. In both cases, the entire confidence interval is contained on just one side of the null value.

# FIGURE 12.10 USING CONFIDENCE INTERVALS FOR NULL HYPOTHESIS SIGNIFICANCE TESTING

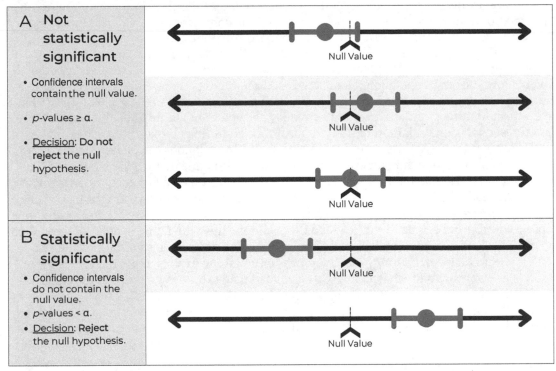

● : Point estimate ⊢⊣ : Confidence intervals

As indicated in **Figure 12.10**, the confidence interval and *p*-value will lead to the same conclusion when using null hypothesis significance testing for a given measure of association and a given alpha.

Let's take a look at what we can (and can't!) learn from the 95% confidence interval around the odds ratio for the estimate of the association between the age of the birthing parent and stillbirth.

What the 95% CI of (1.4, 4.1) tells us:

✓ Based on our data (and assuming the results are unbiased), the true association is unlikely to be 1 (i.e., null).
✓ The study data are not consistent with the null hypothesis.
✓ At an α level of 0.05, there is a statistically significant association between the age of the birthing parent (those aged 40 years and older compared to those aged 20 to 34 years) and stillbirth.
✓ The *p*-value associated with the odds ratio is less than 0.05.

What the 95% CI of (1.4, 4.1) does *not* tell us:

✗ The true odds ratio for the association between the age of the birthing parent and stillbirth is 95% likely to lie between 1.4 and 4.1.
✗ Whether we have identified the true association between the age of the birthing parent and stillbirth.
✗ The exact value of the *p*-value associated with the odds ratio for the association between the age of the birthing parent and stillbirth.
✗ Whether the observed association is meaningfully significant from a public health perspective.

## Common Misinterpretations of Confidence Intervals

A common incorrect interpretation of the confidence interval is that we are 95% confident that the population parameter is contained within the confidence interval. As shown in **Figure 12.7**, each confidence interval either contains the population parameter or does not; thus, confidence intervals are *not* interpreted as the $(1 - \alpha)$% chance that the population parameter is included in the given interval. Rather, confidence intervals provide a range of likely values for the population parameter, based on the data that we have collected and assuming no bias. If we wanted to strictly adhere to the formal definition, we would say that we expect that the population parameter would be contained within 95% of the confidence intervals associated with infinite study replications, assuming no bias.

The difference between the correct and incorrect interpretations can be hard to understand—let's consider a thought exercise to help clarify. Imagine that we flip a fair coin 100 times and that the coin lands heads side up 40 times. Since this is a fair coin, the true probability of heads is 50%; however, the proportion of heads that we observed was 40%. Using the appropriate statistical methods, we can find that the 95% confidence interval around our observed proportion is 30.7% to 49.8%. In this example, the truth (50%) is not contained within the 95% confidence interval; thus, the probability that the truth lies within this interval is 0. It would be incorrect to say that the probability that the truth is in the interval is 95%. However, the probability that an interval calculated using this design will contain the truth is 95%. It is correct to say that if we flipped the coin in sets of 100 an infinite number of times, 95% of the intervals would contain the true value of 50%. We just happen to have generated one of the 5% of the experiments for which the confidence interval did not include the truth.

## Confidence Intervals and Precision (LEARNING OBJECTIVE 12.15)

Confidence intervals also provide information about the precision of our measure of association. Precision is an indicator of how much our results have been influenced by random error and is inversely associated with the width of a confidence interval. Wider confidence intervals are associated with measures that have more random error and are thus said to be less precise. Similarly, narrower confidence intervals are associated with measures that have less random error and are thus said to be more precise. Remember that studies with larger sample sizes have less random error; thus, studies with larger sample sizes will have narrower confidence intervals than studies with smaller sample sizes, all else being equal. **Figure 12.11** illustrates confidence intervals with different degrees of precision. The results shown in **Figure 12.11– Panels A and B** are more precise because they have narrower confidence intervals than the results shown in **Figure 12.11–Panels C and D**. Note that while we generally calculate 95% confidence intervals, if we were to calculate 90% confidence intervals, we would expect that those would be narrower than the 95% confidence intervals since the increase in alpha allows for a greater degree of type I error (i.e., $\alpha$ increases from 5% to 10%).

## Digging Deeper

## Comparing the Width of Confidence Intervals

We can often do an "eyeball" test to ascertain whether one confidence interval is narrower than another; however, we may want to compare confidence intervals in a more systematic way. The method for ascertaining the width of a confidence interval depends on whether you have calculated a difference measure of association or a ratio measure of association.

For difference measures of association, the width of the confidence interval is determined by subtracting the lower limit from the upper limit:

$$\text{CI width}_{\text{difference measure of association}} = \text{Upper limit} - \text{lower limit}$$

To calculate the width of a confidence interval for a ratio measure of association, we take the ratio of the upper and lower limits:

$$\text{CI width}_{\text{ratio measure of association}} = \frac{\text{Upper limit}}{\text{Lower limit}}$$

Of course, we want to make fair comparisons; thus, when comparing the width of confidence intervals, we should only make side-by-side comparisons of confidence intervals calculated using the same value for alpha. That is, we should compare the width of 95% confidence intervals to each other rather than comparing the width of a 95% CI ($\alpha = 0.05$) to a 90% CI ($\alpha = 0.10$).

## FIGURE 12.11 CONFIDENCE INTERVALS: PRECISION AND NULL HYPOTHESIS SIGNIFICANCE TESTING

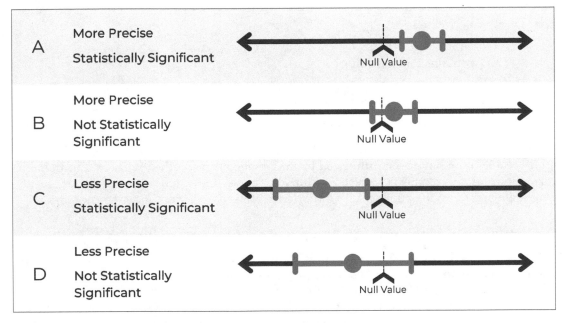

● : Point estimate          ⊢⊣ : Confidence intervals

## Confidence Intervals and the Magnitude and Direction of the Association

Confidence intervals also provide insight into the magnitude (i.e., strength) of an association as well as whether an association is positive or negative. The association observed in **Figure 12.11–Panel A** is stronger than that of **Figure 12.11–Panel B**, as its confidence interval is further away from the null value. Similarly, the association in **Figure 12.11–Panel C** is stronger than that of **Figure 12.11–Panel D**, since its confidence interval is further from the null value. In terms of direction, the associations observed in **Figure 12.11–Panels A** and **B** are both positive as their confidence intervals are entirely or mostly above the null value, respectively. Similarly, the associations observed in **Figure 12.11–Panels C** and **D** are both negative as their corresponding confidence intervals are entirely, or mostly, below the null value, respectively. Even when confidence intervals contain the null value, it is important to note that the confidence interval could lie mostly above or below the null; this information about the likely direction of the measure of association is not apparent from a *p*-value.

# COMPARING AND CONTRASTING CONFIDENCE INTERVALS AND *P*-VALUES (LEARNING OBJECTIVE 12.16)

We now know that *p*-values and confidence intervals are both used to quantify the impact of random error on our study findings. Before concluding our discussion of random error in epidemiologic research, it is important to highlight the key similarities and differences between *p*-values and confidence intervals.

## Similarities Between Confidence Intervals and *p*-Values

Confidence intervals and *p*-values both provide information about the influence of random error and thus are both impacted by sample size. As the sample size increases, random error decreases (all else being held constant), leading to smaller *p*-values and narrower confidence intervals. Conversely, smaller studies are more vulnerable to random error, which leads to larger *p*-values and wider confidence intervals. Both can be used for null hypothesis significance testing:

- Do not reject $H_0$ when:
  - $p \geq \alpha$.
  - $CI_{1-\alpha\%}$ contains the null value.
- Reject $H_0$ when:
  - $p < \alpha$.
  - $CI_{1-\alpha\%}$ does not contain the null value.

Importantly, neither *p*-values nor confidence intervals provide any indication of how the study results may have been influenced by systematic error. Further, without additional information about the context in which the study has been conducted, neither of these measures provide insight into the public health importance of the association under consideration.

## Differences Between Confidence Intervals and *p*-Values

Unlike *p*-values, confidence intervals provide information about the direction, magnitude, and precision of point estimates. For example, risk differences of −0.8 and −0.2, and risk ratios of 1.2 and 6.3, could all be associated with identical *p*-values, yet we would miss the difference in the strength and direction of these associations if we only knew the *p*-values. For this reason, confidence intervals are preferred over *p*-values for quantifying the impact of random error in epidemiologic research.

## Pause to Practice 12.4

### Confidence Intervals, *p*-Values, and Sample Size in the Study of Cross-Sex Estrogen Use and Ischemic Stroke

Previously, we reviewed the data generated from the study of the association between cross-sex estrogen use and ischemic stroke[3] and used the observed two-tailed *p*-value ($p = 0.00066$) for null hypothesis significance testing. We will now take this example a step further to examine the confidence interval around the point estimate and the impact of sample size on measures of random error.

**Table 12.3A** includes the study data that we presented earlier. In **Table 12.3B**, we have decreased the study's sample size by one-tenth and rounded the number of cases and person-years to the nearest integer.

**TABLE 12.3 IMPACT OF SAMPLE SIZE ON THE QUANTIFICATION OF RANDOM ERROR IN THE STUDY OF ISCHEMIC STROKE**

| A. ORIGINAL STUDY DATA | | | | B. ONE-TENTH SAMPLE SIZE | | |
|---|---|---|---|---|---|---|
| | Transfeminine Persons Who Used Hormone Treatment (E+) | Cisgender Men (E−) | | | Transfeminine Persons Who Used Hormone Treatment (E+) | Cisgender Men (E−) |
| Cases of Ischemic Stroke | 17 | 356 | | Cases of Ischemic Stroke | 2 | 36 |
| Person-Years | 2,576 | 122,786 | | Person-Years | 258 | 12,279 |

1. Use the data from the smaller study to calculate the rate ratio that describes the association between cross-sex estrogen use and ischemic stroke (again comparing transfeminine persons who used hormone treatment to cisgender men). How does this measure compare to the one that you calculated for the original study data?

   *Recall that the formula for the IDR rate is given by:*

   $$IDR = \frac{\text{Rate exposed}}{\text{Rate unexposed}} = \frac{\left(\dfrac{\text{Cases among exposed}}{\text{person-time among exposed}}\right)}{\left(\dfrac{\text{Cases among unexposed}}{\text{person-time among unexposed}}\right)}$$

2. Enter these data in OpenEpi using the "Compare 2 Rates" feature[10] to find the two-tailed *p*-values and 95% CIs for the rate ratios using the data from Table 12.3. You should find values that match those noted in **Table 12.4**. Compare and contrast these findings and explain why they differ.

**TABLE 12.4 IMPACT OF SAMPLE SIZE ON MEASURES OF RANDOM ERROR IN THE STUDY OF ISCHEMIC STROKE**

| | A. Original Study | B. One-Tenth Sample Size |
|---|---|---|
| Rate ratio | 2.3 | 2.6 |
| Two-tailed *p*-value | 0.00066 | 0.16 |
| 95% CI | (1.40, 3.70) | (0.43, 9.28) |

3. What is the population parameter that we are trying to estimate?

4. What information does each of the confidence intervals provide us about this population parameter?

5. What conclusions do you draw about the association between cross-sex estrogen use and ischemic stroke from each of these two studies? Think about this from both a statistical perspective as well as a public health perspective.

6. What would have happened to our point estimate, *p*-value, and 95% CI if our sample size had proportionally *increased* instead of decreased?

7. Returning to the results from the original study, how can we interpret these results? What influence might these results have on public health practice?

## Confidence Intervals

- Confidence intervals, like $p$-values, are used to quantify the influence of random error on study results.
- Confidence intervals use the data from a given study to provide a range of plausible values for the population parameter, assuming that the results are not biased.
- Null hypothesis significance testing using confidence intervals:
  - Involves ascertaining whether the null value is included in the confidence intervals:
    - Null value included in the interval → do not reject $H_0$
    - Null value *not* included in the interval → reject $H_0$
  - Leads to the same conclusions about statistical significance as $p$-values
  - Is a widespread practice, but, similar to the use of $p$-values, often leads to misinterpretations of statistical versus meaningful significance
- Confidence intervals provide insight into three important characteristics of the measure of association:
  - **Direction**: positive (above the null) or negative (below the null)
  - **Magnitude**: how far the association is from the null
  - **Precision**: inversely associated with the influence of random error
    - Wider intervals → more random error and measures are less precise
    - Narrower intervals → less random error and measures are more precise
- Confidence intervals are influenced by sample size. Larger samples will typically yield narrower confidence intervals and vice versa.
- Confidence intervals are preferred over $p$-values for quantifying the impact of random error in epidemiologic research.

## WHERE WE'VE BEEN AND WHAT'S UP NEXT

Our final chapter on error in epidemiologic research has focused on the way that random error impacts our study results. Recall that this is but one type of error, and that epidemiologists must also pay attention to the systematic errors of confounding (**Chapter 9**), selection bias (**Chapter 10**), and information bias (**Chapter 11**).

Statistical inference is used to quantify the impact of random error, and is an important tool to have in our epidemiologic toolkit: it is rare to be able to or to need to study an entire source population, and so we use statistical inference to quantify the influence of the error that occurs when we study only a subset of the source population. Although both $p$-values and confidence intervals are used to quantify random error, confidence intervals are more informative as they provide additional insight about the magnitude, direction, and precision around the measure of association that we have calculated.

Null hypothesis significance testing can be appealing because it provides a well-defined decision-making process that can be used to draw conclusions about an epidemiologic study. Unfortunately, the resulting dichotomous decision to either reject or not reject the null hypothesis is not sufficient for drawing a conclusion about whether there is a meaningful association between the exposure and the outcome. We must consider other factors, such as the strength of the association, its precision, how it aligns with similar studies, potential sources of bias, and whether the finding might warrant a change in public health action.

Despite concerns about the misinterpretation of findings based on null hypothesis significance testing,[17] readers can still expect to see it used widely in both scientific literature and popular media. This chapter has provided you with information about what statistical inference can and *can't* tell us, and we hope you will apply these lessons as you read health news and engage in public health work.

Up next is the final chapter in this text, which will revisit and synthesize many of the epidemiologic analysis tools you have learned, as well as take a closer look at how to conduct and interpret more advanced epidemiologic analyses than those already presented.

---

## END OF CHAPTER PROBLEM SET

### Questions 1 to 6 are based on and adapted from:

Jahn JL, Wallace M, Theall KP, et al. Neighborhood proactive policing and racial inequities in preterm birth in New Orleans, 2018–2019. *Am J Public Health*. 2023;113(S1):S21–S28. https://doi.org/10.2105/AJPH.2022.307079. PMID: 36696607; PMCID: PMC9877384.

Investigators undertook a cohort study using historical data to quantify the impact of structural racism on inequities in reproductive health in New Orleans, Louisiana. To do this, they combined publicly available data from the police department with vital statistics data to evaluate whether the association between neighborhood-level proactive policing and preterm birth differed for Black versus White births.

**Proactive policing** is a practice used in urban settings whereby police officers pursue a suspect on the basis of their own discretion. This practice is more common in select predominantly Black neighborhoods and contributes to structural racism in the legal system. Research suggests that the impacts of proactive policing extend beyond those who are stopped by the police. For example, there are health implications associated with chronic stress stemming from persistent concern about the potential for police violence.

**Preterm birth** is defined as the birth of a baby before 37 completed weeks' gestation and is associated with health complications for the newborn, including impaired breathing, hearing, and vision, as well as developmental delays. Louisiana has a particularly high preterm birth rate, with 13% of all babies born preterm in 2018 and 2019.[18] By race, Black babies have the highest preterm birth rate at nearly 17%.[18] Although the reasons for this disparity are multifactorial, they are largely attributed to maternal stress related to the experience of racism.[19]

### Study Findings

Among Black birthing parents, investigators found that the risk of preterm birth among those living in neighborhoods with the highest levels of proactive policing was 1.41* (95% CI: 1.04, 1.93) times the risk of preterm birth among those living in neighborhoods with the lowest levels of proactive policing.

Among White birthing parents, investigators found that the risk of preterm birth among those living in neighborhoods with the highest levels of proactive policing was 0.74* (95% CI: 0.33, 1.66) times the risk of preterm birth among those living in neighborhoods with the lowest levels of proactive policing.

Use the information provided above to indicate whether each of the following statements are true. For statements that are true, provide a brief rationale to describe why. For statements that are false, indicate what would need to be changed for the statement to be true.

---

*Note that these risk ratios have been adjusted to account for potential confounding by individual age, education, Medicaid status, and year, as well as neighborhood-level unemployment, education, poverty, population density, and rate of calls to the police for violence.

1. The associations between proactive policing and preterm birth for both Black and White birthing parents are both statistically significant because neither of the confidence intervals contain zero.

2. These results suggest that race modifies the association between proactive policing and preterm birth.

3. Among Black birthing parents, the population parameter for the association between proactive policing and preterm birth lies somewhere between 1.04 and 1.93.

4. There is less than a 5% chance that these study results have been influenced by bias.

5. The association between proactive policing and preterm birth for Black birthing parents is statistically significant with a $p$-value less than 0.05.

6. The association between proactive policing and preterm birth for White birthing parents is statistically significant with a $p$-value less than 0.05.

### Questions 7 to 13 are based on and adapted from:

COVIDSurg Collaborative; GlobalSurg Collaborative. Timing of surgery following SARS-CoV-2 infection: an international prospective cohort study. *Anaesthesia*. 2021;76(6):748–758. https://doi.org/10.1111/anae.15458. Epub 2021 Mar 9. PMID: 33690889; PMCID: PMC8206995.

Prior to the COVID-19 pandemic, physicians would often delay surgery for individuals who had a respiratory illness around the time of the scheduled surgery to reduce postsurgery mortality. When SARS-CoV-2 emerged, the optimal time interval between having a respiratory infection and surgery was unknown. Investigators undertook an international cohort study to address this important question.

Investigators compared 30-day postsurgery mortality associated with different time intervals, as well as across several different characteristics. Select adjusted risk odds ratios (aRORs) and their associated two-tailed $p$-values are provided in Questions 7 to 9. For each of these, write a sentence that describes what the $p$-value means, and be sure to include which values are considered "as or more extreme" in your response. What do you conclude about the association between each characteristic and 30-day postsurgery mortality from a *statistical* perspective?

7. The risk odds ratio that compares 30-day postsurgery mortality for those aged 70 years or older to those aged 69 years or younger was 1.72, with an associated two-tailed $p$-value less than 0.001.

8. The risk odds ratio that compares 30-day postsurgery mortality for those with respiratory comorbidities to those without respiratory comorbidities was 1.02, with an associated two-tailed $p$-value of 0.77.

9. The risk odds ratio that compares 30-day postsurgery mortality for those whose surgeries were due to trauma to those whose surgeries were for benign issues was 0.91, with an associated two-tailed $p$-value of 0.17.

10. The aRORs for the associations between time since SARS-CoV-2 diagnosis and 30-day postsurgery mortality are shown in **Table 12.5**. Note that each exposure category (time since SARS-CoV-2 diagnosis) is compared to the reference group of individuals who underwent surgery but did not have a SARS-CoV-2 diagnosis. What do these data suggest about the timing of surgery after a SARS-CoV-2 infection?

**TABLE 12.5 ADJUSTED RISK ODDS RATIOS FOR THE ASSOCIATIONS BETWEEN TIME SINCE SARS-CoV-2 DIAGNOSIS AND 30-DAY POSTSURGERY MORTALITY**

| Time Elapsed Between SARS-CoV-2 Infection and Surgery | aROR | 95% CI | p-Value (two-tailed) |
|---|---|---|---|
| No SARS-CoV-2 infection diagnosis | Reference | – | – |
| 0 to 2 weeks | 3.22 | (2.55, 4.07) | <0.001 |
| 3 to 4 weeks | 3.03 | (2.03, 4.52) | <0.001 |
| 5 to 6 weeks | 2.78 | (1.64, 4.71) | <0.001 |
| ≥7 weeks | 1.02 | (0.66, 1.56) | 0.94 |

*Source*: COVIDSurg Collaborative; GlobalSurg Collaborative. Timing of surgery following SARS-CoV-2 infection: an international prospective cohort study. *Anaesthesia*. 2021;76(6):748-758. https://doi.org/10.1111/anae.15458

11. Your colleague (who is not studying epidemiology!) reviews **Table 12.5** and remarks that the finding for those who had their surgeries 7 or more weeks after their SARS-CoV-2 infection isn't important since it doesn't reach statistical significance. Bearing in mind the goal of the study (i.e., to identify the optimal timing after SARS-CoV-2 infection to reschedule surgeries), explain why your colleague's interpretation is misguided.

**Questions 12 and 13 are intended to help you think about the relationship between *p*-values, confidence intervals, and sample size. For each scenario, indicate the expected impact of the change in study protocol on both the *p*-value and the confidence interval. You can assume that the changes described were the *only* deviations from the original study. If you don't have enough information to decide, provide a brief description to explain why.**

12. Study sample size increased by 50% (assume that this increase was proportional, such that all cells of the R×C table were multiplied by 1.5):
    a. Impact on the *p*-value? *Increase, decrease, unknown*
    b. Impact on the confidence interval? *Narrower, wider, unknown*

13. The proportion of people who died in the 30 days after surgery decreased by 20% in all exposure groups:
    a. Impact on the *p*-value? *Increase, decrease, unknown*
    b. Impact on the confidence interval? *Narrower, wider, unknown*

14. As you've learned, there is a direct relationship between sample size and type I error, type II error, and study power. Each row in **Table 12.6** notes a proposed change to one of these elements. Complete **Table 12.6** to indicate what impact the proposed change would have on the remaining elements. The first row has been completed for you.

**TABLE 12.6 PROPOSED CHANGE TO SAMPLE SIZE AND TYPE I ERROR, TYPE II ERROR, AND STUDY POWER**

| Study Power | Type I Error (α) | Type II Error (β) | Required Sample Size |
|---|---|---|---|
| Increase study power | Hold α constant | ↓ | ↑ |
| Hold power constant | Decrease type I error | | |
| Decrease study power | Hold α constant | | |
| | Increase type I error | Hold β constant | |
| | Hold α constant | Increase type II error | |
| Hold power constant | | | Decrease sample size |

15. In no more than two sentences, describe why investigators often choose to construct two-sided versus one-sided alternative hypotheses, even when the likely direction of the association can be assumed.

16. In your own words, describe the limitations of using null hypothesis significance testing for public health decision-making.

## REFERENCES

1. Zhang Q, Goodman M, Adams N, et al. Epidemiological considerations in transgender health: a systematic review with focus on higher quality data. *Int J Transgend Health.* 2020;21(2):125–137. https://doi.org/10.1080/26895269.2020.1753136

2. Institute of Medicine (US) Committee on Lesbian, Gay, Bisexual, and Transgender Health Issues and Research Gaps and Opportunities. *The Health of Lesbian, Gay, Bisexual, and Transgender People: Building a Foundation for Better Understanding.* National Academies Press; 2011. https://www.ncbi .nlm.nih.gov/books/NBK64806

3. Getahun D, Nash R, Flanders WD, et al. Cross-sex hormones and acute cardiovascular events in transgender persons: a cohort study. *Ann Intern Med.* 2018;169(4):205–213. https://doi.org/10.7326 /M17-2785

4. Gregory ECW, Valenzuela CP, Hoyert DL. Fetal mortality: United States, 2020. *NVSR.* 2022;71(4): 1–20. https://www.cdc.gov/nchs/data/nvsr/nvsr71/nvsr71-04.pdf

5. Stillbirth Collaborative Research Network Writing Group. Association between stillbirth and risk factors known at pregnancy confirmation. *JAMA.* 2011;306(22):2469–2479. https://doi.org/10.1001 /jama.2011.1798

6. Sauer MV. Reproduction at an advanced maternal age and maternal health. *Fertil Steril.* 2015;103(5):1136–1143. https://doi.org/10.1016/j.fertnstert.2015.03.004

7. D'Hoore L, T'Sjoen G. Gender-affirming hormone therapy: an updated literature review with an eye on the future. *J Intern Med.* 2022;291(5):574–592. https://doi.org/10.1111/joim.13441

8. Shatzel JJ, Connelly KJ, DeLoughery TG. Thrombotic issues in transgender medicine: a review. *Am J Hematol.* 2017;92(2):204–208. https://doi.org/10.1002/ajh.24593

9. Noordzij M, Dekker FW, Zoccali C, et al. Sample size calculations. *Nephron Clin Pract.* 2011;118(4): c319–c323. https://doi.org/10.1159/000322830

10. Dean AG, et al. OpenEpi: open source epidemiologic statistics for public health. 2013. http:// openepi.com

11. Woloshin S, Schwartz LM, Kramer BS. Promoting healthy skepticism in the news: Helping journalists get it right. *J Natl Cancer Inst.* 2009;101(23):1596–1599.

12. Lash TL, et al. Re: Promoting healthy skepticism in the news: Helping journalists get it right. *J Natl Cancer Inst.* 2010;102(11):829–830; author reply 830.

13. Lappe J, Watson P, Travers-Gustafson D, et al. Effect of vitamin D and calcium supplementation on cancer incidence in older women: a randomized clinical trial. *JAMA.* 2017;317(12):1234–1243. https://doi.org/10.1001/jama.2017.2115

14. Rothman K. JAMA rejected this letter from my colleagues & me ("low priority"), so we're publishing on twitter, hoping JAMA will take it more seriously. May 9, 2017. Accessed May 27, 2023. https://twitter.com/ken_rothman/status/862016511724183553?lang=en

15. Wasserstein RL, Lazar NA. The ASA statement on *p*-values: context, process, and purpose. *Am Stat.* 2016;70(2):129–133. https://doi.org/10.1080/00031305.2016.1154108

16. Poole C. Confidence intervals exclude nothing. *Am J Public Health.* 1987;77(4):492–493. https://doi .org/10.2105/ajph.77.4.492

17. Amrhein V, Greenland S, McShane B. Scientists rise up against statistical significance. *Nature.* 2019;567(7748):305–307. https://doi.org/10.1038/d41586-019-00857-9

18. March of Dimes. Preterm birth. Updated January 2022. https://www.marchofdimes.org/peristats /data?lev=1&obj=1&reg=99&slev=4&sreg=22&stop=60&top=3

19. Kramer MR, Hogue CR. What causes racial disparities in very preterm birth? A biosocial perspective. *Epidemiol Rev.* 2009;31:84–98. https://doi.org/10.1093/ajerev/mxp003

# CHAPTER 13

# INTRODUCTION TO EPIDEMIOLOGIC DATA ANALYSIS

## KEY TERMS

| | | |
|---|---|---|
| Breslow–Day test | linear regression | test for linear trend |
| categorical variables | logistic regression | $t$-test |
| chi-square test | Mann–Whitney test | |
| Fisher's exact test | numeric variables | |

## LEARNING OBJECTIVES

13.1 Understand the importance of the research question and study design in data analyses.

13.2 Understand the initial steps of a basic data analysis.

13.3 Identify the common epidemiologic variable types and the descriptive statistics used to describe them.

13.4 Understand the basic steps in data cleaning.

13.5 Understand when to use and how to interpret the result from a $t$-test or Mann–Whitney test to conduct significance testing for a numeric outcome variable.

13.6 Understand when to use and how to interpret the result from a chi-square test or Fisher's exact test to conduct significance testing for a categorical outcome variable.

13.7 Conduct stratified analyses to assess for effect measure modification and statistical interaction.

13.8 Understand when to use and how to interpret the result from a Breslow–Day test to conduct significance testing for statistical interaction.

13.9 Apply the data-based method for confounding assessment.

13.10 Understand when to use and how to interpret the result from an extended Mantel–Haenszel test of linear trend to conduct significance testing for an ordinal exposure variable.

13.11 Interpret adjusted measures of association generated by linear and logistic regression models.

## MENTAL HEALTH IN THE COVID ERA

The onset of the COVID-19 pandemic took a notable toll on the mental health of individuals around the world, and children and adolescents were uniquely affected.[1,2] The effects of school closures, social isolation, loss of peer interaction and support, delays in healthcare visits, and worsened food security were found to contribute to worsening mental health in young people during the early days of the pandemic.[1,3,4] Moreover, both younger people and adults from racial minority groups were disproportionately at-risk for experiencing negative pandemic-related mental health effects.[5–7]

The good news is that highly effective, evidence-based interventions, including various types of therapy and medication, have been shown to decrease depression, anxiety, and suicidal ideation. Another positive development has been the creation of validated scales for measuring depression and anxiety severity[8] enabling targeting of mental health services. Additionally, awareness of and access to mental health services are increasing, and publication of mental health research has increased over recent years (**Figure 13.1**). This has led to a reduction in mental health-related stigma, which means fewer people are suffering in silence.

Despite these gains, access to mental health services remains unevenly distributed. In particular, more work is needed to increase access to culturally appropriate health services for minority groups.[5] For the field of mental health to continue to have important and lasting success, we must continue to push for equitable mental healthcare including for children and minority groups around the world.

While issues of depression and suicidal ideation can be difficult to discuss, they have become increasingly common and cannot be ignored. As described by a participant in a study about the psychosocial impact of the pandemic in young people: "… during lockdown, I got horrendously depressed. So, I've had stuff going on mentally, but I was finding it tough. The social isolation made everything crash really badly."[9] It is important to normalize these challenges, increase awareness, and continue to address stigma. If you or someone you know is struggling with mental health-related issues, international resources are available through save.org. Additionally, resources may be available for those who are in an academic setting through your institution.

### FIGURE 13.1 NUMBER OF PUBLICATIONS FOUND IN PUBMED USING "MENTAL HEALTH" KEYWORD SEARCH OVER TIME

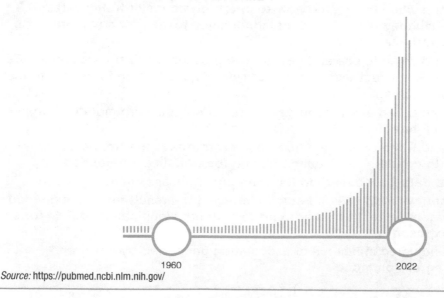

1960          2022

*Source:* https://pubmed.ncbi.nlm.nih.gov/

# INTRODUCTION TO EPIDEMIOLOGIC DATA ANALYSIS

You have now learned about the main epidemiologic study designs, the importance of effect measure modification, and how study results may be influenced by both systematic and random error. In this final chapter, we will synthesize and expand upon what you have already learned, with a focus on epidemiologic data analysis. We will provide a basic overview of data types, data set manipulation, and data analyses, all with the assumption that your data have already been collected. Additionally, we will introduce you to epidemiologic modeling with a focus on interpreting results from published epidemiologic studies.

As we have illustrated throughout this text, data analyses are heavily informed by the study design (Learning Objective 13.1). We have discussed how the study design informs which measures of frequency and association are appropriate to calculate (**Tables M.2** and **M.4**). As you have also learned, data analyses are hypothesis driven, meaning that they are guided by the hypothesized relationship between the exposure and outcome of interest. Thus far, we have presented these concepts using data analysis examples from published studies with the goal of illustrating specific concepts.

We will now take a deeper dive into the epidemiologic data analysis process from start to finish. In this chapter, we will think more holistically about epidemiologic data analysis with a focus on the following considerations (Learning Objective 13.2):

1. Examining the data set and cleaning the data

2. Describing the frequency of outcomes (unless the data come from a case-control study!), exposures, and covariates

3. Calculating unadjusted measures of association between the exposures and outcomes of interest

4. Assessing for effect measure modification by stratifying data by variables hypothesized a priori to modify the association between exposures and outcomes of interest

5. Assessing for confounding using a data-based method and calculating the appropriate measure of association adjusting for meaningful confounders

6. If appropriate, conducting analyses of trends to calculate measures of association between levels of an ordinal exposure and an outcome

7. Interpreting adjusted measures of association from regression models

## TYPES OF VARIABLES AND RELATED DESCRIPTIVE STATISTICS
### (LEARNING OBJECTIVE 13.3)

Before we examine a data set and begin to clean our data, we must first be aware of the different types of variables often found in epidemiologic data sets. It is important to understand the types of variables in our data sets because this determines which statistical tests can be used. A summary of the common epidemiologic variable types and their corresponding descriptive statistics discussed in this chapter is shown in **Figure 13.2**. We will begin with an overview of two different classifications of variables: **numeric** and **categorical**.

### Numeric Variables

**Numeric variables** are those with numeric responses which can be either continuous or discrete.

**Continuous variables** are numeric variables that can take on an infinite set of values bounded by any two values. For example, age is a continuous variable, bounded between 0 and the highest plausible age. Height, weight, total cholesterol, and time are also examples of continuous variables.

## FIGURE 13.2 COMMON TYPES OF QUANTITATIVE EPIDEMIOLOGIC VARIABLES AND THEIR CORRESPONDING DESCRIPTIVE STATISTICS

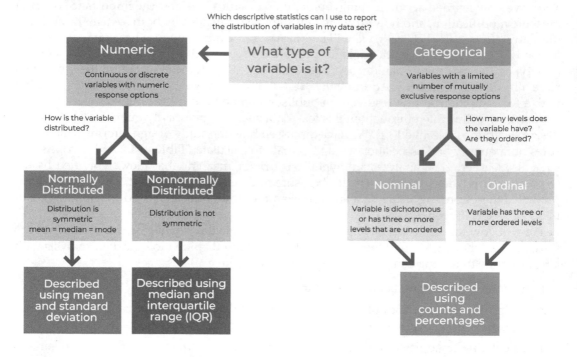

**Discrete variables** are numeric variables that have a limited number of responses. For example, the Patient Health Questionnaire (PHQ-9), a tool used to assess depression severity,[10] is comprised of nine questions, each with four possible answer choices recorded as scores between 0 and 3. Each respondent is assigned a total score, calculated by summing the scores for all nine questions. This results in a discrete variable that can range from 0 to 27, with 0 indicating no depression and 27 indicating the most severe depression.

Numeric variables may be described using **measures of central tendency** in combination with **measures of variability**.

A **measure of central tendency** is a singular value that describes a set of data using the central, or most common, value within those data. Common measures of central tendency include the **mean** (the average value of a set of data), **median** (the middle number in an ordered set of data), and the **mode** (the value that occurs most frequently in a set of data).

A **measure of variability**, related to random error (**Chapter 12, "Random Error in Epidemiologic Research"**), is a value that describes how much the values in a set of data are spread apart. Common measures of variability include the **standard deviation** and the **interquartile range**.

The **standard deviation** is the square root of the **variance**, where variance is a measure of the average spread of the data around the *mean*. Formulae for the standard deviation and variance can be found elsewhere.[11] **Figure 13.3** illustrates examples of two variables in a data set with varying standard deviations. The different values that the variable can take on are presented on the *x*-axes, and the frequency of those values is presented on the *y*-axes. Standard deviation is shown visually in this figure as the spread of the data around the mean, with a low standard deviation implying less variance and therefore less spread around the mean (**Figure 13.3A**) and a high standard deviation implying more variance and more spread around the mean (**Figure 13.3B**).

## FIGURE 13.3 VISUALIZING STANDARD DEVIATION AND THE SPREAD OF A DISTRIBUTION

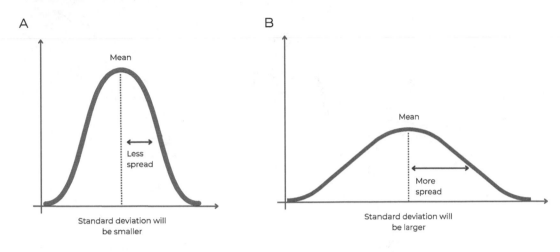

## FIGURE 13.4 ILLUSTRATING THE INTERQUARTILE RANGE (IQR)

The IQR is calculated around the *median* by dividing a set of data into quartiles (meaning dividing ordered data into four equal parts, separated by the value of the data which occurs at the 25th, 50th, and 75th percentiles) and is calculated as the difference between the values associated with the 25th and 75th percentiles. Thus, the IQR describes the range of the middle half of a set of ordered numeric data (**Figure 13.4**).

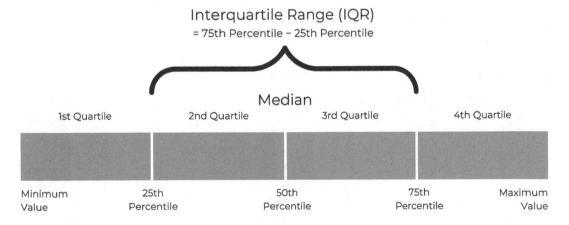

To determine which measures of central tendency and variability to choose, we need to know something about the **distribution** of the variable's responses, which means we need to understand the possible values that the variable could assume and how often each of those values occur in our data set. A distribution that is foundational for numeric variables is the **normal distribution**.[11] Two key features of normally distributed data are that (a) their values are distributed symmetrically around the mean, and (b) the values for the mean, median, and mode are all the same. An example of a normal distribution is shown in **Figure 13.5**. As before, the different values that the variable can take on are presented on the *x*-axis, and the frequency of those values is presented on the *y*-axis.

## FIGURE 13.5 EXAMPLE OF A NORMAL DISTRIBUTION

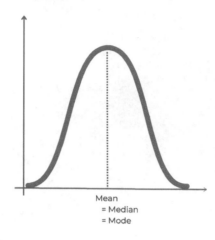

Mean
= Median
= Mode

To determine whether a variable is normally distributed, we can calculate the **skewness** and **kurtosis** of its distribution. Our focus will be to understand how to interpret, rather than generate, these values since these formulae are beyond the scope of this text (though described elsewhere[11]). Additionally, most statistical packages will calculate these measures for you. Briefly, **skewness** is a measure that describes the *lack* of symmetry in a variable's distribution. Skewness values further from zero are indicative of distributions that are more highly skewed (i.e., nonnormal). As shown in **Figure 13.6**, data that are normally distributed will appear symmetric, with a skewness of zero. For nonskewed distributions, the mean, median, and mode are all equal. **Negatively skewed** (also called **left skewed**) distributions contain more data on the left side of the distribution, and the skewness is negative. **Positively skewed** (also called **right skewed**) distributions contain more data on the right side of the distribution, and the skewness is positive. Note that if the data are multimodal (not shown in **Figure 13.6**), meaning the distribution peaks at more than one place, then the data are nonnormally distributed and the sign of the skewness is difficult to interpret.

## FIGURE 13.6 EXAMPLES OF DISTRIBUTIONS WITH VARYING SKEWNESS

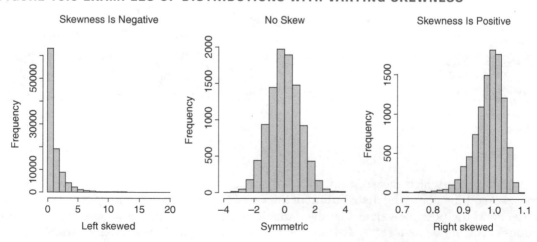

**Kurtosis** is a measure of how the tails of a variable's distribution compare to those of a normal distribution. We can think of this as whether the **tails** of our distribution (meaning the left and right most extreme regions of the distribution) appear above or below the tails of a normal distribution. The solid blue curve in **Figure 13.7** is an example of a **standard normal distribution**

# FIGURE 13.7 EXAMPLE OF DISTRIBUTIONS WITH POSITIVE AND NEGATIVE KURTOSIS

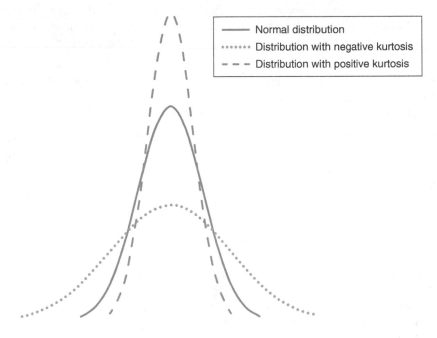

| | |
|---|---|
| —— | Normal distribution |
| •••••• | Distribution with negative kurtosis |
| – – – | Distribution with positive kurtosis |

(which is a normal distribution where the mean is 0 and the standard deviation is 1) which has a kurtosis equal to three. As shown, the tails of a distribution with **negative kurtosis** (shown using a green dotted line) lie above those of the standard normal distribution, and tails of a distribution with **positive kurtosis** (showing using an orange dashed line) lie below those of the standard normal distribution.

A summary of skewness and kurtosis values for normal and nonnormal distributions is shown in **Table 13.1**.

TABLE 13.1 **SUMMARY OF SKEWNESS AND KURTOSIS VALUES FOR NORMALLY AND NONNORMALLY DISTRIBUTED DATA**

| | Normally Distributed Data | Nonnormally Distributed Data |
|---|---|---|
| **Skewness** <br> Measure that describes the lack of symmetry of a distribution | 0 | Negative values: skewed left <br> Positive values: skewed right |
| **Kurtosis** <br> Measure that compares the tails of a given distribution to that of a normal distribution | 3 for a standard normal distribution (mean = 0, standard deviation = 1) | Value >3: positive kurtosis <br> Value < 3: negative kurtosis |

Once you know whether your data are normally distributed, you can determine which measures of central tendency and measures of variability to report. The linkage between a variable's distribution and the corresponding measures of central tendency and variability are summarized in the text that follows, as well as in **Figure 13.2**, which was presented earlier in this chapter.

- Normally distributed numeric variables:
  - measure of central tendency → mean
  - measure of variability → standard deviation
- Nonnormally distributed numeric variables:
  - measure of central tendency → median
  - measure of variability → interquartile range

## Categorical Variables

**Categorical variables** are variables that have a limited number of mutually exclusive response categories. Categorical data are commonly used in epidemiology, particularly for collecting information about health outcomes. Categorical variables are classified as either **nominal** or **ordinal**.

**Nominal variables** are categorical variables with two (**dichotomous**) or more unordered, mutually exclusive categories. For example, different antidepressants categorized into two (or more) mutually exclusive categories would be classified as a nominal variable.

**Ordinal variables** are categorical variables with more than two categories which *do* have an intrinsic order. For example, the educational level (e.g., less than high school, high school, some college, college graduate or higher) is an ordinal variable describing increasing levels of education. As another example, we may categorize the PHQ-9 depression severity score into three mutually exclusive ordered categories as (a) no or mild depression, (b) moderate depression, and (c) moderately severe or severe depression.

Categorical variables are described using **counts** and **percentages**. For example, if we had a sample of individuals who completed the PHQ-9, we may want to describe how many fell into each of the depression severity groups (none; mild depression; moderate depression; moderately severe depression; severe depression), along with the corresponding percentage of respondents in each group. Recall that in order to calculate the percentage of individuals who fall into different depression severity groups, we need a denominator of the total number of people who completed the PHQ-9. Throughout this text, we have described the importance of denominators. Suppose we only knew the count of people who were classified as having severe depression by the PHQ-9. This would not be enough information to understand the scope of the problem of severe depression in the sample population. We would additionally need to know the denominator (i.e., how many total people completed the PHQ-9) to draw any conclusions about the frequency of severe depression using these data.

## DATA EXAMINATION AND CLEANING (LEARNING OBJECTIVE 13.4)

Now that we have described different variable types, we can begin to explore a data set. When approaching an epidemiologic analysis, an important initial step is to closely examine and clean the data set. While it can be tempting to immediately start calculating measures of association, you must first become familiar with your data and ensure that there are not any formatting issues or errors that would bias the results.

To walk you through this process, we will examine, clean, and analyze data from a small hypothetical cross-sectional study about mental health. While data sets from epidemiologic studies are typically much larger, this data set of 15 participants will allow us to perform simple data manipulations and construct R×C (row by column) tables without the use of advanced data analysis packages such as SAS, Stata, or R. The data that we will work with are shown in **Table 13.2**. This data set contains information on participant age, depression severity, mental health service availability, ethnicity, and suicidal ideation for 15 participants, each of whom has a unique study ID.

Let's suppose that this cross-sectional study was conducted to answer two research questions:

1. Is the availability of mental health services in a community associated with decreased depression severity?

2. Are those with moderate to severe depression more likely to report suicidal ideation than those with no or mild depression?

Notice in this cross-sectional study that the outcome in Question 1 is the exposure in Question 2. As we described earlier in the text, it is possible that variables can act as exposures or outcomes, depending on the research question, especially in a cross-sectional study. It is always a good idea to first identify the exposure and outcome for a given research question as you are reading epidemiologic literature.

Before we discuss important considerations in data cleaning, take some time to familiarize yourself with this data set and see if you can spot any potential problems. Unclean data can be a source of selection and/or information bias and the goal of data cleaning is to improve the quality of your data to yield more valid conclusions. Though not exhaustive, we outline some basic steps and considerations for data cleaning in the text that follows. As you work with additional data sets in the future, you will find that there are often other issues that are unique to each study.

**Unwanted observations.** A first, critical step in data cleaning is to make sure the sample size in your data set matches what you expected from the study. Irrelevant or duplicate observations from the same study participant can appear in a data set, often due to errors when data are merged from multiple sources to create the analytic data set. Alternatively, irrelevant or duplicate observations can occur during data collection—for example, if study staff accidently enter participant data multiple times. Looking at **Table 13.2**, note that we have 16 lines (i.e., rows) of data but we were only expecting data for 15 study participants. If you look closely, you'll notice that data from participant ID 1005 is duplicated. This duplicated ID is easily identified by simply looking at this small data set. However, in a larger data set, you can make use of statistical programs which have functions to view and remove duplicate observations. We will remove one line of data for ID 1005. One way to avoid having duplicated study IDs in cross-sectional datasets is to construct the data entry system to flag duplicate ID entry.

**TABLE 13.2 DATA FROM A HYPOTHETICAL, UNCLEAN CROSS-SECTIONAL DATA SET**

| ID | Age | Depression Severity Score[a] | Moderate to Severe Depression[b] | Mental Health Services Available in Community | Ethnicity | Suicidal Ideation |
|---|---|---|---|---|---|---|
| 1001 | 35 | 27 | Yes | Yes | Non-Hispanic | Yes |
| 1002 | 18 | 0 | No | Yes | Non-Hispanic | No |
| 1003 | 28 | 3 | No | Yes | non-Hispanic | No |
| 1004 | 30 | 8 | no | Yes | Non-Hispanic | No |
| 1005 | 31 | 8 | No | Yes | Non-Hispanic | Yes |
| 1005 | 31 | 8 | No | Yes | Non-Hispanic | Yes |
| 1006 | 39 | 19 | Y | No | Non-Hispanic | Yes |
| 1007 | 19 | 26 | Yes | Yes | Hispanic | Yes |
| 1008 | 25 | 1 | N | Yes | Hispanic | No |
| 1009 | 33 | 10 | Yes | No | Non-Hispanic | No |
| 1010 | 500 | 13 | Yes | No | Hispanic | No |
| 1011 | 18 | 23 | Yes | no | Hispanic | Yes |
| 1012 | 20 | 9 | No | No | Hispanic | Yes |
| 1013 |  | 6 | No | No | Non-Hispanic | No |
| 1014 | 31 | 9 | No | No | Non-Hispanic | N |
| 1015 | 33 | 2 | No | No | Hispanic | No |

[a]Depression measured via the Patient Health Questionnaire (PHQ-9).
[b]Moderate to severe depression: Yes (PHQ-9 scores 10–27); No (PHQ-9 scores 0–9).

**Typos and capitalization inconsistencies.** Once we remove our unwanted observations, we can tabulate the frequencies (counts and percentages) of categorical variable responses. This allows for identification and correction of errors such as typos or inconsistent capitalization in the categorical variable responses, which can be a concern when conducting the analysis in some programming languages. See **Table 13.3**, which presents the frequencies of the categorical variables in the data set that we are cleaning. Note that several responses should logically be combined into one response. For example, for the dichotomous variable indicating moderate to severe depression, "N," "No," and "no" should all be combined into one "No" response.

**TABLE 13.3 DATA CLEANING: CALCULATING THE FREQUENCY OF CATEGORICAL VARIABLE RESPONSES AFTER REMOVAL OF DUPLICATE ENTRY**

| Categorical Variable | Count | Percent[c] |
|---|---|---|
| **Moderate to severe depression[a,b]** | | |
| N | 1 | 7% |
| No | 7 | 47% |
| Y | 1 | 7% |
| Yes | 5 | 33% |
| no | 1 | 7% |
| *TOTAL* | *15* | |
| **Mental health services available in community** | | |
| No | 7 | 47% |
| Yes | 7 | 47% |
| no | 1 | 7% |
| *TOTAL* | *15* | |
| **Ethnicity** | | |
| Hispanic | 6 | 40% |
| Non-Hispanic | 8 | 53% |
| non-Hispanic | 1 | 7% |
| *TOTAL* | *15* | |
| **Suicidal ideation** | | |
| N | 1 | 7% |
| No | 8 | 53% |
| Yes | 6 | 40% |
| *TOTAL* | *15* | |

[a]Depression measured via the Patient Health Questionnaire (PHQ-9).
[b]Moderate to severe depression: Yes (PHQ-9 scores 10–27); No (PHQ-9 scores 0–9).
[c]Percentages may not sum to 100% due to rounding

Another way to quickly identify this type of issue is by presenting the data visually using bar plots, as shown in **Figure 13.8**. To correct these issues, we can recode our categorical variable responses within a statistical programming package. Note that many errors related to typos or capitalization inconsistencies can be prevented when constructing the data entry system—for example, by using drop-down menus or checkboxes to capture standardized categorical data, instead of allowing free-text responses.

**Missing data.** As described in **Chapter 10, "Selection Bias,"** missing data can introduce selection bias if the results obtained using incomplete data differ from the results that would have been obtained if we had complete data on everyone who was eligible. In **Table 13.2,**

## FIGURE 13.8 DATA CLEANING: VISUALIZING THE FREQUENCY OF RESPONSES FOR A CATEGORICAL VARIABLE

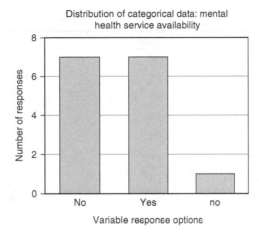

This figure was generated using data from Table 13.3 after removal of the duplicate entry.

there is one cell that does not have any data—ID 1013 does not have a value reported for age. Sometimes, investigators have access to other information in their data set that they could use to derive this information; for example, if there was another variable in the data set that included date of birth, this information could be used to calculate the missing value for age. When such information is not readily available, investigators may decide to conduct data **imputation**, which is a process by which missing data are "filled in." The imputed values are not chosen at random. Rather, investigators may use existing data to explore patterns of responses across several variables and then use this information to predict the most likely value for the missing data. The mechanics and (often rigorous) assumptions needed to apply various imputation strategies are beyond the scope of this textbook and can be found elsewhere.[12] For our purposes, let's assume that we performed data imputation using a statistical software package and found that the most likely age of participant 1013 was 34, and thus this value was imputed for their age. One way to avoid missing data is to construct the data entry system such that certain variables are programed to be required, thereby generating warnings or halting data entry until responses are entered.

**Outliers.** Outliers are responses that are improbable or impossible. It is important to identify outliers and correct data that are likely to be inaccurate because they will otherwise introduce error (information bias!) into your analyses. There is a range of techniques to identify outliers. The simplest of these includes sorting the data to view the highest and lowest values and/or graphing the data to identify extreme or even impossible values. While sorting and graphing your data is often sufficient to identify outliers, statistical approaches are also available and described elsewhere.[11] In our small study, we see that ID 1010 has an age of 500, which common sense tells us is impossible. This is likely to be a data entry error, which should be investigated. Let's suppose that we had access to other study records that indicated that this person was actually 50 years old. In this case, we can assume that the reason for the outlier was an accidental keystroke of an additional 0 during data entry. We should also review PHQ-9 scores, another numeric variable in our data set. Given the description of this scale, we know that possible scores range from 0 to 27. A review of this variable in our data set shows that all of the reported PHQ-9 values are plausible; thus, there are no concerns about implausible values for PHQ-9 scores. To avoid entry of implausible values, some data entry systems are programed to return an error if values are entered that fall outside a previously specified range of plausible values.

A summary of the steps taken during our data cleaning process is shown in **Figure 13.9**.

## FIGURE 13.9 SUMMARY OF DATA CLEANING OF A HYPOTHETICAL CROSS-SECTIONAL DATA SET

| ID | Age | Depression Severity Score[1] | Moderate to Severe Depression[2] | Mental Health Services Available in Community | Ethnicity | Suicidal Ideation |
|---|---|---|---|---|---|---|
| 1001 | 35 | 27 | Yes | Yes | Non-Hispanic | Yes |
| 1002 | 18 | 0 | No | Yes | Non-Hispanic | No |
| 1003 | 28 | 3 | No | Yes | ~~non-Hispanic~~ Non-Hispanic | No |
| 1004 | 30 | 8 | ~~no~~ No | Yes | Non-Hispanic | No |
| 1005 | 31 | 8 | No | Yes | Non-Hispanic | Yes |
| ✗ ~~1005~~ | ~~31~~ | ~~8~~ | ~~No~~ | ~~Yes~~ | ~~Non-Hispanic~~ | ~~Yes~~ |
| 1006 | 39 | 19 | ~~Y~~ Yes | No | Non-Hispanic | Yes |
| 1007 | 19 | 26 | Yes | Yes | Hispanic | Yes |
| 1008 | 25 | 1 | ~~N~~ No | Yes | Hispanic | No |
| 1009 | 33 | 10 | Yes | No | Non-Hispanic | No |
| 1010 | ✓~~500~~ 50 | 13 | Yes | No | Hispanic | No |
| 1011 | 18 | 23 | Yes | ~~no~~ No | Hispanic | Yes |
| 1012 | 20 | 9 | No | No | Hispanic | Yes |
| 1013 | 🔧 34 | 6 | No | No | Non-Hispanic | No |
| 1014 | 31 | 9 | No | No | Non-Hispanic | ~~N~~ No |
| 1015 | 33 | 2 | No | No | Hispanic | No |

✗ Remove duplicate entry for ID 1005    🔧 Impute missing age value for ID 1013    📎 Make responses consistent    ✓ Correct age value for ID 1010

[1]Depression measured via the Patient Health Questionnaire (PHQ-9).
[2]Moderate to severe depression: Yes (PHQ-9 scores 10-27); No (PHQ-9 scores 0-9).

## Highlights

### Variable Types and Data Cleaning

- Common **epidemiologic variable types** include numeric variables (e.g., continuous and discrete) and categorical variables (e.g., nominal and ordinal).

- **Numeric variables** can be described using **means** and **standard deviations** (for normally distributed data) or **medians** and **interquartile ranges (IQRs)** (for nonnormally distributed data).

- **Data cleaning** consists of examining your data for, and correcting, errors that could bias study results. This includes identification of unwanted observations, typos and capitalization inconsistencies, missing data, and outliers.

## DESCRIBING VARIABLE FREQUENCIES

Now that we have examined and cleaned our data set, the next step in our data analysis is to describe the frequencies of the variables of interest. To do this, we will revisit the study design and research questions. Recall that these data came from a cross-sectional study, which means that we will calculate prevalence-based measures.

1. Is the availability of mental health services in a community associated with decreased depression severity?

2. Are those with moderate to severe depression more likely to report suicidal ideation than those with no or mild depression?

Let's first describe the outcomes of interest. Depression severity, the outcome of interest for the first research question, is defined using both numeric and categorical variables in our data set. Since the numeric data are not normally distributed (skewness = 0.7, kurtosis = -0.6, as indicated in **Table 13.4** footnotes), the numeric depression severity score should be summarized using the median and IQR (9 and 16, respectively). A median depression severity scale score of 9 means that half of participants had a depression severity score below 9 (no or mild depression) while the other half had a score above 9 (moderate, moderately severe, or severe depression). Meanwhile, the dichotomous depression severity variable can be summarized using counts and percentages ($n = 6$ participants reported moderate to severe depression, 40%). For the second research question, the outcome of interest, suicidal ideation, is a dichotomous variable. Therefore, it can be described with counts and percentages ($n = 6$ participants reported suicidal ideation, 40%).

All the descriptive statistics for each of the variables in our hypothetical cross-sectional data set after data cleaning are shown in **Table 13.4**. Note that when looking at these descriptive data, we cannot tell whether any two variables are associated with each other. For example, we cannot tell if there is any relationship between categorical depression severity and suicidal ideation just by looking at these descriptive data. Though their distributions are the same, we do not know whether these two health issues are occurring in the same people. We would need to calculate a measure of association to test the hypothesis that there is an association between depression and suicidal ideation.

**TABLE 13.4 DESCRIPTIVE DATA FROM A HYPOTHETICAL CROSS-SECTIONAL DATA SET AFTER DATA CLEANING**

| Variable | *N* (%)[a] |
|---|---|
| Age[b, c] | 28.2 (13.0) |
| Depression severity score[b, d, e] | 9.0 (16.0) |
| Moderate to severe depression[f] | |
| Yes | 6 (40%) |
| No | 9 (60%) |
| Suicidal ideation | |
| Yes | 6 (40%) |
| No | 9 (60%) |
| Mental health services available in community | |
| Yes | 7 (47%) |
| No | 8 (53%) |
| Ethnicity | |
| Non-Hispanic | 9 (60%) |
| Hispanic | 6 (40%) |

[a]Values are *N* (%) unless otherwise noted.
[b]Median (IQR).
[c]Distribution statistics for age: skewness: −0.4, kurtosis: −1.0.
[d]Depression measured via the Patient Health Questionnaire (PHQ-9).
[e]Distribution statistics for depression severity scale: skewness: 0.7, kurtosis: −0.6.
[f]Moderate to severe depression: Yes (PHQ-9 scores 10–27); No (PHQ-9 scores 0–9).
IQR, interquartile range.

## EVALUATING THE ASSOCIATION BETWEEN THE EXPOSURE AND OUTCOME

After cleaning our data set and describing our data using descriptive statistics, we are ready to evaluate the crude (i.e., unadjusted) association between our exposure and outcome. To do this, we will examine the magnitude of the measure of association. Additionally, we will discuss several statistical tests to evaluate whether there is a statistically significant association between the exposure and the outcome. It can be challenging to distinguish between these statistical tests as you are first learning them. A useful guide is to remember that the appropriate analysis is determined by the type of *outcome* data that you have. A description of common statistical tests used to quantify statistical differences in outcome frequency across two independent exposure categories is included in the text that follows and summarized in Figure 13.10.

## FIGURE 13.10 STATISTICAL TESTS TO QUANTIFY DIFFERENCES IN OUTCOME FREQUENCY ACROSS TWO INDEPENDENT EXPOSURE CATEGORIES

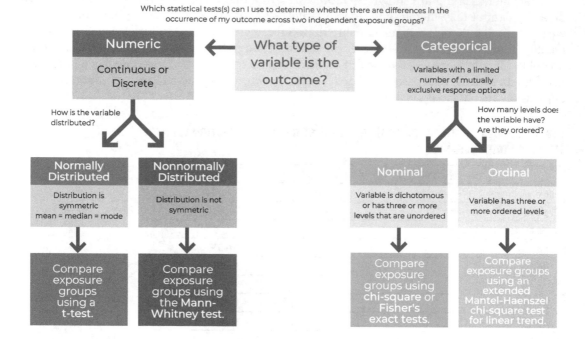

## Numeric Outcomes

The *t*-test or the **Mann–Whitney test** (Learning Objective 13.5) can be used to evaluate whether there is a statistically significant difference in the means or medians of numeric outcomes, respectively, across two independent exposure categories. The *t*-test is appropriate to use when the outcome data are normally distributed; otherwise, the Mann–Whitney test should be used.

The formulae and calculations for these two statistical tests are beyond the scope of this book. However, details of these tests are available elsewhere[11,13] and they can be performed in statistical programs.

Each statistical test will produce a **test statistic** and **p-value**. The test statistic is a number generated from a statistical test that is used to obtain the *p*-value. Recall from **Chapter 12, "Random Error in Epidemiologic Research,"** that the *p*-value is interpreted as the probability of obtaining a result as or more extreme than the result observed in your study, if the null hypothesis ($H_0$) were true and there is no bias. Here, the t-test and the Mann–Whitney test are used to determine whether the means or medians of a variable, respectively, are statistically significantly different across two independent groups. The null hypothesis is that they are not statistically significantly different.

As an example, recall one of our research questions: Are available mental health services in the community associated with depression severity? Let's evaluate this question using depression measured as a numeric outcome variable. The results are shown in **Table 13.5**.

**TABLE 13.5 UNADJUSTED ANALYSIS OF NUMERIC OUTCOME DATA: ARE AVAILABLE MENTAL HEALTH SERVICES IN THE COMMUNITY ASSOCIATED WITH NUMERIC DEPRESSION SEVERITY?**

| | Mental Health Service Availability | | | | *p*-value[a] |
| | Yes | | No | | |
| | Median | IQR | Median | IQR | |
|---|---|---|---|---|---|
| **Depression severity score**[b] | 8.0 | 25.0 | 9.5 | 8.5 | 0.46 |

[a] Two-tailed *p*-value from the Mann–Whitney test.
[b] Depression measured via the Patient Health Questionnaire (PHQ-9).
IQR, interquartile range.

We noted earlier that the numeric depression severity scale data are not normally distributed (skewness: 0.7, kurtosis: -0.6), so we have compared the median scores of the scale (the outcome) across categories of mental health service availability (the exposure). We see in **Table 13.5** that when mental health services are available, the median depression severity score is 8.0 (IQR = 25) while when mental health services are not available, the median depression severity score is 9.5 (IQR = 8.5). We should consult a subject matter expert to ascertain whether these medians are meaningfully different.

Because our data are not normally distributed, we can use a Mann–Whitney test to answer the question of whether those medians are statistically significantly different from one another. The two-sided *p*-value for the Mann–Whitney test is 0.46. Assuming we set our alpha ($\alpha$) at 0.05, we would fail to reject the null hypothesis since the *p*-value is greater than 0.05, meaning that we conclude that the medians are not statistically significantly different. This finding is not surprising given the very small sample size; the observed difference in median depression severity scores between communities with and without mental health services may have reached statistical significance had a larger sample size been enrolled.

## Categorical Outcomes

As we have learned, a first step in the analysis of categorical data is to calculate a measure of association along with its confidence interval and associated *p*-value. Here we will discuss the statistical tests that can be used to evaluate whether a measure of association is statistically significantly different from its null value.

For nominal outcomes, **chi-square tests** or **Fisher's exact tests** (Learning Objective 13.6) can be used to determine whether the frequency of the outcome is significantly different across two or more levels of a categorical exposure. The formulae and calculations for these two tests are beyond the scope of this book and can be found elsewhere.[11,14] Importantly, while the Fisher's exact test may always be used, the chi-square test is only appropriate when there is adequate sample size. Whether the sample size is considered "adequate" is defined as having an R×C table where all the **expected cell sizes** are 5 or greater. The formula to calculate expected cell values using data from an observed 2×2 table is given in **Equation 13.1** and shown in **Figure 13.11**.

$$\text{Expected cell value} = \frac{(\text{Observed row total}) \times (\text{Observed column total})}{\text{Observed table total}} \qquad (13.1)$$

## FIGURE 13.11 CALCULATING EXPECTED 2×2 TABLE CELL VALUES FROM THE OBSERVED 2×2 TABLE CELL VALUES

**Observed data**

| | E+ | E− | TOTAL |
|---|---|---|---|
| O+ | A | B | $A + B = M_1$ |
| O− | C | D | $C + D = M_0$ |
| TOTAL | $A + C = N_1$ | $B + D = N_0$ | $A+B+C+D = N$ |

**Expected data**

| | E+ | E− |
|---|---|---|
| O+ | $\dfrac{M_1 \times N_1}{N}$ | $\dfrac{M_1 \times N_0}{N}$ |
| O− | $\dfrac{M_0 \times N1}{N}$ | $\dfrac{M_0 \times N_0}{N}$ |

Expected cell value

$$= \frac{(\text{observed row total}) \times (\text{observed column total})}{(\text{observed table total})}$$

Note that the decision about sufficient sample size is *not* based on the *observed* cell values, but rather the *expected* cell values. Many statistical packages will provide guidance about which statistical test to use based on the expected cell values.

## Pause to Practice 13.1

### Analysis of Categorical Outcomes: Are Available Mental Health Services in the Community Associated With Moderate to Severe Depression?

We have already answered our first research question when considering depression severity as a numeric variable—now let's evaluate what this relationship looks like if we categorize depression severity into a dichotomous variable (moderate or severe depression vs. mild or no depression). To do this, we can construct a 2×2 table and calculate the prevalence ratio (PR) and its 95% CI. The summary of this analysis is shown in **Table 13.6**; examine this table and answer the following questions.

**TABLE 13.6 ANALYSIS OF CATEGORICAL OUTCOME DATA: ARE AVAILABLE MENTAL HEALTH SERVICES IN THE COMMUNITY ASSOCIATED WITH MODERATE TO SEVERE DEPRESSION?**

| | | Mental Health Service Availability | | PR (95% CI) | p-value[a] |
|---|---|---|---|---|---|
| | | Yes | No | | |
| Moderate to Severe Depression[b, c] | Yes | 2 | 4 | 0.57 (0.15, 2.23) | 0.76 |
| | No | 5 | 4 | | |

[a] Two-tailed p-value from Fisher's exact test.
[b] Depression measured via the Patient Health Questionnaire (PHQ-9).
[c] Moderate to severe depression: Yes (PHQ-9 scores 10–27); No (PHQ-9 scores 0–9).
PR, prevalence ratio.

1. Why was a prevalence ratio calculated?
2. Confirm that you can construct the 2×2 table using corrected data from Figure 13.9 and use this to calculate the prevalence ratio by hand.
3. Use OpenEpi[15] to calculate the PR, confidence interval, and p-value.
4. Are available mental health services in the community meaningfully associated with moderate to severe depression in this study from a public health perspective?

5. The *p*-value is calculated from the Fisher's exact test. Why was the Fisher's exact test used?

6. Is the association between availability of mental health services and depression severity statistically significant at an alpha of 0.05? Why or why not?

## STRATIFIED ANALYSES TO ASSESS FOR EFFECT MEASURE MODIFICATION AND STATISTICAL INTERACTION
### (LEARNING OBJECTIVES 13.7 AND 13.8)

When effect measure modification is of interest for a given research question, we need to stratify the data by the potential effect modifier and calculate stratum-specific measures of association, as described in **Chapter 8, "Effect Measure Modification and Statistical Interaction."** If the stratum-specific measures of association are *meaningfully* different from a public health perspective (e.g., the differences would lead to differences in clinical guidelines or public health policies, as determined by subject matter experts), then the stratified measures of association should be reported.

Recall that the **Breslow–Day test** may be used to assess whether the stratum-specific measures of association are different from one another from a *statistical* perspective on the scale(s) of interest. Evidence of statistical interaction on the **additive** and/or **multiplicative scales** is determined by whether the stratified difference or ratio measures of association, respectively, are statistically significantly different from one another. As described in **Chapter 8, "Effect Measure Modification and Statistical Interaction,"** the Breslow–Day test is a test for homogeneity. The null hypothesis of this test is that the stratified measures of association are the same (homogenous; i.e., the null hypothesis is that there is no statistical interaction). Thus, a *p*-value less than alpha indicates statistically significant heterogeneity of the stratified measures of association, meaning that statistical interaction is present.

Importantly, the decision about whether meaningful effect measure modification is present should *not* rely on the results of a statistical test. Conclusions about whether the measures are meaningfully different should be guided by the judgement of subject matter experts.

## Pause to Practice 13.2

### Assessing Effect Measure Modification and Statistical Interaction: Does the Effect of Mental Health Service Availability of Moderate to Severe Depression Differ by Ethnicity?

Let's extend the analysis that we conducted in **Pause to Practice 13.1** by considering whether the association between availability of mental health services in the community and depression severity (moderate or severe vs. mild or none) is modified by ethnicity. This is a question of effect measure modification: is the association between mental health service availability and moderate to severe depression different for Hispanic versus non-Hispanic individuals? To evaluate this question, we must begin by stratifying the crude 2×2 table by the hypothesized effect measure modifier, as shown in **Table 13.7**.

Examine **Table 13.7** and answer the following questions.

1. Confirm that you can construct the stratified 2×2 tables shown in **Figure 13.10** using the corrected data from **Figure 13.9**, and calculate the stratified prevalence ratios and prevalence differences by hand.

2. Use OpenEpi to calculate the stratified prevalence ratios and differences and their associated 95% CIs.

TABLE 13.7 STRATIFIED DATA FOR ASSESSING EFFECT MEASURE MODIFICATION AND STATISTICAL INTERACTION: IS THE EFFECT OF MENTAL HEALTH SERVICE AVAILABILITY ON MODERATE TO SEVERE DEPRESSION[a,b] DIFFERENT BY ETHNICITY?

| | | Hispanic | | Non-Hispanic | |
| --- | --- | --- | --- | --- | --- |
| | | Mental health service availability | | Mental health service availability | |
| | | Yes | No | Yes | No |
| Moderate to Severe Depression[a,b] | Yes | 1 | 2 | 1 | 2 |
| | No | 1 | 2 | 4 | 2 |

[a]Depression measured via the Patient Health Questionnaire (PHQ-9).
[b]Moderate to severe depression: Yes (PHQ-9 scores 10–27); No (PHQ-9 scores 0–9).

3. Is there statistical interaction on the additive scale (i.e., comparing difference measures of association) at an α level of 0.05?

4. Is there statistical interaction on the multiplicative scale (i.e., comparing ratio measures of association) at an α level of 0.05?

5. Is the effect of mental health service availability on moderate to severe depression severity *meaningfully* different by ethnicity on the additive and/or multiplicative scale? Do you recommend reporting crude (unstratified) or stratum-specific measures of association?

6. Hypothesize some reasons why the effect of mental health service availability on moderate to severe depression may be different by ethnicity.

## STRATIFIED ANALYSES TO ASSESS AND ADJUST FOR CONFOUNDING (LEARNING OBJECTIVE 13.9)

After effect measure modification has been considered, we can proceed to consider whether there are variables that might confound the association between our exposure and outcome of interest. As described in **Chapter 9, "Error in Epidemiologic Research and Fundamentals of Confounding,"** after a review of the literature and consideration of the a priori criteria, we would identify a subset of variables that we hypothesize to be likely confounders. Recall that when using the **data-based criterion** to assess whether a variable is a confounder in our study, we calculate and compare crude and adjusted measures of association. There are several ways to calculate confounder-adjusted measures, including the often-used **Mantel–Haenszel** methods, which are required when the data are sparse. If the crude measure of association is meaningfully different from the adjusted measure (e.g., greater than +/− 10% different), we conclude that confounding is present, and we adjust for the confounder. If the crude and adjusted measures of association are not meaningfully different from one another, there is not evidence of confounding by the factors that were considered, and it is not necessary to adjust for it in the analysis.

Let's now consider our second research question: are those with moderate to severe depression more likely to report suicidal ideation than those with no or mild depression? Assume that we are not interested in effect measure modification, but based on the a priori criteria, we are concerned about the potential for confounding by age. Age is often explored as a potential confounder because it is associated with many health outcomes and exposures of interest. Thinking about the a priori criteria (i.e., the confounding triangle), age could be associated with the exposure of interest (moderate to severe depression) in the source population, it could be a risk factor for the outcome (suicidal ideation) among the unexposed, and it is not caused by either the exposure or the outcome.

## Pause to Practice 13.3

### Using the Data-Based Method for Confounding Assessment: Is the Effect of Moderate to Severe Depression on Suicidal Ideation Confounded by Age?

Let's use the **data-based method** to assess whether age is a confounder of the association between moderate to severe depression and suicidal ideation. The process of using the data-based method to assess for confounding is shown in Figure 13.12. First, we create an unstratified 2×2 table and calculate a crude measure of association. Then we stratify the data by age, which is under consideration as a potential confounder. To simplify this

### FIGURE 13.12 USING THE DATA-BASED METHOD FOR CONFOUNDING ASSESSMENT: IS THE EFFECT OF MODERATE TO SEVERE DEPRESSION[a,b] ON SUICIDAL IDEATION CONFOUNDED BY AGE?

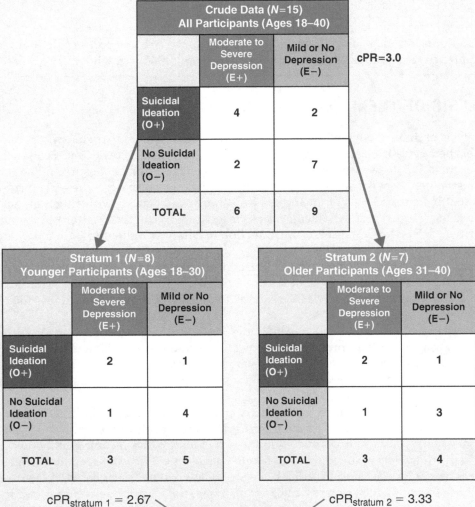

| Crude Data ($N$=15) All Participants (Ages 18–40) | Moderate to Severe Depression (E+) | Mild or No Depression (E−) |
|---|---|---|
| Suicidal Ideation (O+) | 4 | 2 |
| No Suicidal Ideation (O−) | 2 | 7 |
| TOTAL | 6 | 9 |

cPR=3.0

| Stratum 1 ($N$=8) Younger Participants (Ages 18–30) | Moderate to Severe Depression (E+) | Mild or No Depression (E−) |
|---|---|---|
| Suicidal Ideation (O+) | 2 | 1 |
| No Suicidal Ideation (O−) | 1 | 4 |
| TOTAL | 3 | 5 |

| Stratum 2 ($N$=7) Older Participants (Ages 31–40) | Moderate to Severe Depression (E+) | Mild or No Depression (E−) |
|---|---|---|
| Suicidal Ideation (O+) | 2 | 1 |
| No Suicidal Ideation (O−) | 1 | 3 |
| TOTAL | 3 | 4 |

$cPR_{stratum\ 1} = 2.67$   $cPR_{stratum\ 2} = 3.33$

MH-aPR – aPR = 2.98

Percent difference between crude and adjusted prevalence ratios = −1%

[a]Depression measured via the Patient Health Questionnaire (PHQ-9)
[b]Moderate to severe depression: Yes (PHQ-9 scores 10–27); No (PHQ-9 scores 0–9)
cPR, crude prevalence ratio; MH-aPR, Mantel–Haenszel adjusted prevalence ratio

example, we have categorized age into two groups: younger participants (ages 18–30) and older participants (ages 31–40). Next, we calculate a Mantel–Haenszel adjusted prevalence ratio. Finally, we calculate the percent difference between the crude and adjusted measures of association. This process is summarized in Figure 13.12—use this figure to answer the following questions.

1. Use OpenEpi to calculate the Mantel–Haenszel adjusted prevalence ratio.

2. Why did we calculate the Mantel–Haenszel adjusted prevalence ratio as opposed to a different method of adjustment?

3. Calculate the percent difference between the crude and adjusted measures of association and confirm your answer with the result provided.

4. Given your answer to Question 3, is age a confounder of this association in this study? What measure of association should we report?

5. Is there a statistical test to assess for confounding?

6. Recall that residual confounding occurs when a measure of association is still confounded, even after attempting to control for it. Are you concerned about the potential for residual confounding in this example? Why or why not?

## ANALYSIS OF TREND (LEARNING OBJECTIVE 13.10)

An analysis of trend is often of interest in epidemiologic research, particularly for examining whether there have been changes in the frequency of an outcome over time, or to determine whether there is a **dose–response** relationship between an ordinal exposure and an outcome of interest. When there is a dose–response relationship between an exposure and outcome, this means that increasing levels of the ordinal exposure are associated with either an increasing or decreasing frequency of the outcome. Dose response is one of the Bradford-Hill guidelines supportive of causality (**Chapter 3, "Introduction to Analytic Epidemiologic Study Designs and Measures of Association"**).

Variables can exhibit different types of trend in relation to other variables (e.g., linear, parabolic, logarithmic); however, our focus will be on **linear trends**, which occur when there is a consistent increase or decrease in the frequency of the outcome across the ordinal exposure categories.

Suppose we adapt our second research question to evaluate whether there is a trend between *increasing* levels of depression severity and suicidal ideation. To answer this question, we can use the numeric depression severity variable to construct an ordinal depression severity variable with three categories: moderately severe/severe (scores 15–27), moderate (scores 10–14), and none/mild (scores 0–9).

The 2x3 R×C (row x column) table shown in **Table 13.8** presents the distribution of the dichotomous outcome (suicidal ideation) across the three levels of the ordinal exposure (depression severity). We can assess whether there is evidence of a meaningful increase or decrease in the frequency of suicidal ideation with increasing depression severity by calculating measures of association for each ordinal category relative to one designated reference group. We will use the depression severity category of "none/mild" as the reference group for each of these calculations:

$PR_{\text{moderately severe/severe vs. none/mild}}$

$= \dfrac{\text{Prevalence of suicidal ideation among those with moderately severe or severe depression}}{\text{Prevalence of suicidal ideation among those with no or mild depression}}$

$= \dfrac{3/4}{2/9} = 3.38$

**TABLE 13.8 ASSESSING TREND: IS THERE A LINEAR TREND BETWEEN ORDINAL LEVELS OF DEPRESSION SEVERITY AND SUICIDAL IDEATION?**

| | Depression Severity[a] | | |
|---|---|---|---|
| | Moderately Severe or Severe (E = 2) | Moderate (E = 1) | Mild or No Depression (E = 0) |
| Suicidal Ideation (O+) | 3 | 1 | 2 |
| No Suicidal Ideation (O−) | 1 | 1 | 7 |
| TOTAL | 4 | 2 | 9 |

$PR_{2 \text{ vs.} 0}$ = 3.38 95% CI: (0.35–14.28)
$PR_{1 \text{ vs.} 0}$ = 2.25 95% CI: (0.88–12.98)
$p$-value[b] = 0.14.
[a] Depression measured via the Patient Health Questionnaire (PHQ-9).
[b] Two-sided $p$-value from the extended Mantel–Haenszel chi-square test for linear trend.
PR, prevalence ratio.

$$PR_{\text{moderate vs. none/mild}}$$
$$= \frac{\text{Prevalence of suicidal ideation among those with moderate depression}}{\text{Prevalence of suicidal ideation among those with no or mild depression}}$$
$$= \frac{1/2}{2/9} = 2.25$$

Examining these data, there appears to be a trend between increasing levels of depression severity (compared to no or mild depression) and a higher likelihood of suicidal ideation. These PRs appear quite different from one another, and this trend may be meaningful. We can also assess whether there is a statistically significant linear trend at an alpha of 0.05 using the **extended Mantel–Haenszel chi-square test for linear trend**. The null hypothesis for this test is that there is no linear trend. Thus, a $p$-value lower than alpha would indicate the presence of a statistically significant linear trend. It is important to note that this is a test of *linear* trend, and nonlinear trends may not be detected. This test can be calculated in OpenEpi. From the main OpenEpi menu (www.openepi.com/Menu/OE_Menu.htm), select "Dose Response," select "Enter New Data," and then enter the appropriate number of exposure levels (i.e., 3). Review the table orientation and enter in the data. Select "Calculate." You should have calculated a $p$-value of 0.14 which is also shown in the footnote of **Table 13.8**. This statistical test indicates that there is no statistically significant linear trend, which is not surprising given the very small sample size.

## Summary of Analyses

We've reviewed several analytic techniques associated with the research questions outlined at the beginning of the chapter—let's take a look back to summarize what we found. Recall that these are hypothetical data; thus, these results should not be thought to apply to a real-world public health setting.

**Research question #1**: Is the availability of mental health services in a community associated with decreased depression severity?

- Regardless of whether depression severity was considered as a numeric or categorical variable, we found that depression severity was lower in communities where mental health services were available, compared to those without such services.

  - **Numeric:** The median depression severity scores in communities with and without mental health services were 8.0 and 9.5, respectively (Mann–Whitney two-sided $p$-value = 0.46).

- **Categorical:** The prevalence of moderate to severe depression is lower in individuals with access to mental health services (PR = 0.57, 95% CI = 0.15–2.23, Fisher's exact test two-sided $p$-value = 0.76).

- It appears that there may be a meaningful association between mental health service availability and moderate to severe depression. Note that these results did not reach statistical significance (both $p$-values were greater than 0.05); however, this is not surprising given the small sample size ($N$ = 15).

• Additional analyses considered whether the association between mental health service availability and depression severity was modified by ethnicity.

- While mental health service availability is protective for depression among non-Hispanic study participants (PR = 0.4, PD = -30%), there is no effect of mental service availability among Hispanic study participants (PR = 1; PD = 0%).

- The effect of mental health service availability on moderate to severe depression is meaningfully different by ethnicity.

- The stratum-specific results should be reported, even though the Breslow–Day tests did not indicate statistically significant interaction at an alpha level of 0.05 ($p$-values for additive and multiplicative interaction were both > 0.05).

**Research question #2:** Are those with moderate to severe depression more likely to report suicidal ideation than those with no or mild depression?

• Analysis of confounding by age

- Age is not a confounder of these data because the confounder-adjusted measure of association is roughly the same (i.e., within ±10%) as the crude measure of association.

- Age does not need to be adjusted for in this analysis.

• Analysis of trend

- The prevalence of suicidal ideation increases with increasing depression severity (moderately severe to severe depression vs. none/mild depression [PR = 3.38]; moderate depression vs. no/mild depression [PR = 2.25]; extended Mantel–Haenszel chi-square test for linear trend $p$-value = 0.14).

- There may be a meaningful linear trend between moderate to severe depression and suicidal ideation, even though the $p$-value did not indicate a statistically significant association at an alpha level of 0.05 ($p$-value was > 0.05).

## Highlights

## Common Epidemiologic Data Analyses

• **Statistical tests to quantify differences in outcome frequency across two independent exposure categories for:**

- Numeric outcome variables:

  ▪ t-test (for normally distributed outcome variables)

  ▪ Mann–Whitney (for nonnormally distributed outcome variables)

- Categorical outcome variables:

  ▪ Chi-square or Fisher's exact test if sample size is large enough (e.g., all expected 2×2 cell counts are ≥ 5)

  ▪ Fisher's exact test if sample size is sparse (e.g., at least one expected cell of a 2×2 table is < 5)

- **Effect measure modification assessment**

  - Effect measure modification assessment can be accomplished by looking for meaningful differences in stratum-specific measures of association.

  - Testing for statistical interaction can be accomplished in stratified analyses using the Breslow–Day test.

  - Whether effect measure modification is present should be based on an assessment of meaningful differences across strata and should *not* rely on findings from statistical tests.

- **Confounding assessment**

  - Confounding assessment is conducted using data-based methods by comparing crude and adjusted measures of association.

  - There are many options for calculating adjusted measures of association. If the data are sparse, the Mantel–Haenszel method is required.

  - Recall that there is no statistical test for confounding.

- **Testing for linear trend** is possible when the exposure can be expressed as an ordinal variable and is accomplished using the extended Mantel–Haenszel test of linear trend.

## INTRODUCTION TO REGRESSION MODELING
### (LEARNING OBJECTIVE 13.11)

Thus far, we have used R×C tables to evaluate crude (i.e., unadjusted), stratified, or adjusted associations between exposures and outcomes of interest. These simple analyses lay the groundwork for more robust epidemiologic data analyses which can accommodate effect measure modification and control of multiple confounders. The stratified analyses that we have conducted thus far cannot easily accommodate such analyses and additionally cannot be used to control for numeric variables.

An alternative to stratified analyses, and the analytic method of choice for most epidemiologists, is **regression modeling**. This is an analytic tool whereby mathematical formulae are used to describe how an outcome variable (the **dependent variable**) is associated with exposure(s) and other covariates (the **independent variables**). The key strengths of regression modeling are that it allows for estimation of measures of association that control for many confounders, including numeric variables, *and* there are fewer limitations related to sparse data. Regression models can also be used to assess for the presence of effect measure modification and statistical interaction.

In generic terms, unadjusted (crude) regression models are structured like this:

*Outcome* (dependent variable) = intercept + *exposure*

Adjusted regression models are structured like this:

*Outcome* (dependent variable) = intercept + *exposure* + confounder 1 + confounder 2
(… + additional confounders)

Although regression modeling is a powerful analytic tool, it is not without limitations. There are a number of different types of models, and some of these require assumptions that may not be met by your study data. Additionally, it may not always be clear which model to choose. We recommend consulting with epidemiology methodologists or biostatisticians regarding model assumptions, decisions about what model to use, and construction of multivariable models.

TABLE 13.9 **WHICH REGRESSION MODEL IS APPROPRIATE GIVEN THE TYPE OF OUTCOME DATA?**

| Outcome Variable Type | Regression Type | Model Output |
|---|---|---|
| **Numeric** | | |
| Continuous | Linear regression | Yields estimated β coefficients |
| Discrete | Linear regression<br>Poisson regression | Yields estimated β coefficients<br>Yields estimated IDRs, RRs, or PRs |
| **Categorical** | | |
| Nominal: Dichotomous | Logistic regression<br>Log binomial regression | Yields estimated ORs<br>Yields estimated RRs or PRs |
| Nominal: More than two levels | Polytomous (multinomial) logistic regression | Yields estimated ORs |
| Ordinal | Ordinal logistic regression | Yields estimated ORs |
| **Time-to-event** | Survival analysis | Yields estimated HRs |

HR, hazard ratio; IDR, incidence density ratio (i.e., rate ratio); OR, odds ratio; PR, prevalence ratio; RR, risk ratio.

In brief, the type of mathematical model you choose is determined by the type of *outcome* data that were collected. **Table 13.9** provides a list of common epidemiologic outcomes and the corresponding types of regression models that may be appropriate. Note, this listing is not exhaustive; however, this table highlights that the choice of mathematical model is driven by the type of *outcome* data that you have. Notice that there are two options listed for the analysis of dichotomous outcomes: **logistic regression**, which estimates odds ratios (ORs), and log binomial regression, which estimates risk ratios (RRs) and prevalence ratios (PRs). Thus, while knowing the type of outcome data is important, it is also critical to be familiar with the study design so that you obtain the correct measure of association (e.g., ORs for case-control studies, RRs for cohort studies in which there is no loss to follow-up or competing risks, PRs for cross-sectional studies). The mathematical formulae and assumptions underlying these models are beyond the scope of this textbook and can be found elsewhere.[11,16–18] The remainder of our discussion of regression modeling will focus on interpreting results obtained from these models.

## INTERPRETING FINDINGS FROM REGRESSION MODELS

In this section, we will provide a framework for interpreting results from the most common regression models you are likely to encounter in the published literature. Much of this material should feel familiar because it will focus on interpreting measures of association, confidence intervals, and *p*-values; however, we will add some additional considerations related to regression models. While we focus on interpreting findings from linear and logistic regression models, the basic principles that you will learn broadly apply to most regression models.

We encourage readers to approach these interpretations keeping in mind a recurring theme in this textbook, which is that one should not rely on statistical significance testing to make decisions about whether associations are meaningfully important from a public health perspective. This is an easy trap to fall into, particularly when a publication includes *p*-values associated with each of the comparisons made in their study. It is much easier to scan a column of *p*-values to find those that are less than a certain threshold than it is to holistically evaluate the study findings based on subject matter expertise. Interestingly, some journals are moving away from the practice of calculating and relying on *p*-values to interpret the importance of study results and will not allow inclusion of *p*-values in manuscripts that they publish. If you train yourself to avoid drawing conclusions from study results using null hypothesis significance testing from the beginning of your epidemiologic journey, you will find that you are much better prepared to evaluate, understand, and describe the nuances in epidemiologic research.

## Interpreting Results From Linear Regression

**Linear regression** is often the first type of model that new learners of epidemiology are exposed to, in part because it is closely aligned with what you learned in algebra when plotting lines on a coordinate plane. However, the output of these models is a departure from what you have learned previously in this text, because linear regression models do not output the ratio or difference measures of association that you are already familiar with. Instead, linear regression models estimate **beta (β) coefficients** and their confidence intervals. When the outcome is numeric, we want to know how the value of the outcome changes as the exposure changes, adjusting for any confounders that we have identified—this is exactly the information the β coefficient provides. Formally, the β coefficient for a given exposure in a linear regression model is interpreted as the average change in the outcome for every unit change in the exposure variable, controlling for all of the other independent variables in the model. The 'unit change' for an independent variable can be thought of as the difference between one level of the variable and the next. For a numeric variable, a unit change is determined by how the variable has been measured (e.g., a unit change in age may be 1 month for babies or 1 year for adults). For an ordinal variable, a unit change represents the change between one level of the variable and the next level (e.g., low versus moderate, or moderate versus severe). For a dichotomous variable, a unit change represents the comparison of the two levels of the variable (e.g., cancerous versus benign tumors). Linear regression models also estimate confidence intervals around the β coefficients and $p$-values. The null hypothesis is that $β = 0$ (i.e., there is no statistically significant association between the exposure and outcome) whereas the alternative two-sided hypothesis is that $β ≠ 0$ (i.e., there *is* a statistically significant association between the exposure and outcome).

As an example, consider a study that used a series of cross-sectional surveys to evaluate outcomes of depressive symptoms, mental well-being, and substance use during the COVID-19 pandemic in 59,701 adolescent (aged 13–18 years) girls and boys in Iceland.[19] The investigators evaluated differences in the prevalence of depressive symptoms reported in 2016, 2018, and 2020, and also considered whether there were differences by gender. Depression-related questions on the Symptom Checklist-90 (SCL-90)[20] were used to measure depressive symptoms. Participants responded to 10 questions about depressive symptoms that were assessed using four-point Likert scales. Depressive symptoms scores ranged from 0 (none) to 40 (most often). Overall, depressive symptoms increased from a mean of 17.96 (SD = 7.53) in 2016 to a mean of 20.30 (SD = 7.98) in 2020. Results from the linear regression model are shown in **Table 13.10**. Be sure to note what the models adjusted for in the table footnote.

**TABLE 13.10 THE EFFECTS OF TIME (PRE-COVID-19 PANDEMIC AND COVID-19 ERA) ON DEPRESSIVE SYMPTOMS (2016-2020)**

|  | Total | | Girls | | Boys | |
|---|---|---|---|---|---|---|
|  | β | 95% CI | β | 95% CI | β | 95% CI |
| Time | 0.57 | 0.54–0.61 | 0.64 | 0.59–0.70 | 0.41 | 0.36–0.46 |

Model results are adjusted for household status, primary language spoken at home, and residency.
*Source*: Adapted from Thorisdottir IE, Asgeirsdottir BB, Kristjansson AL, et al. Depressive symptoms, mental wellbeing, and substance use among adolescents before and during the COVID-19 pandemic in Iceland: a longitudinal, population-based study. *Lancet Psychiatry*. 2021;8(8):663–672. https://doi.org/10.1016/S2215-0366(21)00156-5
CI; confidence interval

From the results presented in **Table 13.10**, we can interpret the effect of time on depressive symptoms for all study participants accordingly: after controlling for household status, primary language spoken at home, and residency, depressive symptoms increased an average of 0.57 points per two-year increase (e.g., 2020 versus 2018) (95% CI: 0.54–0.61, $p$-value < 0.0001) on the SCL-90. The authors also presented linear regression model results stratified by gender, allowing us to evaluate whether there were meaningful differences by gender (i.e., did gender modify the association between the pandemic and depressive symptoms?). Indeed, the data show that the association was stronger among girls ($\beta$ = 0.64) than among boys ($\beta$ = 0.41) during the study period. Assuming these results are meaningfully different (a determination which should be made after consulting with subject matter experts), the stratified results should be reported. And in fact, the study authors conclude: "Our results suggest that COVID-19 has significantly impaired adolescent mental health. ... Population-level prevention efforts, especially for girls, are warranted."[18]

## Common Misinterpretations of Linear Regression Models

Since there are often several things being presented in a single table of results, it can be easy to overlook some of the important elements that inform the interpretation of the results. The text that follows shows two common mistakes when interpreting the results of the linear regression models presented in **Table 13.10**.

*Forgetting the reference group*

✗ After controlling for household status, primary language spoken at home, and residency, depressive symptoms were higher by an average of 0.64 points (95% CI: 0.59–0.70) on the SCL-90 in 2020 (the COVID-19 era) among girls.

– This interpretation fails to describe that this represents the average change in depressive symptoms relative to the pre-COVID-19 era.

*Forgetting confounders*

✗ Among boys, depressive symptoms increased an average of 0.41 points (95% CI: 0.36–0.46) on the SCL-90 comparing pre-COVID-19 era versus COVID-19 era.

– This interpretation fails to describe the confounding factors which were controlled for. The $\beta$ estimate is calculated controlling for these factors and therefore needs to be interpreted by describing confounders were included in the regression model.

## Interpreting Results From Logistic Regression

Logistic regression is often the next regression type that new learners of epidemiology will encounter. Similar to linear regression, logistic regression provides information about how the occurrence of a health outcome changes with every unit increase in the exposure variable, controlling for confounders of interest. However, logistic regression estimates odds ratios along with their corresponding confidence intervals.

For example, a cross-sectional study used logistic regression to investigate the association between racial discrimination and delaying or forgoing healthcare during the COVID-19 pandemic among 2,552 U.S. study participants.[21] A total of 64% of study participants self-reported delaying or forgoing healthcare during the COVID-19 pandemic. Two exposures of interest were considered: coronavirus-related racial bias and race-related cyberbullying. Consider **Table 13.11**, which presents data from logistic regression models that evaluated these two outcomes, stratified by race and ethnicity. Stratification was used to assess whether the association between these exposures and delayed or forgone healthcare was modified by race or ethnicity.

**TABLE 13.11 ASSOCIATION OF EXPERIENCED CORONAVIRUS RACIAL DISCRIMINATION AND RACE-RELATED CYBERBULLYING WITH THE OUTCOME OF DELAYING OR FORGOING HEALTHCARE DURING THE COVID-19 PANDEMIC**

| | aOR | 95% CI |
|---|---|---|
| **Coronavirus-related racial bias (yes vs. no)** | | |
| Non-Hispanic Black | 1.37 | 0.97–1.92 |
| Hispanic | 1.24 | 0.85–1.80 |
| Non-Hispanic Asian: East/Southeast | 1.55 | 1.16–2.07 |
| Non-Hispanic Asian: South | 1.47 | 0.81–2.65 |
| **Race-related cyberbullying (yes vs. no)** | | |
| Non-Hispanic Black | 1.34 | 1.02–1.77 |
| Hispanic | 1.22 | 0.87–1.73 |
| Non-Hispanic Asian: East/Southeast | 1.51 | 1.19–1.90 |
| Non-Hispanic Asian: South | 1.00 | 0.57–1.75 |

East/Southeast Asian includes Burmese, Cambodian, Chinese, Filipino, Hmong, Indonesian, Japanese, Korean, and Vietnamese.
South Asian includes Asian Indian, Bangladeshi, Nepalese, and Pakistani.
Models adjusted for age, sex, educational attainment, marital status, region, urban/rural status, insurance status before pandemic, employment status before pandemic, score of personal protective behaviors, and self-rated health.
aOR, adjusted odds ratio; CI, confidence interval.
*Source*: Adapted from Zhang D, Li G, Shi L, et al. Association between racial discrimination and delayed or forgone care amid the COVID-19 pandemic. *Prev Med*. 2022;162:107153. https://doi.org/10.1016/j.ypmed.2022.107153

You may notice that the measures of associations are labeled "aOR" for adjusted odds ratio. As we described in **Chapter 6, "Case-Control Designs,"** investigators may report ORs for some cohort or cross-sectional studies—this is one such example. Though labeled "aOR," the more precise term for this measure of association is adjusted *prevalence* OR (aPOR), since these data are from a cross-sectional study.

Let's take a close look at the measures of association that describe the association between both exposures and delayed or forgone healthcare among East and Southeast Asians:

- East or Southeast Asians who experienced coronavirus-related racial bias were 1.55 times as likely to report delaying or forgoing healthcare compared to East or Southeast Asians who did not experience coronavirus-related racial bias (aOR = 1.55, 95% CI = 1.16–2.07), adjusting for age, sex, educational attainment, marital status, region, urban/rural status, insurance status before pandemic, employment status before pandemic, score of personal protective behaviors, and self-rated health.

- East or Southeast Asians who experienced race-related cyberbullying were 1.51 times as likely to report delaying or forgoing healthcare compared to East or Southeast Asians who did not experience race-related cyberbullying (aOR = 1.51, 95% CI = 1.19–1.90), adjusting for age, sex, educational attainment, marital status, region, urban/rural status, insurance status before pandemic, employment status before pandemic, score of personal protective behaviors, and self-rated health.

The aPORs appear to be meaningfully higher for non-Hispanic East/Southeast Asian populations than for other racial and ethnic groups. The authors conclude: "… domains of racial discrimination were consistently associated with delayed or forgone health care among East/Southeast Asians during the COVID-19 pandemic; some of the associations were also seen among non-Hispanic Blacks and Hispanics. These results demonstrate that addressing racism is important for reducing disparities in healthcare delivery during the pandemic and beyond".[21]

## Common Misinterpretations of Logistic Regression Models

Let's review some common misinterpretations of the results from the logistic regression models presented in **Table 13.11**.

✗ Study participants identifying as non-Hispanic Black had higher odds of experiencing coronavirus-related racial bias (aOR = 1.37, 95% CI = 0.97–1.92), controlling for age, sex, educational attainment, marital status, region, urban/rural status, insurance status before pandemic, employment status before pandemic, score of personal protective behaviors, and self-rated health.

  – This interpretation fails to describe the referent group, which is not experiencing coronavirus-related racial bias. Remember, it is critical to ask yourself "compared to what?" to interpret analytic study data.

  – This interpretation also fails to describe the outcome of interest, which is delaying or forgoing healthcare during the COVID-19 pandemic.

✗ Study participants identifying as non-Hispanic Black who delayed or forwent healthcare during the COVID-19 pandemic had higher odds of experiencing coronavirus-related racial bias (aOR = 1.37, 95% CI = 0.97–1.92) relative to those who did not delay or forgo healthcare during the COVID-19 pandemic.

  – This interpretation fails to describe the confounding factors which were controlled for. The odds ratio is calculated controlling for these factors and therefore needs to be interpreted by describing which factors were controlled for in the regression model.

## SENSITIVITY ANALYSES

Since there is always concern about the potential influence of bias on our study results, investigators often employ **sensitivity analyses** to explore how study results could be impacted by different assumptions. When conducting sensitivity analyses, investigators re-analyze their data using different sets of assumptions to evaluate whether the results meaningfully change. Sensitivity analyses are often used to explore how variables measured with uncertainty or missingness may influence the study results, or the impact of biases due to selection processes or loss to follow-up.

Some examples of how we may use sensitivity analyses include:

• **Use hypothetical extreme values for a variable that is measured with uncertainty to understand the impact of information bias**. For example, in a study in which the exposure of interest is participant self-reported pain, study investigators may be interested in evaluating how different assumptions about pain misclassification may impact the study results since assessments of pain are rather subjective.

• **Conduct analyses with and without data imputation to understand the impact of missing data**. For example, in a study with a high level of missingness of participant income, investigators may conduct a sensitivity analysis in which they impute all the missing income data to see how their results may change compared to an analysis in which those data were not imputed.

• **Conduct analyses under varying assumptions about participant loss to follow-up to understand the impact of selection bias**. For example, investigators may choose to conduct one sensitivity analysis assuming that all the study participants who were lost to follow-up would have gotten the outcome of interest, and a second sensitivity analysis assuming that all of the study participants who were lost to follow-up would *not* have gotten the outcome of interest. This strategy can help to understand the potential impact of loss to follow-up on the study results.

## Thoughts on Reading Published Scientific Papers

Scientific papers are often structured with the following sections: abstract (which is an overview of the manuscript), introduction, methods, results, discussion, conclusion, and references. One strategy for reading scientific papers is to read the abstract and then review the tables and figures. Each table and figure is the result of a specific set of analyses, and all aspects of the manuscript should be connected to the data that are presented in these tables and figures. After you are familiar with the "story" that the tables and figures present, it often becomes easier to critically read the manuscript text and ask questions like:

- Are the study methods described adequate for generating the presented data?

- Are there concerns about bias in how the data were generated?

- Do the data described in the results section reflect what is presented in the tables and figures?

- Are the conclusions supported by the presented data?

## Highlights

### Introduction to Regression Modeling and Sensitivity Analyses

- **Regression models** can examine the association between an exposure and an outcome while simultaneously controlling for one or more other factors, including numeric variables. These models can also be used to assess effect measure modification and statistical interaction.

- The choice of regression model depends on the type of outcome data that were collected.

- If the outcome is numeric, use **linear regression** where β coefficients reflect the average change in the outcome when exposure changes by one unit while controlling for all other variables in the model.

- If the outcome is dichotomous, **logistic regression** may be used. Logistic regression models estimate ORs along with their corresponding confidence intervals and $p$-values.

- **Sensitivity analyses** explore how study results may be impacted by different assumptions.

## CONCLUDING THOUGHTS

Now that you have concluded this textbook on the fundamentals of epidemiology, we would like to call attention to how much you have learned. You now have a strong foundation in descriptive epidemiology and surveillance, analytic epidemiology, study designs, effect measure modification, systematic and random error, and basic data analysis strategies. You have also been introduced to each of the core disciplines of public health, grounded in an epidemiologic lens. Your understanding of core epidemiologic concepts better positions you to critically interpret data from published studies and to be better consumers of health-related media.

As the COVID-19 pandemic has shown us, our health is interconnected, and there is much work to be done to achieve optimal and equitable health around the world. By detecting patterns in data, and effectively communicating the results of those patterns, epidemiology holds one of the keys to improving public health. As we conclude, we also want to remind students to keep the "so what" from a public health viewpoint in mind as you conduct epidemiologic studies or read the literature. As the cover art on the text reminds us, every data point reflects a real person with a real story, and we must not lose the people in the numbers.

We hope this textbook has laid a solid foundation for whatever comes next for you. If you do pursue additional studies in epidemiology, you will quickly learn that many of the concepts that we have presented are more nuanced than they may initially appear. We have tried to distill these concepts in a way that is both accessible and accurate but know that you will find ample areas where there is far more to learn.

For readers who will pursue other avenues, whether in medicine, business, the arts, or any other endeavor, we hope that you will carry the lessons learned here with you as well. Epidemiology provides a foundational framework for critical thinking that is applicable to many facets of life and provides a toolkit of skills that will make you better poised to evaluate the health-related data which impact your life, the lives of everyone you know, and the world at large.

## END OF CHAPTER PROBLEM SET

**Questions 1 to 10 are based on and adapted from:**

Robb CE, de Jager CA, Ahmadi-Abhari S, et al. Associations of social isolation with anxiety and depression during the early COVID-19 pandemic: a survey of older adults in London, UK. *Front Psychiat.* 2020;11:591120. https://doi.org/10.3389/fpsyt.2020.591120

A study published in 2020 examined the effects of social isolation on anxiety and depression among older adults in London during the COVID-19 pandemic. The investigators designed a cross-sectional study among 7,127 study participants (mean age = 70.1, SD = 7.4) and collected data using a survey.

1. The following quote describes how the authors collected information about their outcomes of interest. Given this information, what type of variables were these?

*"Depression and anxiety levels were assessed with the Hospital Anxiety and Depression Scale (HADS) which includes 14 questions on feelings related to anxiety and depression (seven items for each), rated on a 4-level Likert scale from 'most of the time' to 'not at all' ..."*(p. 3).

  a. Continuous
  b. Discrete
  c. Categorical
  d. Nominal
  e. Ordinal

2. The following quote describes an important epidemiologic concept. What concept is it, and what are the corresponding null and alternative hypotheses?

*"Interaction terms by sex and exposure were included in each model to determine if the effect of exposure on the outcome measure significantly varied as a function of sex"*(p. 4).

3. The following is another quote from the manuscript—what epidemiologic concept does this quote refer to?

*"Less than 7% of data were missing for any one variable; hence, we did not compute missing values"*(p. 4).

  a. Data imputation
  b. Outliers
  c. Selection bias
  d. Sensitivity analysis
  e. Confounding

4. The following is another quote from the manuscript–what epidemiologic concept does this quote refer to?

*"Models were controlled for confounding effects of age and sex (model 1), and additionally for hypertension, hypercholesterolemia, diabetes, cardiovascular disease, chronic obstructive pulmonary disease (COPD) and any mental health conditions, pre-lockdown (model 2). These common chronic conditions were included as subjectively reported poor health is a known risk factor for depression and anxiety"* (p. 4).

    a. Data imputation

    b. Outliers

    c. Selection bias

    d. Sensitivity analysis

    e. Confounding

5. The authors indicated that several variables were included in the model as potential confounders since *"These common chronic conditions were included as subjectively reported poor health is a known risk factor for depression and anxiety"* (p. 4). Per the a priori criteria, what are the other considerations for identifying possible confounders?

**Table 13.12** is adapted from an evaluation of the association between age, sex, and loneliness as independent variables and the outcome of worsened depression. The aPORs reflect the relationships between each of the variables listed and the dichotomous outcome of worsening depression, controlling for the other variables in the model. The authors state: *"Results are presented as odds ratios (ORs) and 95% confidence intervals (CI)"* (p. 4).

**TABLE 13.12 LOGISTIC REGRESSION RESULTS[a]: ASSOCIATIONS BETWEEN AGE, SEX, AND FEELING LONELY AND WORSENED DEPRESSION[b]**

|  | aPOR (95% CI) |
|---|---|
| Age (per 5-year increase) | 2.43 (2.07–2.84) |
| Sex assigned at birth (vs. male) | |
|    Female | 1.02 (1.00–1.04) |
|    Male | 1.00 (Reference) |
| Feeling lonely (vs. not ever) | |
|    Rarely | 1.65 (1.32–2.07) |
|    Sometimes | 4.77 (3.91–5.82) |
|    Often | 11.27 (8.75–14.51) |
|    Not ever | 1.00 (Reference) |

[a]Not an exhaustive presentation of all variables included in the final published model.
[b]Reference group is those with no change in depression.
aPOR, adjusted prevalence odds ratio; CI, confidence interval.

6. Using the findings in **Table 13.12**, interpret the aPORs associated with age and sex assigned at birth. Assume the only variables included in the model are those shown in the table. Recall that we have discussed interpreting measures of association for numeric exposures per unit increase. Here, note that the aPOR for age is reported for the association with the outcome per 5-year increase in age (i.e., the "unit" is 5 years).

**TABLE 13.13 LOGISTIC REGRESSION RESULTS[a]: ASSOCIATION BETWEEN FEELING LONELY AND WORSENED DEPRESSION,[b] CONTROLLING FOR AGE AND STRATIFIED BY SEX ASSIGNED AT BIRTH**

|  | Men | Women |
|---|---|---|
|  | aPOR (95% CI) | aPOR (95% CI) |
| Feeling lonely |  |  |
| Rarely | 2.86 (1.97–4.16) | 2.68 (2.00–3.60) |
| Sometimes | 7.53 (5.28–10.74) | 7.17 (5.49–9.37) |
| Often | 11.60 (6.86–19.62) | 19.74 (14.28–27.29) |
| Not ever | 1.00 (Reference) | 1.00 (Reference) |

[a]Not an exhaustive presentation of all variables included in the final published model.
[b]Reference group is those with no change in depression.
aPOR, adjusted prevalence odds ratio.

7. Without conducting a test of statistical significance, do these data appear to indicate a meaningful linear trend (i.e., dose response) for the effect of feeling lonely on worsened depression?

8. Consider the study data in **Table 13.13,** which are adapted from the analysis that was stratified by sex assigned at birth. Do these data suggest meaningful effect measure modification by sex?

9. The following is another quote from the manuscript—what epidemiologic concept does this quote refer to?

*"The use of cross-sectional data in this study precludes causal inferences. We are unable to establish the direction of the association between various factors such as changes in alcohol consumption, cigarette smoking, sleep quality, and worsened levels of anxiety or depression"*(p. 9).

   a. Loss to follow-up
   b. Effect measure modification
   c. Generalizability
   d. Temporality
   e. Confounding

10. The following is another quote from the manuscript—what epidemiologic concept does this quote refer to?

*"The CCRR cohort are healthier with fewer comorbidities than would be expected for this age group, are predominantly Caucasian and living within the West London region, an area typically associated with higher socioeconomic status"*(p. 10).

   a. Loss to follow-up
   b. Effect measure modification
   c. Generalizability
   d. Temporality
   e. Confounding

**Questions 11 to 15 are based on and adapted from:**

Jewell JS, Farewell CV, Welton-Mitchell C, et al. Mental health during the COVID-19 pandemic in the United States: online survey. *JMIR Form Res*. 2020;4(10):e22043. https://doi.org/10.2196/22043

A study published in 2020 evaluated the association between various demographic characteristics and mental health outcomes, including self-reported well-being, among U.S. adults during the COVID-19 pandemic. Data from 1,083 U.S. adults were collected using a cross-sectional survey. The Short Warwick-Edinburgh Mental Wellbeing Scale (SWEMWBS) was used as a numeric measure of well-being. The SWEMWBS has a range of 7 to 35, with higher scores indicating higher well-being. Linear regression models were used to evaluate associations between demographic variables and well-being outcomes.

11. Adapted results from the linear regression models for the association between several of the demographic variables and well-being scores are presented in **Table 13.14**. Interpret the findings that are significantly significant at an α of 0.05, assuming the only variables included in the model are those shown in **Table 13.14**.

**TABLE 13.14 LINEAR REGRESSION RESULTS: ASSOCIATION BETWEEN DEMOGRAPHICS AND SELF-REPORTED WELL-BEING**

|  | β |
|---|---|
| **Age (per decade increase)** | 1.86* |
| **Race** | |
| White | 1.00 (Reference) |
| Black | 2.62 |
| Native American or American Indian | 2.18 |
| Asian | 1.94 |
| **Work status** | |
| Working remotely before and after COVID-19 | 1.00 (Reference) |
| Unemployed prior to COVID-19 | −2.81 |
| Work outside home | 0.03 |
| No longer working due to COVID-19 | −3.90* |
| Working remotely due to COVID-19 | −0.33 |
| **Insurance** | |
| Full coverage | 1.00 (Reference) |
| Partial coverage | −2.20 |
| Medicare/Medicaid | −1.77 |
| None | −9.59* |
| **Sex** | |
| Female | Ref |
| Male | 1.61 |

*$p$-value less than 0.05.
Adapted: not an exhaustive presentation of all variables included in the final published model.
*Source*: Adapted from Jewell JS, Farewell CV, Welton-Mitchell C, et al. Mental health during the COVID-19 pandemic in the United States: online survey. *JMIR Form Res*. 2020;4(10):e22043. https://doi.org/10.2196/22043

12. Provide a hypothesized explanation for the association between age and well-being.

13. The following is a quote from the manuscript—what epidemiologic concept does this quote refer to?

*"Data cleaning included testing of assumptions, exploration of outliers, and missingness for all key variables. As all key variables had less than 10% missing data and data were missing completely at random…, listwise deletion was used in all analyses"*(p. 3).

    a. Data imputation

    b. Outliers

    c. Selection bias

    d. Sensitivity analysis

    e. Confounding

14. The following is a quote from the manuscript—what epidemiologic concept(s) does this quote refer to?

*"Minority populations tend to experience the effects of trauma to a greater degree than others. Given the results seen in this study in a non-Hispanic White population that is primarily insured, it is reasonable to assume that minority populations may be impacted to an even greater degree than what was demonstrated in this study"*(p. 9).

    a. Loss to follow-up

    b. Effect measure modification

    c. Generalizability

    d. Temporality

    e. Confounding

15. The following is a quote from the manuscript—what epidemiologic concept does this quote refer to?

*"In addition, due to the small number of African Americans in this sample, we were not able to explore the relationship between race and mental health, a limitation that should be prioritized for exploration in follow-up research"*(p. 9).

    a. Loss to follow-up

    b. Effect measure modification

    c. Generalizability

    d. Temporality

    e. Confounding

## REFERENCES

1. Benton TD, Boyd RC, Njoroge WFM. Addressing the global crisis of child and adolescent mental health. *JAMA Pediatr*. 2021;175(11):1108–1110. https://doi.org/10.1001/jamapediatrics.2021.2479

2. Racine N, McArthur BA, Cooke JE, et al. Global prevalence of depressive and anxiety symptoms in children and adolescents during COVID-19: a meta-analysis. *JAMA Pediatr*. 2021;175(11):1142–1150. https://doi.org/10.1001/jamapediatrics.2021.2482

3. Lee J. Mental health effects of school closures during COVID-19. *Lancet Child Adolesc Health*. 2020;4(6):421. https://doi.org/10.1016/S2352-4642(20)30109-7

4. Patrick SW, Henkhaus LE, Zickafoose JS, et al. Well-being of parents and children during the COVID-19 pandemic: a national survey. *Pediatrics*. 2020;146(4):e2020016824. https://doi.org/10.1542/peds.2020-016824

5. McGuire TG, Miranda J. New evidence regarding racial and ethnic disparities in mental health: policy implications. *Health Aff (Millwood)*. 2008;27(2):393–403. https://doi.org/10.1377/hlthaff.27.2.393

6. Snowden LR, Snowden JM. Coronavirus trauma and African Americans' mental health: seizing opportunities for transformational change. *Int J Environ Res Public Health*. 2021;18(7):3568. https://doi.org/10.3390/ijerph18073568

7. Fante-Coleman T, Jackson-Best F. Barriers and facilitators to accessing mental healthcare in Canada for Black youth: a scoping review. *Adolesc Res Rev*. 2020;5(2):115–136. https://doi.org/10.1007/s40894-020-00133-2

8. Kroenke K, Wu J, Yu Z, et al. Patient Health Questionnaire anxiety and depression scale: initial validation in three clinical trials. *Psychosom Med*. 2016;78(6):716–727. https://doi.org/10.1097/PSY.0000000000000322

9. McKinlay AR, May T, Dawes J, et al. 'You're just there, alone in your room with your thoughts': a qualitative study about the psychosocial impact of the COVID-19 pandemic among young people living in the UK. *BMJ Open*. 2022;12(2):e053676. https://doi.org/10.1136/bmjopen-2021-053676

10. Kroenke K, Spitzer RL, Williams JB. The PHQ-9: validity of a brief depression severity measure. *J Gen Intern Med*. 2001;16(9):606–613. https://doi.org/10.1046/j.1525-1497.2001.016009606.x

11. Weiss NA. *Introductory Statistics*. 9th ed. Addison-Wesley; 2011.

12. Sterne JAC, White IR, Carlin JB, et al. Multiple imputation for missing data in epidemiological and clinical research: potential and pitfalls. *BMJ*. 2009;338:b2393. https://doi.org/10.1136/bmj.b2393

13. Sundjaja JH, Shrestha R, Krishan K. *McNemar and Mann–Whitney U Tests*. StatPearls; 2022. https://www.ncbi.nlm.nih.gov/books/NBK560699

14. Nowacki A. Chi-square and Fisher's exact tests (From the "Biostatistics and Epidemiology Lecture Series, Part 1"). *Cleve Clin J Med*. 2017;84(9 suppl 2):e20–e25. https://doi.org/10.3949/ccjm.84.s2.04

15. Dean AG, et al. OpenEpi: open source epidemiologic statistics for public health. 2013. http://www.openepi.com/SampleSize/SSPropor.htm

16. Kleinbaum DG, Klein M. *Logistic Regression: A Self-Learning Text*. 3rd ed. Springer Science + Business Media; 2010.

17. Kleinbaum DG, Klein M. *Survival Analysis: A Self-Learning Text*. 3rd ed. Springer Science + Business Media; 2012.

18. Kleinbaum DG, Kupper LL, Nizam A, et al. *Applied Regression Analysis and Other Multivariable Methods*. 5th ed. Cengage Learning; 2014.

19. Thorisdottir IE, Asgeirsdottir BB, Kristjansson AL, et al. Depressive symptoms, mental wellbeing, and substance use among adolescents before and during the COVID-19 pandemic in Iceland: a longitudinal, population-based study. *Lancet Psychiatry*. 2021;8(8):663–672. https://doi.org/10.1016/S2215-0366(21)00156-5

20. Derogatis LR, Unger R. Symptom Checklist-90-revised. In: Weiner IB, Craighead WB (Eds.). *The Corsini Encyclopedia of Psychology*. Wiley; 2010:1–2. https://doi.org/10.1002/9780470479216.corpsy0970

21. Zhang D, Li G, Shi L, et al. Association between racial discrimination and delayed or forgone care amid the COVID-19 pandemic. *Prev Med*. 2022;162:107153. https://doi.org/10.1016/j.ypmed.2022.107153

# GLOSSARY

**Adjusted Measure of Association:** Measures of association calculated after adjusting (also called controlling) for potential confounders.

**Allocation Concealment:** A process employed in controlled trials whereby the order in which participants (or groups of participants) are assigned to the trial arms is hidden until the moment of assignment. The purpose of allocation concealment is to prevent bias in the allocation of participants to study arms.

**Alternative Hypothesis:** In the context of statistical inference, the alternative hypothesis is a statement that posits that the population parameter *is* statistically significantly different from the null value. Alternative hypotheses can be two-sided (where the hypothesized direction of the association *is not* stated) or one-sided (the hypothesized direction of the association *is* stated).

**Analytic Epidemiology:** A branch of epidemiology used to investigate the association between exposures and health outcomes, with the goal of understanding *why* outcomes occur. These associations are measured by quantitatively comparing measures of frequency across two or more groups to calculate measures of association.

**Bias:** Also called systematic error, bias results from a flaw in the design, conduct, or analysis of a study that leads to incorrect conclusions.

**Biologic Interaction:** Occurs when two (or more) factors must both (all) be present to cause an outcome to occur.

**Breslow–Day Test:** An assessment used to determine whether stratum-specific measures of association are different from one another from a statistical perspective on the scale(s) of interest (additive and/or multiplicative).

**Case Definition:** Criteria that must be met for an individual to be classified as having the outcome of interest.

**Case Report:** A detailed description of a single person with a noteworthy health-related outcome of interest.

**Case Series:** A collection of case reports for multiple individuals with the same noteworthy health-related outcome.

**Categorical Variables:** Variables that have a limited number of mutually exclusive response categories.

**Chi-Square Test:** A statistical test that is used to determine whether the frequency of the outcome is statistically significantly different across two or more levels of a categorical exposure. The chi-square test is only appropriate when there is adequate sample size.

**Closed Cohort:** Closed cohorts are defined by a common start time, and no one is added to the cohort during the follow-up period. Individuals only exit the cohort when they get the outcome of interest, the study ends, or they die.

**Cohort:** A group of individuals who are followed or traced over a period of time, and for which membership is defined by some common criteria.

**Cohort Design:** An observational study design in which, an at-risk group of individuals with different exposures are followed to see who develop(s) the outcome of interest.

**Cohort Studies Conducted in Real-Time:** A cohort design in which investigators identify and enroll a cohort of at-risk individuals and follow them forward in real-time. Outcomes occur at some point in the future relative to when the study was conceived.

**Cohort Studies Conducted Using Historical Records:** A cohort design in which investigators make use of historical records to understand what has happened to a cohort of individuals in the past. Thus, both the exposure and outcome have already occurred before the investigators begin the study.

**Confidence Interval:** Given the data observed in the sample population, the confidence interval is a range of values that are more plausible for the population parameter than those outside the range. Confidence intervals can be used for statistical inference to quantify the impact that random error may have had on study results, including null hypothesis significance testing.

**Confounder:** A confounder is an "extraneous factor" that causes an imbalance between comparison groups, which leads to bias in the measure of association of interest.

**Confounding:** A type of systematic error (bias) that occurs when the association of interest is mixed with the effect of an extraneous factor (a confounder) that is not balanced between comparison groups.

**Continuous Variables:** Numeric variables that can take on an infinite set of values bounded by any two values.

**Cross-Sectional Design:** An observational study design in which investigators measure the exposure(s) and outcome(s) at the same time. The cross-sectional design provides a "snapshot" of the health status of the study population at a single point in time.

**Crude Measure of Association:** The measure of association that only considers the relationship between the exposure and the outcome. In the context of confounding, crude measures of association are also called unadjusted measures of association.

**Descriptive Epidemiology:** A branch of epidemiology used to investigate the distribution of health-related outcomes or events, often using person, place, and time characteristics.

**Determinants:** Factors that cause a health-related outcome or event to occur; also called exposures.

**Diagnostic Tests:** Assessments used in individuals with abnormal signs or symptoms (or individuals with a positive screening test) to either establish or rule out a disease which would then go on to be treated or managed.

**Differential Misclassification:** Occurs when the extent of misclassification of the exposure or outcome depends on the status of the other variable.

**Discrete Variables:** Numeric variables that have a limited number of responses. In epidemiology, these are often scales used to identify select health conditions that have a fixed set of possible scores.

**Effect Measure Modification:** Sometimes referred to as stratum-specific heterogeneity, effect measure modification occurs when the measure of association meaningfully differs across values of a third variable. This third variable is called an effect modifier.

**Effect Modifier:** In the presence of effect measure modification, the effect modifier is the third variable by which the data are stratified.

**Effectiveness:** In a controlled trial, effectiveness is a measure of the ability of an intervention to prevent or treat the health outcome it was designed for among people who are randomized to the intervention, *whether or not they actually receive the intervention.*

**Efficacy:** In a controlled trial, efficacy is a measure of the ability of an intervention to prevent or treat the health outcome it was designed for *among those who use the intervention according to the study protocol.*

**Endemic:** Diseases that regularly occur with some expected frequency in a particular population. This expected frequency is called the endemic level of disease.

**Epidemic:** Occurs when the frequency of a disease exceeds the expected (endemic) level in a particular population.

**Epidemiologic Transition:** A change characterized by a shift from relatively high mortality among infants and children (largely attributable to communicable diseases—diseases that can be transmitted from one individual to another) to a higher morbidity and mortality among older adults (largely attributable to noncommunicable diseases—diseases that cannot be transmitted from one individual to another).

**Equipoise:** A prerequisite for conducting controlled trials, which occurs when none of the exposure conditions in a trial are already known to be inferior or superior prior to the start of the study.

**Experimental Studies:** A branch of epidemiologic study designs in which the study investigators assign the exposure status to participants.

**Exposures:** Factors that cause a health-related outcome or event to occur; also called determinants.

**Exposure Odds Ratio (EOR):** In the case-control design, the exposure odds ratio is the measure of association compares the frequency of the exposure in cases to the frequency of the exposure in controls. The exposure odds ratio is calculated by taking the ratio of the odds of exposure among cases and the odds of exposure among controls. The exposure odds ratio is unitless.

**External Validity:** Is achieved when the point estimates calculated in a sample population are applicable to populations of interest other than the source population (i.e., target populations). External validity is also called generalizability.

**Fisher's Exact Test:** An assessment used to determine whether the frequency of the outcome is statistically significantly different across two or more levels of a categorical exposure. The Fisher's exact test does not require a minimum sample size, and thus can always be used for this assessment.

**Generalizability:** Is achieved when the point estimates calculated in a sample population are applicable to populations of interest other than the source population (i.e., target populations). Generalizability is also called external validity.

**Health-Related Outcome:** Any event that impacts population well-being, also called health-related states or events, or simply outcomes. In epidemiology, health-related outcomes are often but not always diseases.

**Human Subjects:** People who are included in the sample population for a research study.

**Hypothesis:** A statement that posits that an exposure of interest is associated with an outcome of interest. An epidemiologic hypothesis additionally includes information about the population of interest, and may or may not include the expected direction of the association.

**Induction Period:** The time it takes for an outcome to occur *due to an exposure of interest.*

**Information Bias:** A type of systematic error (bias) that occurs when there is error in the measurement of the exposure and/or outcome that leads to a measure of association that is meaningfully different from what would have been obtained if all variables had been measured correctly. Information bias is often referred to as measurement error.

**Intention-to-Treat Analysis:** An analysis for a controlled trial in which all study participants who underwent randomization are analyzed in their respective assigned arms, regardless of whether they actually receive the intervention.

**Interaction:** An umbrella term that may refer to effect measure modification, statistical interaction, or biologic interaction.

**Internal Validity:** Is achieved when point estimates calculated in a sample population are close to their corresponding population parameters. Internal validity is influenced by systematic error (or bias).

**Interrater Reliability:** The reproducibility of test results by two or more raters; also known as interobserver reliability.

**Latency Period:** The time during which an outcome exists but is not clinically or otherwise detectable.

**Levels of Prevention:**

- *Primary prevention:* Public health efforts designed to keep negative health outcomes from occurring at all; primary prevention can be passive or active.

- *Secondary prevention:* Public health efforts designed to address the health of those who are already affected by a negative health outcome but are not yet experiencing symptoms. The goal of secondary prevention is to decrease morbidity or mortality using interventions such as screening for early detection.

- *Tertiary prevention:* Public health efforts designed to reduce long-term complications and death from health-related outcomes in those with established disease. Interventions that focus on treatment, management of comorbidities and complications, rehabilitation, and palliative care are all considered tertiary prevention strategies.

**Linear Regression:** An analytic technique that uses a mathematical formula to describe how a numeric outcome variable (the dependent variable) is associated with exposure(s) and other covariates (the independent variables).

**Logistic Regression:** An analytic technique that uses a mathematical formula to describe how a dichotomous outcome variable (the dependent variable) is associated with exposure(s) and other covariates (the independent variables).

**Mann–Whitney Test:** An assessment that is used to evaluate whether there is a statistically significant difference in the medians of numeric outcomes across two independent exposure categories when the outcome data are nonnormally distributed.

**Masking:** A process employed in controlled trials that involves withholding exposure status information from certain groups including study participants, investigators, and/or data analysts. The purpose of masking is to prevent bias in the measurement of key variables of interest.

**Matching in a Case-Control Study:** Controls are matched to cases on one or more factors (e.g., age, calendar year, sex) that are thought to be strong confounders of the relationship between the exposure and the outcome.

**Matching in a Cohort Study:** Unexposed study participants are matched to exposed participants on one or more factors (e.g., age, calendar year, sex) that are thought to be strong confounders of the relationship between the exposure and the outcome.

**Meaningful Significance:** A term used to describe whether study findings have important implications for public health—this could include leading to a change in clinical care, policy, or public health resource allocation.

**Measurement Error:** A type of systematic error (bias) that occurs when there is error in the measurement of the exposure and/or outcome that leads to a measure of association that is meaningfully different from what would have been obtained if all variables had been measured correctly. Measurement error is also referred to as information bias.

**Measures of Association:** Measures that quantify the association between an exposure and a health outcome. Measures of association are calculated by comparing measures of frequency across two groups.

**Measures of Frequency:** Measures that quantify the occurrence of a health outcome such as risk, rate, and prevalence.

**Misclassification:** A subset of information bias (or measurement error) that occurs when there is error in the measurement of categorical variables.

**Negative Predictive Value (NPV):** The proportion of those who test negative who truly *do not* have the disease. NPV can be reported as either a decimal or a percentage.

**Nondifferential Misclassification:** Occurs when the extent of misclassification of the exposure or outcome does not depend on the status of the other variable.

**Null Hypothesis:** In the context of statistical inference, the null hypothesis is a statement that posits that the population parameter is *not* statistically significantly different from the null value.

**Null Hypothesis ($H_0$) Significance Testing:** A method to test whether study results differ from the null hypothesis from a statistical perspective.

**Numeric Variables:** Variables with numeric responses that can be either continuous or discrete.

**Observational Studies:** A branch of epidemiologic study designs in which the exposure is not assigned by the study investigators; rather, the study investigators observe the exposure status that has occurred or will occur anyway.

**Open Cohort:** Cohorts in which members can enroll and leave at different times. These are also called dynamic cohorts.

**Pandemic:** An epidemic that occurs across geographically distant populations; for example, across international borders.

**Per-Protocol Analysis:** An analysis for a controlled trial that only includes data from individuals with perfect adherence to their assigned trial arm.

**Placebo:** An inert or "fake" exposure condition, such as a sugar pill or sham procedure, that sometimes used as the control condition in controlled trials.

**Point Estimate:** Study results calculated using data collected from the sample population.

**Population Parameter:** The unobserved true values in the source population.

**Positive Predictive Value (PPV):** This represents the proportion of those who test positive who truly *do* have the disease. PPV can be reported as either a decimal or a percentage.

**Precision:** An indiciation of how much study results have been influenced by random error; it is inversely associated with the width of a confidence interval.

**Prevalence:** A measure of frequency that is used to describe the proportion of individuals in a specified population who have an existing outcome at a particular point in time.

**Prevalence Difference (PD):** A measure of association used in cross-sectional studies that is calculated by subtracting the prevalence of the outcome in the unexposed group from the prevalence of the outcome in the exposed group. The prevalence difference is expressed as a decimal or percentage.

**Prevalence Ratio (PR):** A measure of association used in cross-sectional studies that is calculated by dividing the prevalence of the outcome in the exposed group by the prevalence of the outcome in the unexposed group. The prevalence ratio is unitless.

**Public Health:** An art and science that is broadly dedicated to promoting and protecting the health of human populations.

**Public Health Research Ethics:** Guidelines for the responsible conduct of public health research to ensure the protection of human subjects.

*p*-**Value:** This indicates the probability of obtaining a result as or more extreme than the result observed in a study, if the null hypothesis is true and there is no bias.

**Random Error:** Also called sampling error, random error occurs because we typically make inferences about a population using an estimate obtained from a sample of that population.

**Randomization:** A process employed in controlled trials in which every individual (or groups of individuals) in a study has an equal chance of being assigned to each exposure condition.

**Rate:** A measure of frequency that is used to describe how quickly new health-related outcomes occur in at-risk persons during a specified follow-up period.

**Rate (Incidence Density) Ratio (IDR):** A measure of association used in controlled trials and cohort designs that is calculated by dividing the rate of the outcome in the exposed group by the rate of the outcome in the unexposed group. The rate ratio is unitless.

**Rate (Incidence Density) Difference (IDD):** A measure of association used in controlled trials and cohort designs that is calculated by subtracting the rate in the unexposed group from the rate in the exposed group. The rate ratio is expressed per units of person-time.

**Risk:** A measure of frequency that is used to describe proportion of at-risk individuals who develop a newly occurring outcome during a specified time-period.

**Risk Ratio (RR):** A measure of association used in controlled trials and cohort designs that is calculated by dividing the risk of the outcome in the exposed group by the risk of the outcome in the unexposed group. An interpretation of the risk ratio must be accompanied by information about the length of the follow-up period. The risk ratio is unitless.

**Risk Difference (RD):** A measure of association used in controlled trials and cohort designs that is calculated by subtracting the risk in the unexposed group from the risk in the exposed group. An interpretation of the risk difference must be accompanied by information about the length of the follow-up period. The risk difference is expressed as a decimal or percentage.

**Sample Population:** Also called the study population, the sample population is the subset of the source population that is enrolled in a study, and for whom exposure and outcome data are measured.

**Scale-Dependence:** An indication that effect measure modification and/or statistical interaction may be present on the multiplicative scale (i.e., differences in the stratified ratio measures of association), additive scale (i.e., differences in the stratified difference measures of association), both scales, or neither scale.

**Screening Tests:** Assessments that are used in individuals who appear to be healthy but may be at-risk for a disease of interest, with the goal of classifying them with respect to their likelihood of having that disease.

**Selection Bias:** A type of systematic error (bias) that occurs when the measure of association calculated from the sample population is meaningfully different from the measure of effect that would have been estimated if data had been available for all eligible subjects in the source population.

**Selection Probability:** This is the probability of being selected from the source population and providing data in the sample population.

**Sensitivity:** This represents the proportion of those *with* the outcome or exposure who are correctly classified. Sensitivity can be reported as either a decimal or a percentage.

**Sensitivity Analyses:** These data analyses use explore how different sets of plausible assumptions affect study results.

**Social Determinants of Health:** These are defined by the U.S. Centers for Disease Control and Prevention as "conditions in the places where people live, learn, work, and play that affect a wide range of health risks and outcomes." These determinants include access to quality healthcare and education, social and community context, and socioeconomic status.

**Source Population:** The population of eligible individuals from which the study participants are sampled. In a cohort study, it is the population from which the cohort is selected based on the eligibility criteria defined by the investigators. In a case-control study, it is the population that gave rise to the cases.

**Specificity:** This measures the proportion of those *without* the outcome or exposure who are correctly classified. Specificity can be reported as either a decimal or a percentage.

**Statistical Interaction:** Occurs when stratum-specific measures of association are statistically significantly different from one another.

**Statistical Significance:** Describes whether measures are different from one another from a statistical perspective.

**Stratified Analysis:** The process of stratifying (i.e., splitting) data into mutually exclusive strata (i.e., groups) and conducting data analysis using the stratified data.

**Surveillance:** The systematic, ongoing collection of health-related data in a specified population that is disseminated in a timely manner to improve the health of the population.

**Systematic Error:** Also called bias, systematic error results from a flaw in the design, conduct, and/or analysis of a study that leads to incorrect conclusions.

**Target Population:** The group of individuals for whom the study results will be relevant. The target population is often an external population to which investigators want to generalize their findings. The target population could be the same as the source population, slightly broader than the source population, or completely external from the source population.

**t-Test:** An assessment used to evaluate whether there is a statistically significant difference in the means of numeric outcomes across two independent exposure categories when the outcome data are normally distributed.

**Test for Linear Trend:** An assessment used to determine whether there is a statistically significant linear trend that occurs when there is a consistent increase or decrease in the magnitude of the measure of association across ordinal exposure categories.

# INDEX

Note: Page numbers in *italics* denote tables and figures.

active prevention, 7
active surveillance, 30
additive scale
   effect measure modification (EMM) on, 206
   statistical interaction on, 206
adjusted measures of association, 231–232, 378
   calculation using stratified analysis,
     246–248, *246*
   compared to crude measures, 232, 235, 236–239
   interpreting, 239
   reporting, 239
adjusted odds ratio (aOR), 232
adjusted prevalence odds ratio (aPOR), 387
adjusted prevalence ratio (aPR), 236
adjusted risk odds ratio (aROR), 358
adverse childhood experiences (ACEs), 222,
   234–235, 236–237, 238, 250
allocation concealment, 103, 105, 110
alpha, 200, 202, 336, 375
alternative hypotheses, 92, 199, 332, 385
analytic epidemiology, 55–56, *217*
   cycle of, 56–57, *57*
   versus descriptive epidemiology, *24*, 25
   developing study hypotheses, 57–59
   exploratory, 60–61
   study designs, 62–69
   *see also* measures of association
a priori criteria, for confounding assessment,
   233–235
asymptomatic, 7
at risk, 32, 34–35, 63, 120
audio computer-assisted self-interviewing
   (ACASI), 311
autism spectrum disorder (ASD), 48, 67,
   80, 188


Behavioral Risk Factor Surveillance
   System (BRFSS), 182–183
Berkson's bias, 279, 291
beta coefficients, 385
bias
   away from the null, 228
   direction of, 227–230, 237–239, *238*, *298*
   switchover, 228
   towards the null, 227–228, 269
   *see also* systematic error
biological interaction, 195
biological sex, 42
birth cohort, 120
Black Women's Health Study, 120, 125
blinding. *See* masking
Bradford Hill's guidelines for causality,
   83, *84*
Breslow–Day test, 200, 202, 377

caliper matching, 161
case-control designs, 65–66, 140–141
   case selection in, 281
   data layout and measure of association in,
     143–152
   hypothesis development in, 142–143
   incident versus prevalent cases, sampling of, 157
   limitations of, 165
   matching in, 162–164
   participant identification and selection into,
     154–161
   primary versus secondary base, 152–154
   reporting study findings from, 166
   sampling cases with enumeration of source
     population, 155–156
   sampling cases without enumeration of source
     population, 155–156
   schematic of, *65*, *141*, *155*
   selection bias in, 273–276
   strategies to identify controls, 157–159
case definition, 3, 26–28, *28*
case reports, 28–29
case series, 29
categorical variables, 251, 295, 368
category matching, 161
causality, 66–67, 68–69, 96, 133
chi-square test, 375
climate change and health, 44–45
clinical trial. *See* controlled trial
closed cohort, 121–122, *122*
   comparison with open cohort, 123
cluster randomization, 98–99, 100–101
cluster sampling, 281
cohort
   defining, 120–121
   open and closed, 121–123
cohort designs, 64, 118–119
   basics of, 118–119
   data layouts and measures of frequency
     and association calculated in, 130–133
   exposure and reference group and, 126–127
   hypothesis development in, 119–120
   induction and latency periods and, 128–130
   limitations of, 133–134
   real-time and historical, 123–126
   schematic of, *64*, *118*
   strengths of, 133
communicable diseases, 7
competing risk, 34
confidence intervals (CIs), *203*, *249*, 348–356,
   *349–351*, *353*, 385
   calculation of, 349–350
   comparing the width of, 352–353
   comparison to *p*-values, 354
   conceptualization of, 349

confidence intervals (CIs) (*contd.*)
  magnitude and direction of association and, 353
  misinterpretations of, 352
  null hypothesis significance testing and, 350–352
  precision and, 352
confounders, 158, 161, 223, 231, 254
confounding, 223, 230–233, *234*, 240–241
  addressing, 232, 241–253
  a priori criteria for assessment, 233–235
  assessing, 232–241, 378–380, *379*
  compared to effect measure modification, 254–258
  data-based method for assessment, 235–241, 378–380, *379*
  examples, 232
  triangle, 233, *234*
CONSORT statement, 110
contact tracing, 30
contingency tables. *See* R×C tables
continuous variables, 363
controlled trials, 61, 90–91
  ethics of, 109–110
  example of, 63
  exposure definition in, 91–92
  FDA phases of, 107–109
  limitations of, 110–111
  masking and, 102–103
  objectives and hypotheses of, 92–95
  schematic of, *63*
  strengths of, 110
  types of, 99–102
  *see also* randomization; randomized controlled trial designs
convenience sampling, 282
COVID-19 vaccine trial, 104, 106–107, 111
crossover trial, 100
cross-sectional designs, 172–173
  data layout and measures of frequency and association calculated in, 176–181
  for descriptive and analytic analyses, 173–175
  example of, 67
  hypothesis testing for, 174–175
  limitations of, 183–185
  measures of frequency and association calculation in, 181
  schematic of, *66, 173*
  selection bias in, 276–278
  serial, 182–183
  source and sample population identification for, 175–176
  strengths of, 183
crude measures of association, 232, 235, 236–239, 378
cumulative incidence, 32–34, 38
  *see also* risk

Danish Cancer Registry, 155, 167
data analysis, 363
  data examination and cleaning and, 368–372
  descriptive statistics and, 363–368
  exposure and outcome association evaluation and, 373–377
  regression modeling and, 383–388

sensitivity analyses and, 388–389
stratified analyses for effect measure modification and statistical interaction and, 377–378
stratified analysis for confounding and, 378–380
trend analysis and, 380–382
variable frequencies and, 372–373
data examination and cleaning, 368–372
data imputation, 371
death, leading causes of, 8–9
Declaration of Helsinki, 13, *15–16*, 92
dengue, 49
dependent variable, 383
descriptive epidemiology, 4, 23–48
  compared to analytic epidemiology, *24*, 25
  meaning and significance of, 24–25
  measures of frequency and, 32–41
  outcome frequency description and, 42–47
  public health surveillance and, 29–31
  study designs of, 28–29
descriptive statistics, 363–368
diagnostic tests, 312–313
dichotomous exposure, 131
differential loss to follow-up, 268, *269*, 270, 273
differential misclassification, 299–300, 301, 304–306
differential participation
  in case-control studies, 274–275
  in cross-sectional studies, 277–278
  *see also* self-selection bias
differential selection, 268
directed acyclic graphs (DAGs), 240–241
discrete variables, 364
dose–response relationship, 380
double-masked trial, 103, 105
Down syndrome, 231
dynamic cohort. *See* open cohort

ecologic designs, 67–68
ecologic fallacy, 68
effect heterogeneity. *See* effect measure modification
effectiveness of an intervention, 106
effect measure modification (EMM), 192–196, 247
  assessment of, 196–204
  biological interaction and statistical interaction and, 205
  compared to confounding, 254–258
  examples of, *193*
  OpenEpi for, 200–201
  public health importance of, 209–210
  scale dependency of, 206–208, 255
  statistical tests to assess, 199–204
  study hypotheses and, 194
  visualizing assessment of, *197*
effect modifier, 192, 196, 209
efficacy of an intervention, 106
endemic, 4–5, 10
Enhancing QUAlity and Transparency of Health Research (EQUATOR) Network, 28–29
epidemic, 4–5
epidemic curves, 45–46
epidemiologic transition, 7–9
epidemiologic triangle, 46

epidemiology, 1–6, *3*
   achievements in public health and, 9–11
   classification of studies of, 61–82, *61*
   social determinants of health and, 17–18
equipoise, 109
equivalence trials, 93–94
error, in epidemiologic research, 222–227, *223*
expected cell size, calculation of, 375–376, *376*
experimental study, 61
   *see also* controlled trials
exploratory analytic epidemiologic studies, 60–61
exposure, 5, *56*, 58
   defining exposure groups, 126–127, 131
exposure and outcome association,
      evaluating, *374*
   categorical outcomes and, 375–377
   numeric outcomes and, 374–375
exposure misclassification, 297–298, *298*, 299
   differential, 299–300, 301, 304–306
   nondifferential, 299–301, 304–306, 308
   quantifying, *302*
   tables, 301, *301*
exposure odds ratio (EOR), 80–82, 143–144,
      146–148, 150, 162, 273–274, 333
   calculating and interpreting, 81–82, 151
   calculation, in pair-matched analysis, 162–164
   common mistakes in interpreting, 148
extended Mantel–Haenszel chi-square test
      for linear trend, 381
external reference group, 127
external validity, 225, 286
   *see also* generalizability

factorial trials, 101–102, 104
   schematic illustration of, *101*
false negatives, 295, 301
false positives, 301
Fisher's exact tests, 375
Flint water crisis, 55–56, *58*
follow-up period, 33, 95–96, 100, 110, 120–122, 129
Ford, S., 23
Framingham Heart Study, 117, 120, 121,
      125, 127, 288
frequency matching. *See* group matching

gender-affirming hormone therapy (GAHT), 333
generalizability, 111, 225, 245, 281
   *see also* external validity
general population cohort, 120, 123
gestational diabetes, 211
gestational weight gain (GWG), 210
gold standard, 142, 143, 294, 313
gonorrhea, 26
group matching, 244, *244*

Hanna-Attisha, M., 55–56
health equity, 18
Health Professionals Follow-Up Study, 120–121
   data analysis in, 131–132
   design considerations in, 126

health-related states and events. *See* outcome
heart disease, 77, 261, 304–305
Herpes zoster, 52
Hippocratic Oath, 13
historical cohort study, 123–124, *124*, 125
   comparison with real-time cohort study,
      125–126
HIV, 11, 29, *40*
human papillomavirus (HPV), 193, *198*
   vaccination study of, 210, 257
human subjects research, ethical foundations of,
      12–17
hypotheses in epidemiologic studies, 57–59, *58*, 199
hypothetical study replications, 329

imputation, 285
incidence, measures of
   rate, 34–38
   risk, 32–34, 37
incidence density difference (IDD),
      76, 77, 206
incidence density ratio (IDR), 75, 344, 355
incidence rate, 34–38
incubation period, 129
independent variable, 383
individual matching, 244, *244*
individual randomization, 98
induction period, 128–129, *129*
infectious diseases. *See* communicable
      diseases
influenza, 46, *46*
information bias, 223, 294, *294*
   conceptualizing, *220*
   correction opportunities, in study
      analysis stage, 306–310
   differential and nondifferential misclassification
      and, 299–301
   misclassification impact on R×C tables,
      297–300
   misclassification tables and, 304–306
   quantifying, 301–303
   reduction opportunities, in study design stage,
      311–312
   sources of, 295–297
Institutional Review Boards (IRBs), 16
intention-to-treat analysis, 106
interaction. *See* effect measure modification
internal reference group, 127
International Classification of Diseases
      (ICD), 26, 27
interobserver reliability, 319–320
interquartile range (IQR), 364, 365, *365*
interrater reliability, 319–321
inverse probability weighting, 285
investigator error, 296

Jenner, E., 9–10

Kelsey, F. O., 13
kurtosis, 366

latency period, 128–129, *129*, 135
lead time bias, 318
left skewed data. *See* negatively skewed data
length time bias, 318–319, *319*
leprosy, 261
linear regression, 385–386
linear trends, 380
log binomial regression, 384
logistic regression, 384, 386–388
longitudinal studies
  maximizing follow-up in, 280
  selection bias in, 268–273
  selection probabilities for, *283*
loss to follow-up, 34, 121, 267
  differential, 268, *269*, 270, 273
  nondifferential, 272
lower limit, of confidence intervals, 348

malaria, 10, 44–45, *45*
Mann–Whitney test, 374, 375
Mantel–Haenszel adjusted measure of
  association, 248, 380
marginal totals, 71
masking, 102–103, 105, 110, 311
matching, in case-control studies, 162–164,
  243–244, 253
  advantages of, 162
  data layout and measures of association for, *162*
  limitations of, 162
matching, in cohort studies, 243, 253
maximizing participation, 280
meaningful differences, 204–205, 235, 237–238,
  247, 249, 266, 270, 289, 345, 346
measure of central tendency, 364
measurement error. *See* information bias
measures of association, 59, 224
  calculating and interpreting, 70–82
  case control studies and, 65–66, 81
  causality and interpreting, 83
  clinical trials and, 62–63
  cohort studies and, 64, *78*, 130–133
  cross-sectional studies and, 66–68, 79, 176–181
  to evaluate study hypotheses, 82–84
  exposure odds ratio and, 80–82
  formulae and features of, *218*
  magnitude and direction of, 82–83
  prevalence-based, 78–80
  *p*-values and, *339*
  rate-based, 75–78
  risk-based, 72–75
  statistical significance and, 337
  *see also* analytic epidemiology
measures of effect, 224, 266
measures of frequency, 24, 32, 56
  of incidence, 32–38
  of prevalence, 38–42
misclassification. *See* information bias
misclassification tables, 304–306
  for differential and non-differential
    determination, 304–306
  exposure and outcome, 301–302, *301*
missing data and data cleaning, 370–371

morbidity, 3
mortality, 3, 7–9
multiplicative scale
  effect measure modification (EMM) on, 206
  statistical interaction on, 206

National Health and Nutrition Examination
  Survey (NHANES), 43
National Health Interview Survey (NHIS), 67,
  176, 186
National Research Act (1974), 16
negative associations, 5
negative kurtosis, 367, *367*
negatively skewed data, 366
negative predictive value (NPV), 313, 315
nominal variables, 368
nondifferential loss to follow-up, 272
nondifferential misclassification,
  299–301, 304–306
non-inferiority trials, 93
nonprobability sampling, 282
nonsteroidal anti-inflammatory drugs
  (NSAIDs), 290
normal distribution, 365–366, *366*
notifiable conditions, 31
Notifiable Conditions Surveillance System, 31
*n*-to-one matching, 161
null hypothesis significance testing, 334–348
  confidence intervals and, 350–352
  *p*-values and, 338–348
  type I and type II errors and, 336–338
null value, 199
numeric variables, 251, 363
Nuremberg Code, 13, *15*
Nurses' Health Study, 120, 125, 126, 289

observational study, 61–62, 118, 123, 133,
  140, 152, 166, 172, 181
observer bias. *See* investigator error
odds, 146–147
  definition of, 146
  of exposure, 145
one-sided alternative hypothesis, 332
one-tailed *p*-value, 340, 342, *345*
open cohort, 122
OpenEpi, 200–201, *201*, 248, *249*, 341, 349, 381
open-label trial, 103
opioid crisis, in United States, 265–266
oral contraceptives, 192–193
ordinal variables, 131, 368
outcome, 3–4, 24
outcome frequency
  by person, 42–44
  by place, 44
  by time, 45–46
outcome misclassification, 298–299, *299*
  differential, 300, 304
  nondifferential, 304, 308
  quantifying, *303*
  tables, 301–302, *301*
outliers, 371

pair-matched odds ratio, 162–164
pair-matching, 161
    exposure odds ratio calculation in, 162–164
pandemic, 5
parallel controlled trials, 90–91, 99
    schematic of, 90
participant barriers, 296
participant nonresponse, 279
passive prevention, 6
passive surveillance, 30
Patient Health Questionnaire-9 (PHQ-9),
        93, 364, 368, 371
people who inject drugs (PWID), 275
percent agreement, 320–321
period prevalence, 41
per-protocol analysis, 105–106
person, place, and time characteristics, 4
person-time, 34–36
    epidemiologic studies with varying
        person-time, 35
phenylketonuria (PKU), 195–196
placebo, 91, 92
placebo control groups, 109
placebo effect, 92
pneumocystis pneumonia, 23–24, 29
point estimates, 223, 224, 329–330, 334,
        340, 346, 348–350, 354
point prevalence, 38, 41
political variables, 241
population-based controls, 158
population parameters, 223, 224, 228–229, 348
positive associations, 5
positive kurtosis, 367, 367
positively skewed data, 366
positive predictive value (PPV), 313, 315
power, 336
precision, 223, 330
Pregnancy Risk Assessment Monitoring
        System (PRAMS), 224
preterm birth, 357
prevalence, 38–41, 39, 177–179
    in cross-sectional studies, 174
    period prevalence, 41
    point prevalence, 38, 41
prevalence-based measures of association, 78–80
    calculating and interpreting, 80
prevalence difference (PD), 79–80, 178–179
prevalence odds ratio (POR), 149, 179
    and prevalence ratio (PR) compared, 180–181
prevalence ratio (PR), 78, 179, 235–236, 376, 380, 381
    and prevalence odds ratio (POR) compared,
        180–181
prevention, in public health, 6
    levels of, 6–7, 6
preventive exposures in controlled trials, 91
primary base case-control study, 152–154
primary prevention, in public health, 6–7
probability density functions (PDFs), 344
probability sampling. See random sampling
        strategies
prospective cohort study. See real-time
        cohort studies
publication bias, 335

public health, 2
    core disciplines of, 2
public health preparedness, 11–12
public health surveillance, 29–31
    characteristics of, 30
p-value, 200, 338–341, 374–375
    calculation of, 341
    factors influencing, 346–348
    interpretation of, 342–346
    for null hypothesis significance testing, 342

qualitative research, 10

R×C tables, 70, 271, 283
    example of, 70
    orientation of, 71
random error, 223, 328–330
    confidence intervals and, 348–356
    null hypothesis significance testing and,
        334–348
    precision and sample size and, 330–331
    statistical inference and, 332–333
    and systematic error compared, 226–227
randomization, 62, 95, 104, 109, 110, 127, 155
    attempts to approximate the counterfactual
        ideal, 96
    compared to random sampling, 282–283
    confounding and, 242, 253
    rationale for, 95–96
    techniques of, 96–98
    units of, 98–99
    see also controlled trials; randomized controlled
        trial designs
randomized controlled trial designs, 89
    analysis of, 105–107
    efficacy and effectiveness estimation in, 105
    intervention effectiveness and intention-to-treat
        analyses and, 106
    intervention efficacy and per-protocol
        analyses and, 105–106
    measures of frequency and association and, 105
    see also controlled trials; randomization
randomized controlled trials (RCTs), 288
random sampling strategies, 281
rare outcomes and cohort studies, 133, 134
rate, 34–38
rate-based measures of association, 75–78
    see also incidence density difference (IDD),
        incidence density ratio (IDR)
rate difference. See incidence density
        difference (IDD)
rate ratio. See incidence density ratio (IDR)
real-time cohort studies, 123–124, 124
    comparison with historical cohort studies,
        125–126
recall bias, 296
reference group, 126–127
regression modeling, 383–388
    adjusting for confounding using, 250–251, 254
    interpreting findings from, 384–388
representative sampling strategy, 281

residual confounding, 251
  causes of, 252–253
retrospective cohort study. *See* historical
    cohort study
restriction, 245, 246, 254
right skewed data. *See* positively skewed data
risk, 32–34, 37
  calculation challenges, 34
risk-based measures of association, 72–75
  *see also* risk difference (RD), risk ratio (RD),
    risk odds ratio (ROR)
risk difference (RD), 73–74
  calculating and interpreting, 74
  comparison with risk ratio, 74–75
  positive and negative, interpreting, 73
  statistical interaction and, 207
risk odds ratio (ROR), 149
risk period, 128
risk ratio (RR), 72–73, 74, 269, 270, 272
  calculating and interpreting, 74
  comparison with risk difference, 74–75
  OpenEpi to assess, *203*
  as undefined, 72
  as unitless, 76

sample population, 118, 141, 175–176,
    223, 224, 266, *287*
sample size, determination of, 337–338
sampling error. *See* random error
screening and diagnostic testing, 312–317
  interrater reliability and, 319–321
  screening program considerations and, 317–319
secondary base case-control study, 153
secondary prevention, in public health, 7
selection bias, 110, 133, 157, 165, 223, 266–268
  addressing, 279–286
  in case-control designs, 273–276
  compared to generalizability, 287
  conceptualizing, *220, 266*
  in cross-sectional designs, 276–278
  impact on 2×2 table, 269–270, *270*
  internal validity and external validity and,
    286–289
  in longitudinal designs, 268–273
  sources of, *267*, 278–279
  strengths of, 165
selection probabilities, 271, 283
  for selection bias correction, 284
self-reported data, 296, 311
self-selection bias, 318
  *see also* differential participation
sensitivity, 301–302
sensitivity analyses, 270, 284–285,
    308–309, *310*, 388–389
sentinel surveillance, 31
severe acute respiratory syndrome
    coronavirus-2 (SARS-CoV-2), 31, 63
sexually transmitted infections (STIs),
    27, 228, 303
Short Warwick-Edinburgh Mental Wellbeing
    Scale (SWEMWBS), 393
significance level, 336

simple randomization, 96–97
  schematic illustration of, *97*
simple random sampling, 281
single-masked trial, 102–103, 105
skewness, 366, *366*
Snow, J., 9, 56
snowball sampling, 282
social desirability bias, 296
social determinants of health, 17–18
socioeconomic status (SES), 42, 43, 44
source population, 118, 140, 223, 266, 283–284,
    *287*, 328–330, 332, 356
  in case-control studies, 154
  in epidemiologic research, 224
  sampling cases with enumeration in, 155–156
  sampling cases without enumeration in,
    155–156
special exposure cohort, 121
specific exposure cohort, 123
specificity, 301–302
standard deviation (SD), 364
  visualization, and distribution spread, *365*
standard normal distribution, 366–367
standard of care, 109
statistical inference, 328, 332–333, 356
statistical interaction, 195, 199
  basics of, 199–204
  Breslow-Day test for, 200
  meaningful differences and, 204–205
  scale dependency of, 206–209
statistical significance, 200, 202, 332, 334, 337, 342,
    345–346, 350
statistical testing, 226
Stillbirth Collaborative Research Network
    (SCRN), 143, 151, 160, 345–346
strata, significance of, 192
stratified analysis
  confounding and, 246–250, 254, 256, 378–380
  for effect measure modification and statistical
    interaction, 377–378
stratified randomization, 97
  schematic illustration of, *97*
stratified random sampling, 281
stratum-specific heterogeneity. *See* effect
    measure modification
stratum-specific measure of association,
    195, 196
STROBE Statement, 133, 166, 186
study design hierarchy, rethinking of, *69*
study population. *See* sample population
study power. *See* power
superiority trials, 92–93
survival bias, 185, 267, 274, 276–277
  impact assessment, in case-control studies, 274,
    *275*
  impact assessment, in cross-sectional studies,
    277
Symptom Checklist-90 (SCL-90), 385
syndemic, 5
systematic error, 222, 296, 321, 328
  compared to random error, 226–227
  relationship with internal validity, *225*
  *see also* bias

tails of distribution, 366
target population, 286, *287*, 288
temporality, 66–67, 133, 165, 183–184
tertiary prevention, in public health, 7
test statistic, 374
therapeutic exposures in controlled trials, 91
time-varying exposures, analysis of, 132–133
trend analysis, 380–382
triple masked trial, 103, 105
true negative data, 301
true positive data, 301
t-test, 374
two-sided alternative hypothesis, 332
two-tailed *p*-value, 340, 342, *345*
type I and type II errors, 335–338
   power and sample size and, 337–338
typos and data cleaning, 370

underserved populations, trials in, 109
unexposed group, definition of, 58–59
United States Food and Drug Administration
   (FDA), 11, 107–109
United States Preventive Services Task Force
   (USPSTF), 313

upper limit, of confidence intervals, 348
U.S. Belmont Report, 16
U.S. Centers for Disease Control and
   Prevention (CDC), 3, 6, 9–12, 17, 23,
   26, 58, 67, 204, 265
U.S. Common Rule, 17
U.S. Kafauver–Harris Amendments, 13
U.S. National Research Act, 16
U.S. Public Health Service, 16

vaccination, 9–10
validation studies, 306–307
validity
   external, 111, 225, 229, 245, 254,
      286–289
   internal, 222, 223, *225*, 229, 235, 245,
      286–289
   meaning of, 225
variable frequencies, 372–373
variance, 364
voluntary response sampling, 282

World Health Organization, 174, 204